FROM INNER SPEECH TO DIALOGUE

From Inner Speech to Dialogue

Psychoanalysis, Linguistics & Development

Theodore Shapiro, MD

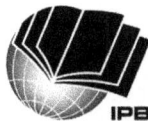

IPBOOKS.net
International Psychoanalytic Books

International Psychoanalytic Books (IPBooks)
New York • http://www.IPBooks.net

From Inner Speech to Dialogue

Published by IPBooks, Queens, NY
Online at: www.IPBooks.net

ISBN: 978-1-949093-66-7

To Joan, my wife of many years
My love and best friend
And my wisest critic

ACKNOWLEDGMENTS

This volume comprises twenty-two essays and studies, of which three were coauthored. I wrote "On Psychoanalytic Listening" (Section I: 11) with George Makari, who brought his extensive historical knowledge and modern clinical psychoanalytic experience to the text. I first met George in a medical-student tutorial in linguistics at Cornell Medical College. The essay "Latency Revisited" (Section IV: 18), was coauthored by a resident and then colleague, Richard Perry, who went on to be an expert in the field of early infantile autism, and a Child-and-Adolescent psychiatrist at NYU School of Medicine. The study grew out of a newly formed seminar in which I encouraged residents to read the new burgeoning literature on developmental psychopathology. He combed the literature and joined me in the formatting of the arguments concerning this developmental landmark, and in writing the essay. The research report on "Children's Conceptions of Ghosts" (Section IV: 18) was co-authored with Miriam Sherman, whom I first met as a resident when I moved to the Payne Whitney Clinic at Cornell Medical College in 1976. She helped gather data, reviewed results, and integrated a prior study I had done on the figure-drawings of toddlers. She became a friend and colleague at Cornell until she moved on to San Diego before the millennium.

These coauthors are but a few of the many students, residents, and colleagues whom I encountered and worked with these many years in academia, and which complemented my exposures at the New York Psychoanalytic institute and the Columbia Clinic for Psychoanalytic Research, as well as the Sackler Institute for Developmental Psychobiology at Cornell, where I serve as Director of the Infant Psychiatry Program. I owe much to these academic institutions that allowed me to interact and learn from students, candidates, and a rich array of faculty throughout my academic career at NYU Medical College (1958–1976), and at Weill Cornell Medicine (1976–present). These colleagues and friends broadened the scope of my intellectual curiosity and allowed me to become conversant with border disciplines to psychiatry and psychoanalysis, and to stimulate many students and residents to expand their interests to include psychoanalysis. I believe the shrinking number of physician candidates in our Institutes is a direct result of the failure of psychoanalysts to keep their feet in the door of the Medical Colleges.

The fact is, I supervised with analysts of many stripes during residency and my Residency Director, John Frosch (who was Editor of *JAPA*), was an especially inspiring and a lively—teacher. They were the spurs to extending my learning at an Institute. This volume does not cover the breadth of my writing, which was accomplished largely at both Medical Colleges. I wish to mention a few of the other areas of work that could not be included in this volume, stimulated by a rich collaboration with others:

Barbara Fish was my mentor in Child Psychiatry at NYU. She taught me research methodology and child-psychopharmacology as well as how to communicate with children. She was a gifted and devoted educator, and we wrote many peer-reviewed articles together until she departed to UCLA. During my residency at NYU, I met Bill Frosch, who coauthored two papers with me in response to social upheavals: student uprisings in the sixties, and then a clinical study of the effect on young men of the sexual liberation of women during the seventies. These timely presentations appeared in major journals. Bill has been a close colleague and friend throughout my career at NYU and Cornell, and was a classmate at New York Psychoanalytic Institute.

I cannot leave my NYU experience without acknowledging my years of coauthorship with Margaret Hertzig, whom I met at Bellevue as a student. She then joined me on the Cornell Faculty as a clinician and research colleague. She and I studied and wrote together about children with developmental disorders and autism for 40-plus years, and she enriched my understanding of development and served me well as an outspoken critic, keeping my judgements plausible. We have written more than 20 papers and chapters together that do not appear in this compendium.

Arnold Cooper, a Cornell co-faculty member, and I were enlisted by a young resident, Barbara Milrod, to perform dynamically oriented interviews with panic-disorder patients. This early encounter led to many years of systematic study and writing about anxiety disorders in adults, children, and adolescents. Barbara's diligence to task and zeal were infectious, and fostered a long cooperation that produced many peer-reviewed articles, as well as three books and training manuals. She, too, shared training at New York Psychoanalytic Institute. Regrettably, none of our work could appear in this volume.

Jack Barchas and Robert Michels, Chair and former Chair of Psychiatry, invited me to lead the search for a Director of the Sackler Institute of Developmental Psychobiology. As the Director of the Infant Psychiatry Program of that Institute, I met a young postdoc, Amir Raz, who engaged me in a project concerning hypnosis and neuroscience, drawing on my early-career collaboration 30 years before with a NYU physiologist. We produced at least four reports of research on hypnosis, using behavioral and fMRI techniques. This was somewhat off- course, but proved to be a major thrust into the neural basis of top-down influence of psyche on the brain. Indeed, what is psychoanalysis but a top-down modulator of behavior based on linguistic translation? Amir moved on to McGill, and then to California, where he has directed two very productive laboratories. We remain friends and colleagues.

Directly related to the current volume is the relationship to a teacher and colleague at the New York Psychoanalytic Institute, Victor Rosen, who introduced me to the literature of linguistics, and its relevance to clinical psychoanalysis. His devotion to integrative science and zeal for teaching inspired a whole career change that I hope illuminates this volume. I regret that I never coauthored a paper with him, but I am proud that I was asked to coedit a post-mortem volume of his essays, including the introductory tribute and guide to this new integrative science. I hope that these remarks expound my conviction that good thinking and creative inquiry is done in communion with others who may be students or mentors in a non-hierarchic collegial interactive search for new knowledge.

CONTENTS

PART I.

TALKING TO CURE
(THEORY AND PROCESS)

Anna O, Freud's first case described in the *Studies on Hysteria*, referred to her treatment as the "Talking Cure." Another Freudian shorthand aphorism adds, "hysterics suffer from reminiscences." Later in his long and productive career Freud's paper "Remembering, Repeating and Working Through" provides the encompassing framework that earmarks matters I address in this section. I review the theoretical and clinical issues that I encountered during the treatment process of patients during the 50-plus years of my clinical career and active writing.

My initial paper in this section, written in 1981, concerns how we remember what happened and how those memories color our relationships and our lives. Freud initially described a metapsychology of infantile reminiscences in accord with the sequence of bodily excitements and disruptions due to out-of-phase actual trauma. He focused on phase- and stage- constellations that determine symptom specificity. Erikson paraphrased that idea from the vantage of ego adaptation as "the tragedies and comedies surrounding the orifices of the body." My paper was stimulated by an interdisciplinary challenge from developmental researchers who study emerging infant and child behavior and further prompted by Jeffrey Masson, who revived Freud's original premise of actual trauma, as opposed to the virtual reorganization of mental content during the Oedipal phase of development. The late-20-th century arguments regarding "false memories" became a public issue that led to a revival of the idea of repeated intrapsychic reorganization, which could be accounted for on the basis of a new cognitive concept of memory reconsolidation that does not necessitate actual abusive trauma.

This reorganization of mind gained credence from the data of developmental psychologists who also posited "hierarchic reorganization" during the same period that Freud referred to his

Oedipus constellation as the Nuclear Conflict of Psychoanalysis. This nuclear constellation could now viewed as the most recent ontogenetic iteration of fantasies that could be appreciated in terms of the active and passive aims directed toward the father and mother who nurtured maturation. These fantasies moved forward from earliest stages to a time when the child could fully grasp the triadic nature of her family. This reorganization received explicit notice in Anna Freud's *Ego and the Mechanisms of Defense* (1937), where she posits that the listening therapist's retrospective stance can only see the influences of the id dimly through the latest fantasy reorganization, and never in pure form. Thus, my first contribution in this section is an application of a modern cross-disciplinary developmental concept that enhances our position about the way the mind structures experience. Deep earlier structures can be triangulated from retrospective and prospective investigation. I was impressed that by introducing extra-psychoanalytic empirical developmental models I could gain credence for psychoanalytic proposals that would further permit dialogues with adjacent disciplines, such as developmental sciences.

The paper concerns reminiscences, and how experience is preserved in the mind over time, and how such memories may be recovered during an analysis. The paper reviews the models that reference the experiential origins of ideas and narratives. I then address the contribution of perceptual reorganization, adding the contributions of poignance and affective valence that are included in how memories are structured and then affect later behavior. As described, the idea is a variant of the posited nuclear constellation as it emerges during clinical exposure.

My next contribution, "Representational World and the Linguistic Idiom" (1999), appeared as a tribute to Joseph Sandler.

It amplifies the role of memories in neuroses in terms of repetition during the life cycle, driven by symbolic transformations. Sandler's quip that "there are no immaculate perceptions" is echoed throughout the psychoanalytic corpus. Freud insisted in *Constructions in Analysis* that there are no memories of the past . He was followed by Loewald, who indicated "The patient, instead of having a past, is his past"(1986). These alterations in description of how the mind stores memories were stimulated by a number of incursions on psychoanalytic thought and practice during the latter part of the 20th century, such as the rise in interpersonal and dyadic models of the relationists, Masson's revival of real actual trauma, the early rise in consideration of intersubjectivity, and the hermeneutic turn.

I was concerned that the latter relational movements threatened the earlier focus on depth analysis and interpretation in psychoanalytic practice. I thought this view diminished the importance of the study of mind and the role of compromise formation as the precursor of symptom formation with a model that was recklessly headed toward relativism and surface behavioral paraphrasing, rather than the analysis of stored anachronistic personal memories anxiously buried by defense and continuing to distort behavior and belief systems. The listening for unconscious themes seemed to be in free fall, as the relationships between analyst and patient were analyzed without a view toward how the mind was actively creating the narratives told and the symptoms experienced, as well as the dyadic templates.

At this time, I was embarked on a study of the new linguists stimulated by participation in a Linguistic Study Group at the New York Psychoanalytic Institute under the leadership of Victor Rosen and Henry Edelheit. The linguistic turn was stimulated by Noam Chomsky and others who had created an intellectually stimulating upheaval within linguistics and psychology and developmental psychology. Applying these ideas to psychoanalysis seemed an exciting opportunity. This turn found expression in many papers on mental organization by me and other group members. Parenthetically, upon Rosen's departure from New York, I assumed the leadership of this lively group ,which continued for almost a decade, and I was instrumental in inviting Chomsky to run a workshop at the annual meeting of the American Psychoanalytic Association and later invite him to offer the keynote address.

In the paper "Naming the Unamable" (2005), I revisit the unconscious fantasy that had preverbal roots and had never been encoded in words. I revived Freud's construct that thing representations and word representations could only be conceived consciously when given a cipher and a representational code in a language, i.e. something requiring naming. This makes way for section II with a paper on ""Naming and Interpretation written much earlier—in 1979—and appears as the lead paper of the next section.

The final contribution, written most recently, on Now Moments (2018) is a tribute to Daniel Stern and his role in the Boston Process Study Group, who introduced the concept of Now Moments derived from mother infant observation and its application to the dyadic therapeutic dance. Simply stated, they posit that the " something more" that is necessary for therapeutic effect is the timing and ambience during the presentation of words of the analyst. The reader will recognize that my discussion of this posited phenomenon as a revisit to the powerful role of memory. The thesis must be questioned as a simplistic reiteration of the past. Rather we must be ever careful not to believe that it is a full regression to another time, but rather an incorporation of early intimacies in redacted later narratives, nonetheless facilitating communication. In the words of Stern himself, early infantile sense of mother-infant communing is not the same as the communication that takes place during the stage of the verbal-self.

During the late 1970s, throughout the next decade, and more Dan Stern and I shared a common faculty home at Cornell University College of Medicine, where we collaborated in thinking and mentoring our students and colleagues, focused on developmental issues as they can be encountered clinically, normatively and personally.

On the Quest for the Origins of Conflict

(1981). *Psychoanalytic Quarterly* 50:1–21.

The psychoanalytic genetic point of view was developed initially to account for choice of symptom in terms of points of regression and the conflict that developed around the expression of drives formerly unopposed. Later, clinical problems gave rise to positing an earlier and earlier anlage for conflict and symptom formation. The data on direct observation of preverbal infants and rules for validation of retrospective constructs are reviewed. The psychoanalyst's interpretation of symbols is emphasized as the most cultivated skill of our science. A restraint on genetic theory formation derives from the discontinuities in method between the task of analyzing and that of infant observation.

Piaget was fond of referring to what he called the American Question: "Can the child do it earlier?" His response is perhaps more interesting: "Chimpanzees at three months are far ahead of human infants of similar age, but where do they go from there?" I would like to suggest that there is a similar ubiquitous psychoanalytic question which occupies our theorists and parallels Piaget's American

Question: "To how early a period in the ontogenetic past can we track current clinical psychopathology? When did it begin?" This race into the past that parallels the American Question has become a competition for the laurel of primacy among practicing and theorizing analysts. To those who are swift and crafty enough to denote an ever earlier anlage for a current derivative or disposition goes the crown of victory. How this race began and what its relationship is to the irrationality of our rational, intellectual work is very difficult to answer. However, some of the answers may be divined from a study of the history of ideas in our discipline. There we will find ample preparation of the track for such a thrust backward, and perhaps denote how our history foreshadows our current stance. The reader will note how embedded we are as human beings in the historical: even in my critique I yield to the method that I may finally decry. I will help anticipate my conclusion by stating that it is similar to Piaget's—i.e., I am not sure that how early a conflict arises matters as much as how far we go as human beings in mastering the conflict. It is not difficult to see that Freud's earliest excursions into the mental life of his hysterical patients already tempted him to name traumatic events as precursors for the later outbreak of neurotic symptoms. While he infrequently penetrated into childhood in these early case histories, he certainly was able to see causes at a distance, and he began to think of hysterics as those who *"suffer mainly from reminiscences"* (Breuer and Freud, 1893–1895, p. 7). The moment one postulates that reminiscences are the core constellations for current behavior, then current behavior must be tracked to that core, and the conflicts that arise at such junctures must be laid open and divested of their abscess walls so that pus and the foreign body may both be evacuated. Trauma, as we know, occurs when the organism is overwhelmed by stimuli, and memories have to be sealed over by repression of the drives that are organized in a sequence of memories.

While Freud intermittently alluded to a variety of way stations along the developmental path, it took Abraham's (1924) embryological interest to permit him to construct a theory of developmental sequence that described the zonal content of conflict and the associated qualities that were essential to each drive position: passive and active forms of libidinal attachment; ambivalent, preambivalent, and postambivalent relations to the object of the drives. These way stations came to be viewed as the sites of origin for later psychopathology and character type in accord with the vicissitudes of the expression of derivatives. Everything was so neat then: psychopathology could be traced to clearly designated polymorphous perverse beginnings, which then had their expressions in adult perversion, neurosis, or character type. Indeed, Freud (1911) sharpened his reasons for the quest in the past by stating that "the form taken by the subsequent illness (the *choice of neurosis*) will depend on the particular phase of the development of the ego and of the libido, in which the dispositional inhibition of development has occurred" (pp. 224–225). Thus, it was a matter of accounting for the choice of neurosis that created the demand for developmental staging in the past.

The march backward received an important thrust when Ferenczi (1913) responded to Freud's *Two Principles of Mental Functioning* (1911) by elaborating the stages in the development of the sense of reality, which included a description of the author's speculations regarding antenatal and preverbal reality organization (again, to make current phenomenology correspond to a postulated past). Then libido theory came under significant attack when Jung (1912) insisted that the phenomenology of the schizophrenias could not be accounted for on the basis of a variety of libidinal fixation points. Freud (1914) responded with his idea of narcissistic libidinal distribution, pushing his own genetic theory even further back into the early history of the individual to find an anlage for the behavior of psychotics.

The origin of anxiety itself then became a theme that might define choice of symptom and quality of psychopathology. Otto Rank (1924) sought to use this theme and win the race backward when he postulated birth anxiety as the core of human variation. Freud saw this move as a breach of his developmental principles because, if everything depended upon birth, what then depended upon the interplay of accident and life events at varying developmental stages that could be analyzed and understood by patients? What chance did we have as human beings—unless we were to "rip everyone untimely" from the mother's womb in order not to create an overwhelming birth anxiety, which would dispose us toward psychopathology?

Thus challenged in his seventieth year, Freud (1926) responded with his most masterly developmental document, *Inhibitions, Symptoms and Anxiety,* which turned psychoanalysis from its biological emphasis into a psychological science postulating stage- and phase-characteristic psychological signals that determine the dangers and the resolutions required to move along the epigenetic ladder. Freud recognized in Rank's position the potential demise of a truly developmental view and fought hard during the late 1920s and the 1930s, along with others, to emphasize that the first five years of life were central, but not to the exclusion of later developmental events that also had their impact on pathology. At the same time, Melanie Klein and her London followers were condensing and telescoping the significant events of mind into the first year, and they became the champions of backward-looking by espousing the view that our relationship to the breast made or broke us in one fell swoop on

10

our path. However, when Anna Freud (1936) and Heinz Hartmann (1939) began to elaborate the role of the ego during the late 1930s and the early 1940s, the human being's external appearance and overt behavior took on increasing interest. They reaffirmed the importance of the depth psychology which had occupied psychoanalysis, but also reminded us that the id was inferred and seen only through the ego's mediation; that primary process was always relative and modified by secondary process. They even suggested that the earliest *anlagen* of ego development postulated by Freud (1937) as nuclei did not just emerge from the id, but might be distorted, deviant, and responsible for later deviation and variation in ego presentation.

Under this broader mandate, psychoanalysts began to study children. They also began to study children with severe disorders, such as autism. Mahler renamed a group of developmental problems as distortions of the relationship to internalized objects (Mahler & Gosliner, 1955), and, with that, she infused a new vocabulary into psychoanalysis. She was careful to suggest, however, that the autistic syndrome is not the same as normal autism. Perhaps a concept closer to that of normal autism is found in Freud's (1914) postulation of a period in which there is no evident relation to the object, and narcissistic cathexis reigns over object cathexis. Ferenczi, Freud, and Mahler cohere well on this juncture. Each is circumspect, however, and reminds us of his or her speculative base. For instance, in *Civilization and Its Discontents* Freud (1930) writes, "...the adult's ego-feeling... must have gone through a process of development, which... admits of being constructed with a fair degree of probability" (p. 66).

Mahler, Pine, and Bergman (1975) write, "The question of the kind of inferences that can be drawn from direct observation of the preverbal period is a most controversial one" (p. 13) and, writing about "coenesthetic empathy," they add, "although we cannot ultimately prove the correctness of such constructions, we, nonetheless, believe that they can be useful" (p. 14).

Ferenczi is somewhat less circumspect and seems more confident and emboldened in his assertiveness.

Abraham's timetable may have said it all by referring to preambivalent relations' giving way to ambivalent relations to the object, but it took the object-relations theorists, who trace a complex route from Klein, Jacobson, Mahler, and Freud, to suggest that it is in relation to the object itself that the initial conflicts of life begin and that affects are somehow joined stage-by-stage with each varying object level. These then have their profound effects on the way that conflict determines later psychopathology.

After this brief review, the answer to the question of why we push backward may seem evident. We have been instructed by our intellectual fathers that the etiology of adult neurosis lies in childhood conflict. Thus, our history, as recounted, indicates we need to track that conflict to its roots. Kris (1950) even ventured the suggestion that psychoanalysis is human nature seen from the standpoint of conflict. Arlow (1979), discussing the genesis of interpretation, echoes this view, indicating that psychoanalysis is essentially a psychology of conflict that requires the principles of psychic determinism, the dynamic interplay of forces, and topographic considerations. From a somewhat different vantage point, Otto Kernberg (1979), an object-relations theorist, disavows a breach with classical psychoanalysis and suggests that psychoanalytic object- relations theory is a special approach or focus within psychoanalysis. He goes on to elaborate the important features of the analytic view of the human being in the dyadic aspects of internalized objects which he sees as the focus of a set of polarities that essentially end up in conflictual opposition to each other. Thus, conflict is central to Kernberg's view as well. Having turned now from our history and its lessons to our *task* in analysis, we see that the role of conflict in our work becomes more prominent. We study the symbolic transformations and resolutions of human mental conflicts as they emerge in fantasy, behavior, and character.

If, as analysts, we study that which is symbolic, we perforce are involved in an enterprise which entails the process of how one thing may come to stand for something else and the rules by which such transformations come about. Our study of these processes permits us to say that it is not *what is remembered* that is dealt with in the present just as it had occurred in the past, but that *what was experienced* in a certain way is then telescoped and restructured in a new memorial signifier that becomes apparent as a derivative form in current life. In the sense mentioned, psychoanalysts have adopted and espoused a genetic vantage point, as well as structural, dynamic, topographic, and economic vantage points, as part of their theoretical credo. This genetic vantage point was as much a part of Freud's early theorizing as it was of his later theorizing. Thus, it was he who invited us on our trip backward into the past.

Even though he invited us, however, Freud always maintained the possibility that the human being builds new structures out of old materials. New mental structures are not simple replays of early developmental events or impressions, but also may include the encroachment of later events and pressures, which appear as emergent derivatives in the current analysis. When the Wolf Man's dream permitted the discovery of primal-scene influence, Freud (1918) was cautious enough to speculate that the event referred to may have occurred at six months, but was more likely to have occurred at eighteen months; but most important was that the Wolf

Man might have reinterpreted his early impressions on the basis of later having seen animals at coitus and thus created a conglomerate memory upon which form was imposed later. Greenacre's (1950) discovery that prepuberty traumata organized prior experiences in a new symbolic expression is also relevant.

This object lesson is important insofar as our science depends upon early impressions that are reorganized and transformed, while the process of analysis means breaking down anew the synthetic products, thoughts, that pass through our minds—i.e., we break the whole of human ideas and behavior with others into varying components of wish, defense, adaptation to reality, and superego demands, in accordance with their roles as part of a system of overdetermination and multiple function (Waelder, 1930). These elements were, it seemed, forced together as a psychic adaptation to a phase-specific need or crisis in the resolution of a conflict. Such matters were already in the air for Freud as far back as 1897 when he suggested in a letter to Fliess, "The choice of neurosis... probably depends on the nature (that is, the chronological relation) of the step in development which enables repression to occur, i.e., which transforms a source of internal pleasure into one of internal disgust" (Freud, 1887–1902 p. 234). This interesting starting point for the concept of conflict is an idea which corresponds to Hartmann's later rephrasing as "the change of sign." Thus, conflict and the need for repression arise because of the experience of potential unpleasant judgments and affects related to an idea that formerly was considered to be pleasurable.

It is the result of these forces, the wish for pleasure and defense, that emerges as a representation in symptomatic behavior, in character traits, or in other derivatives. We now look not only for an anlage of a drive, but for a possibility that a drive may meet opposition by other agencies within. However, what we do, in fact, is see a symptom in the present, analyze its components, and then suggest that its form and content indicate a time in the past, childhood, when it began. We then venture a genetic interpretation, not being certain if the patient's response is a genuine recall or a wish to flatter our narcissism for having arrived at that conclusion. Lest we think that this is a new idea, Waelder was similarly skeptical about our model in his critical discussion in 1936, called "The Problem of the Genesis of Psychical Conflict in Earliest Infancy." He wrote, regarding Melanie Klein and her school, "By devoting their attention to the experiences of early infancy and deriving from these initial processes the later phases in the evolution of the infantile psyche—these writers place great weight on certain early processes, the existence of which they have inferred or conjectured" (p. 124). I would elaborate upon Waelder's comments now by asking: Have we reified conjecture about the past to explain the present and then used it as our theoretical basis and guidepost? After all, at the point in history when Waelder was writing, infant observation and childhood observation were indeed sparse. Now I might add that, although we have looked at children with greater frequency, I am not sure we are further ahead in our quest for certainty. The model of finding states of mind in the past that parallel current adult states of mind, which are inexplicable on other grounds, and using that past as the reason that those states occur now, by virtue of either regression or fixation, is a circular path of reasoning that leads us to a "no-win," nonverifiable proposition.

In reading Waelder I was struck by the thought that, if one substituted for the Kleinians, whom he criticizes, those groups that are currently in vogue in psychoanalysis, one might visualize other sets of binary oppositions that include the innatists versus the environmentalists or the drive theorists versus the ego psychologists;

the Freudians versus the interpersonal Sullivanians; the Anna Freudians versus the Melanie Kleinians; the Oedipal regressionists versus the developmental arresters. I am puzzled about where to put some of the object relationists, because they clearly disavow the claim that they are Kleinians, and yet at other times they place clear emphasis upon the preOedipal beginnings of life as the anlage for later stages of mind and defensive operations such as splitting.

If we examine our current set of institutional oppositions and intramural conflicts, we may view it as a regressive trend in psychoanalysis itself, unless, of course, we postulate that it is an arrest. Were I called in as a consultant to examine a sick child—i.e., according to our science—I would find it very difficult to know the difference between regression and fixation, because I can see within the current situation these early discussions preserved in form, but I am not sure from whence they derive. Do they represent no movement, or a repetitious conflict? Are they the result of a property of mind seen projected onto a group phenomenon? Are they a property of human dialectic with hope of successive resolutions at higher synthetic levels? I am sure that some may even diagnose the problem as eternal recurrence, in the Nietzschean sense, or perhaps it is not recurrence at all, or re-experiencing, but rather some of the old fantasies recast in the current *Zeitgeist*.

We have yet another way of examining our conflict: we can call in a consultant who knows us well, but who also uses other methods that may complement our self-analysis. Psychoanalytic and nonpsychoanalytic developmental observers and biological baby-watchers come to mind. But the hope that practitioners in these fields will offer more certainty about how early conflict occurs also has its problems. They seem to provide us with parallel theories to lie alongside our own theories and sometimes create new problems that paraphrase the old problems in new languages. Let us look at some of the developmental curiosities of such observations, first from those within our field.

The idea has been advanced that perhaps we can build a new set of railroad stops for aggression, just as we did for libido; we can outline the stages in the development of the ego and make them as important as the stages in the development of the drives. Certainly Spitz's (1959) genetic-field theory, based upon the concept of organizers, was one such idea. Mahler's enterprise (Mahler, et al., 1975) concerns normal observed developmental landmarks, and she recasts ego psychology in the new language of the separation/individuation process. As to the issue of conflict, she has certainly elaborated the notion that there are crucial developmental stages in which conflict becomes more evident and possible. Lichtenberg (1979) suggests that Mahler is not alone, but is joined by Kohut, Kernberg, Sandler, and Winnicott in a "subtle to significant shift of emphasis from mental functioning to an emphasis on experiencing" (p. 376). This shift leaves us in a difficult therapeutic position with respect to how to consider the transference as evidence of prior conflict. Concepts have been proffered, such as reliving, resymbolizing, re-experiencing. Schafer (1977)suggests that transferences are new experiences and can become the creative road to better understanding.

Investigators who follow Mahler's particular position are notable in their continued efforts to build a developmental observational core, around which they can put phase-specific experiences and build a new hierarchy of sequential settings for conflict. Roiphe and Galenson (1973) have used direct observation, too, in order to establish new timetables for castration concerns. McDevitt (1979) feels that children must be capable of having symbolic objects as a necessary step prior to conflict. Ambivalence and the struggle around ambivalence are said to lead to a more active type of imitation between twelve and eighteen months of age, at the end of the practicing subphase and the beginning of the rapprochement subphase. He sees brief absences of the mother as promoting internalization and claims that the resolution of distress at loss of the early phases can be evinced by imitation. At yet a later period, in the fourth subphase (twenty-four to thirty-six months), identification appears as a means of attaining object constancy. McDevitt describes this landmark in terms of "actual and intrapsychic conflicts between [the toddler's] own wishes and his parents' prohibitions, as well as his feelings of helplessness and his wish to please his parents, by selectively identifying with them" (p. 333).

Also using a Mahlerian frame of reference, Parens (1979) has written an extended essay that elaborates the development of ambivalence and its relation to conflict. He marks as the two conditions for ambivalence an intrapsychic libidinal object as a remembered object; and the emergence of love and hate by the self in relation to that object. There are many descriptions of observed interactions that he uses as evidence for these intrapsychic states. I mention the circumstance of demonstration in order to raise some questions about the adequacy of such demonstration, despite the utilitarian function already suggested by Mahler, Pine, and Bergman. It must be clear by now that I hold suspect the point of view that such concepts as "hallucinatory wish fulfillment," or that conflict exists because of opposing actions such as biting and sucking, are self-evident rather than inferred. Each is subject to doubt because of what Werner (1940) calls the "constancy fallacy." That activities carried out by phylogenetically lower or ontogenetically younger organisms resemble activities of mature or higher order organisms is no reason to assume a linear continuous path or identity of substructure that subsumes such behaviors.

Parenthetically, we have an apt example of this proviso from Freud himself. When he disavowed Rank's idea about birth trauma, he did not disavow the idea that birth itself served as a biological prototype for later psychological problems; but it was not a phenomenon of the same dimensions or structure as later behaviors. My own question in regard to our activity as analysts is: What does it avail us if we know that something has a biological prototype, unless we use that biological prototype as a means of influencing the biology, or unless the biological beginning in some way has a significant influencing continuity with psychology and is usable for our analytic understanding later on?

Some psychoanalysts have become baby-watchers because they wished to penetrate the questions of the origin of conflict firsthand. However, because they all engage in new techniques and new instrumentation with the restraints of a new discipline, they arrive at data which has been variably interpreted by other psychoanalysts. Their field of operation at the current time tends to be either biophysiological or interpersonal, or, as they are fond of saying, "ethologic" or "interactional." Some patterns do emerge which seem consonant with what analysis has said about early life, but sometimes the data are contradictory. At best, we should watch for method discontinuity as the biggest problem.

Shapiro and Stern (1980) have recently discussed some of the implications of this baby research in the first year of life, and I will review but a few of the conclusions. These have to do with the fact that psychoanalysis has directed developmental attention to objects in an affective field while prior work concerned the cognitive object. Moreover, recent work suggests that the concept of the development of part-objects now has to be complemented by a body of information that indicates prestructured, prewired propensities already in the child for receiving sensory impressions, which become incorporated into representations as wholes. The concept of the stimulus barrier must also be complemented by knowledge about the infant's stimulus-seeking propensity within specific limits of intensity. Judgments regarding whether the data gathered have any value in terms of a transfer to later developmental stages, where conflict accrues, are still moot.

Peter Wolff (Panel, 1965) makes the most explicit critique about the discontinuities in observations of the early developmental period in relation to later developmental periods and the lack of relationship to what analysts do. He essentially calls on psychoanalysts to re-examine their propositions about infancy in light of principles of validation propounded by Steven Pepper. He elaborates distinctions between: (1) the descriptive and the explanatory; (2) corroborative evidence and compatible evidence; and (3) multiplicative corroboration and structural corroboration. Descriptions are not explanations, and explanations applied to descriptions only serve within certain frames of reference. Not only is a cigar sometimes only a cigar, but trucks and towers of blocks are not always phallic. That we find something in childhood that we expect from examining adults is simply compatible, but not necessarily corroborative. Multiplicative corroboration by repeated observations is not available to sciences like psychoanalysis because we cannot repeat experiments. Our discipline more closely resembles anthropology or paleontology, in which structural corroboration constitutes the proof. A similar approach uses the rule of coherence, namely, a "best fit" hypothesis. On these grounds Wolff contests the idea of applying propositions derived from psychoanalysis to the data of infant observation. He does this, he says, because psychoanalytic interpretation presupposes symbolic activity.

I sympathize with these propositions in regard to our quest for the origins of conflict in psychic life. In fact, I do not believe that we have progressed much further in our nomenclature than the original words utilized in developmental psychology, *amentia* and *dementia*—that is, children suffer either from arrests or from tendencies to recapitulate that which they have gone through in the past, in an updated form. Such a model, by the way, leaves us only fixation and regression. My impression is tempered, however, by remembering that Freud and his followers were interested in points of fixation and regression as a route to understanding *choice of symptom*. In that sense, the influence of Darwin marked Freud's quest. The current symbol must have had earlier origins, *but* the level of the fantasy may not have determined the form of the symptom. Within the narrow scope of the neuroses, conflict clearly plays a role. Moreover, patients in the extended group of psychopathologies also have a fantasy life and structured psyches—and we can even detect conflict. However, we trip over the etiological significance of fantasies when we find similar constellations of ideas across all pathologies. Rather than paying attention to the similarities, we might better attend to the mental structures and organizations in which the fantasies are embedded. In short, anal fantasies alone are no longer thought to provide the total-drive component of compulsive symptoms; neither do we now consider oral fantasies as the basis of depression, or Oedipal fantasies as the sole source of hysterical outcomes. The important developmental questions for us as psychoanalysts today are: Why is there so much symptomatic variation that some children are deviant, and how much of that deviance may be secondary to incursions of accident rather than biological necessity? What are the biological distorting forces on ego development, if you will, and what are the environmental influences—and how do the two interact?

I much admire the extended notion espoused by psychoanalysts like Hartmann, who has provided us with the idea of "average expectable environment" interacting with "average expectable biological equipment" and Winnicott's "good-enough mothering." I have admired these because they have lessened our anxiety that psychopathology is rampant among us. Not that I believe we are all very healthy—but health, at best, has many variants. In other words, I think what we deal with in the development of psychopathology is a spectrum of possibilities, against which there are certain circumstances of interaction with biological equipment that are good enough to make a reasonably adaptive life. In this light the crucial issue is: What are the limits of caretaking, such that a specific infant will or will not yield to an anaclitic depression? What are the sources of excess anger or love that lead to expression of drive derivatives in a way that is destructive rather than helpful? These questions, interestingly enough, lead us into a study of the interactional field rather than of the intrapsychic organizations which give rise to certain sets of symbols.

Margaret Mahler's studies have implications for interactive family research. Her work has already led us to study, for example, how mothers interact with children and how that interaction seems to have a determining effect on affect disposition, as well as on psychological disposition, in relation to self and object differentiation. The most-studied area thus far seems to be the rapprochement subphase. What we need, however, is a prospective study, in order to see how those externally observed interactions are later symbolized—if they are at all. We do have some data from the Yale developmental studies to suggest that prediction is a problem. Again, the question is one that Freud seemed to be alluding to in his earliest exposition: How does conflict between the principles guiding pleasure and reality adjustment become represented as internal conflict? Let us try a thought experiment as a way to consider the question and define the limits of the problem of internalized conflict intellectually.

A toddler at the onset of speech—between twelve and eighteen months—wanders into the street. His mother retrieves him. We can assume that she does it to protect him from danger and is not punitive. However, her action provides a counter to his exuberance and "will" and, perforce, may be seen as a conflict between him and his caretaker. We can envision various extremes of response. The conflict with the environment is re-enacted within as a conflict between self and object images. The conflict is forgotten and requires repetition in actuality to become fixed. The child stores the memory and anticipates he will be countered at every point that he attempts to exert his will. The three extremes refer to a variety of onsets of symptom formation: repetitive new experience-seeking, impulsiveness without internal inhibition, and, finally, inhibition. Interestingly, thus far a behaviorist vantage might serve as explanation if we could dispense with our internal image superstructure, i.e., in some way what we do to a child in life as a stimulus becomes the sole influence on what the child himself does. This view says we contract conflict within as a result of conflict with the environment. Strange as it seems, I see the concepts of those analysts who insist that the transference is a direct replay of the past, or that re-experiencing is what happens in analysis, or that countertransference is the analyst's response to the other side of the object dyad, or that nonempathic responses are mimicries of nonempathic parents, as *neobehaviorist,* and therefore interpersonalist, assumptions that do not attend to what psychoanalysis does best—i.e., the analysis of conflict as drive representation in opposition to moral prohibition that sets an executive agency into action.

Although our hypothetical toddler may experience his first "no" in the way mentioned, its meaning is layered on by other experiences and recast through innumerable developmental transformations, which only emerge as dimly related to that first encounter. I regretfully admit to those who espouse earliness as next to truth that my position emerges more clearly: I do not think it matters in the least who has discovered the earliest conflict; I do not believe the practice of analysis can deal with this issue, except as an intellectual analogy. The derivatives we analyze are too far from that earliest past, and I do not believe we still search for the choice of symptom in the content of the conflict, but rather in the warp of the ego.

This position does not negate Freud's notion that in order to have conflict we have to determine a point in the history of the individual where what was pleasurable suddenly became unpleasurable. I do not presume to know what a baby thinks, and I do not know what role biological drive disposition plays in the structure of wishes. I can only conceive of it as adding to the intensity of a wish, and perhaps as having an influence on what becomes a leading zone of interest. However, there are those who then shift from this desultory endeavor to look at the role of the mother in the patterning of wishes and behaviors as central to psychoanalytic propositions. Gedo (1979) takes the strong position that we need to find a substitute for the death instinct because its functional component, the repetition compulsion, was at the motivational core of Freud's psychology. Current conceptions of early object relations, he believes, may become a new source for a theory of human motivation which is designed to fill what he considers to be a metapsychological void. He cautions that we may again see alternation between nature and nurture in such an explanatory idea, and yet it might be possible to see motivation as deriving from how the early mothering actually occurred. Perhaps he is correct, but this is an empirical question, and no one has yet solved the longitudinal methodology by which such an experiment could be carried out.

A final problem concerns hierarchic reorganization of mental structure. Once conflict takes hold in the mind and is structured, how is it possible to see the past as a true reflection of events through the current organizations? Freud's insistence that the oedipus is the nuclear conflict is, I think, his paraphrase of the idea that conflicts are hierarchically organized. I have taken the position elsewhere (Shapiro, 1977) that the oedipus is at the center of severe ego pathology as well as neurosis. Indeed, I would even emphasize that in severe psychopathology we see the oedipus too clearly rather than less clearly. Even in psychosis, these matters are more transparent, because of the failure of the defensive role of the ego.

In a recent article, while espousing early object relations as a significant factor in borderlines, Kernberg (1979) also insists that the oedipus has a central symbolic role in these patients. He states: "Not even in nonanalyzable borderline conditions or in cases with severe pathology of object relations, such as the narcissistic personality, have I ever been able to find a patient without evidence of crucial Oedipal pathology" (p. 219). He then goes on to qualify, however, by suggesting that preOedipal features distort the Oedipal constellation. He is in good company here, for Freud (1931) himself focused to some degree on preOedipal influences but suggested that they become somewhat "shadowy" and "gray" with age. Anna Freud (1936) wrote, in *The Ego and the Mechanisms of Defence,* that the drives themselves are never seen except as they filter through the ego. It is in that sense that the essential analytic task remains the understanding of these hierarchic reorganizations, which appear as syntheses of conflicts. If what we are analyzing are symbolic transformations of mental traces, they must be broken into their component parts. The components are not self-evident—they are products of our model. The real problem concerning us today is not in the origin of conflict. It seems to me that any child growing up in the human condition will necessarily be confronted with conflict during his development, not only between self and others, but within himself. The more significant question is: Are there disorders that we can say are essentially developmental and nonconflictual? A related subquestion is: Are there developmental disorders that occur not on a biological maturational basis, but are environmentally induced? Is it possible, for example, to identify with regressive parental images in order not to take the next developmental step? Moreover, if these disorders are not analyzable as conflictual, what has psychoanalysis to say about them? This has to do, of course, with the concept of the widening scope of psychoanalysis, or whether analysts do more or different things than what has traditionally been involved in psychoanalysis.

The free-wheeling, unexamined use of concepts such as empathy and projective identification has become part of the repertoire of the working models of many analysts. These ideas presuppose certain fundamental axioms that are not held to by everybody in our field. Freud's psychoanalysis has many roots in romanticism. Indeed, Freud is looked at by some as using a model of mind which is fraught with romantic imagery: love against hate, man in conflict with himself. On the other hand, Hartmann calls Freud a true mechanist. Freud (1930) himself wrote, regarding the oceanic feeling that Romain Rolland suggested was the inescapable origin of religious feeling, "From my own experience I could not convince myself of the primary nature of such a feeling. But this gives me no right to deny that it does in fact occur in other people" (p. 65). He goes on to suggest that the idea of receiving such immediate knowledge of the world "sounds so strange" that one must endeavor to seek a "psycho-analytic—that is, a genetic—explanation of such a feeling" (p. 65).

My reading of Freud, in that mood at least, is that he was, above all, a rationalist who founded a method of inquiry that explained that which was formerly thought to be ineffable, romantic, and mystical. In the latter sense he was also a thoroughgoing empiricist, in that nothing was excluded from exploration.

Freud's model, however, relied on fantasies about childhood and on a metapsychology that he called his mythology. The analysis of the past as recast in the present as the result of the forces of conflict was and remains the central, most precise tool of Freud's method. The origins of conflict are most certainly earmarked, but we need not make it a developmental holy ground subject to the competition of crusaders in varied forays into the past. What we analyze are symbols made by mind. Our paradigms are not precise, but they are precise enough to do our work without knowing if our own Wolf Man saw or heard animals or people making love—or were they fighting?

REFERENCES

Abraham, K. (1924) A short study of the development of the libido, viewed in the light of mental disorders In *Selected Papers of Karl Abraham, M.D.* New York: Basic Books, 1953 pp. 418–501.

Arlow, J. A. (1979) The genesis of interpretation *Bull. Am. Psychoanal. Assoc.* 27:193–206.

Breuer, J. & Freud, S. 1893–1895 Studies on hysteria S.E. 2.

Ferenczi, S. (1913).. Stages in the development of the sense of reality In *Sex and Psychoanalysis* New York: Basic Books, 1950 pp. 213–239.

Freud, A. (1936).. *The Ego and the Mechanisms of Defence* New York: Int. Univ. Press, 1946.

Freud, S. (1887–1902).. *The Origins of Psychoanalysis. Letters to Wilhelm Fliess, Drafts and Notes, 1887–1902* ed. M. Bonaparte, A. Freud & E. Kris. New York: Basic Books, 1954.

———— 1911 Formulations on the two principles of mental functioning. *Standard Edition* 12.

———— (1914). On narcissism: an introduction. *Standard Edition* 14.

———— (1918). From the history of an infantile neurosis. *Standard Edition* 17.

———— (1926). Inhibitions, symptoms and anxiety. *Standard Edition* 20.

———— (1930). Civilization and its discontents. *Standard Edition* 21.

———— (1931). Female sexuality. *Standard Edition* 21.

———— (1937). Analysis terminable and interminable. *Standard Edition* 23.

Gedo, J. E. (1979). Theories of object relations: a metapsychological assessment *J. Am. Psychoanal. Assoc.* 27:361–373.

Greenacre, P. (1950). The prepuberty trauma in girls. *Psychoanal. Q.* 19:298–317.

Hartmann, H. (1939). *Ego Psychology and the Problem of Adaptation.* New York: Int. Univ. Press.

Jung, C G. (1912). Wandlungen und Symbole de Libido. Beiträge zur Emtwick-lungsgeschichte des Denkens Leipzig & Vienna: Deuticke.

Kernberg, O.F. (1979). Some implications of object relations theory for psychoanalytic technique. *Bull. Am. Psychoanal. Assoc.* 27:207–239.

Kris, E. (1950). On preconscious mental processes. *Psychoanal. Q.* 19:540–560.

Lichtenberg, J.D. (1979). Factors in the development of the sense of the object. *J. Am. Psychoanal. Assoc.* 27:375–386.

Mahler, M.S. & Gosliner, B.J. (1955). On symbiotic child psychosis: genetic, dynamic and restitutive aspects. *Psychoanal. Study Child* 10:195–212.

———. Pine, F. & Bergman, A. (1975). *The Psychological Birth of the Human Infant. Symbiosis and Individuation.* New York: Basic Books.

Mc Devitt, J B. (1979). The role of internalization in the development of object relations during the separation-individuation phase. *J. Am. Psychoanal. Assoc.* 27:327–343.

Panel (1965). Contributions of longitudinal studies to psychoanalytic theory. R. Schafer, reporter *J. Am. Psychoanal. Assoc.* 13:605–618.

Parens, H. (1979). Developmental considerations of ambivalence. Part 2 of an exploration of the relations of instinctual drives and the symbiosis-separation-individuation process. *Psychoanal. Study Child* 34:385–420.

Rank, O. (1924). *The Trauma of Birth* New York: Robert Brunner, 1952.

Roiphe, H. & Galenson, E. (1973). Object loss and early sexual development *Psychoanal. Q.* 42:73–90.

Schafer, R. (1977). The interpretation of transference and the conditions for loving .*J. Am. Psychoanal. Assoc.* 25:335–362.

Shapiro, T. (1977). Oedipal distortions in severe character pathologies: developmental and theoretical considerations. *Psychoanal. Q.* 46:559–579.

———. & Stern, D. (1980). *Psychoanalytic contributions to the study of infancy In Infancy and Early Childhood Vol. 1* ed. S. I. Greenspan & G. H. Pollock. Washington, D.C.: U.S. Government Printing Office.

Spitz, R.A. (1959). *A Genetic Field Theory of Ego Formation. Its Implications for Pathology.* New York: Int. Univ. Press.

Waelder, R. (1930). The principle of multiple function: observations on over-determination. *Psychoanal. Q.* 1936:5 45–62.

——— (1936). The problem of the genesis of psychical conflict in earliest infancy. In *Psychoanalysis: Observation, Theory, Application; Selected Papers of Robert Waelder* ed. S. A. Guttman. New York: Int. Univ. Press, 1976 pp. 121–188.

Werner, H. (1940). *Comparative Psychology of Mental Development.* New York: Int. Univ. Press, 1957.

On Reminiscences

(1993). *Journal of the American Psychoanalytic Association* 41:395–421.

Recently, psychoanalysts have focused on narrative truth and hermeneutics with diminished attention to the role of remembering in symptom formation and treatment. This shift has tended to remove us from prior status as a motivational and cognitive science with potential for causal inferences. At the same time, psychiatry and cognitive science have moved toward a vigorous study of reminiscences and their role in pathology. Arguments for a revival of Freud's position on the central role of memory are cited. A case example is offered to show that Freud and his psychoanalytic progeny have never taken a simplistic view of archeological truth, but were among the original group to bring to light the distorting effect of mind on remembering, and actually led the way for other scientific approaches.

Freud's earliest formulation about psychoneuroses was, "Hysterics suffer mainly from reminiscences" (Breuer and Freud, 1895, p. 7), This notion soon became the shibboleth for all neuroses. He could as well have said that neurotics suffer from difficulties in remembering, or from repression or motivated forgetting. All of these represent two sides of the same coin (Erdelyi, 1990), but he specifically focused on reminiscences, because he believed in the traumatic effect of certain early experiences, and because he believed his patients' tales about episodes of sexual assault that reached back into middle childhood—no earlier than eight years of age in the cases cited in *Studies on Hysteria* (Breuer and Freud, 1895).

Psychoanalysis, since that time, has taken a turn that might be paraphrased in parallel form—that *neurotics suffer from narratives.* It is said that these narratives do not permit us to reach for reminiscences as etiologic agents. Those who espouse this view recommend instead an approach to analysis that has been compared to interpretations of texts (Spence, 1982), (1987). Schafer (1988) writes: "... interpretation of texts, especially Freud's texts, is interminable. Readings of written texts are necessarily interpretive, and the same applies to what can be called readings of texts patients present verbally and nonverbally in the course of analysis" (p. 296). This view has contributed to the shift in the focus to the here-and-now relational frame between analyst and patient. I shall argue that to simply nod to this or similar hermeneutic formulations without reconsidering issues of *how we remember* is not only unwise, but renders our existing theories and models of mind useless, and will, if logically and consistently applied, lead to the abandonment of certain key concepts which I believe hold psychoanalytic theory together. While we may remember imperfectly, we do remember. I shall argue that the psychoanalytic dependence on concepts of repression, defense, splitting, transference, and construction are in fact logically irrelevant in a hermeneutic scheme, and also that recent nonpsychoanalytic advances in understanding of the role of memory in the human mind and brain are relevant to psychoanalysis. But first I shall follow a path of inquiry about Freud's discoveries as they apply, and then reach for the larger issues.

Freud listened to his patients' tales about seductions, but also recorded an early graphic note about a hypnotized patient in his autobiography in 1925: "As she woke up on one occasion, she threw her arms around my neck. The unexpected entrance of a servant relieved us from a painful discussion, but from that time onwards there was a tacit understanding between us that the hypnotic treatment should be discontinued. *I was modest enough not to attribute the event to my irresistible personal attraction, and I felt that I had now grasped the nature of the mysterious element* that was at work behind hypnotism" (p. 27; italics added). The moment he asserted, "this has little to do with me," Freud opened the door to a new view of a treatment variable that would ultimately evolve into the concept of transference (G. Makari, 1991, unpublished). Earlier in that same paragraph, Freud noted, "... the personal emotional relation between doctor and patient was after all stronger than the whole cathartic process, and it was precisely that factor which escaped every effort at control." Thus, actions performed in the present became *current empirical reference points derived from prior relationship*. Current interactions became emblematic of how patients present their past experiences with others. Experiences described in *Studies on Hysteria* include dissociation of affect, giving up hypnotic suggestion for voluntary expanded narratives, and the invocation of repression or motivated forgetting as a way of keeping unpleasant past events or ideas defensively away. Thus, forgetting was dynamically motivated. Over the next years, with the establishment of the concept of psychic reality and growing attention to the intrapsychic variables of thought formation, Freud began to narrow his field of interest, and his theories were correspondingly directed to *the way the mind works*. He developed a series of models to illuminate pathology, and then normality as well, that included the proposition that childhood was important to adulthood, that the ills of adulthood ranging from perversion through foreplay to neurosis were all related to polymorphous perverse infantile sexuality and the reformulation of experience under the sway of the Oedipus complex. That is, the early stages of wish formation came to be structured around the loving and hating attitudes around the two initial caretakers, and mental operations and fantasies were well structured by nuclear conflict resolution (Shapiro, 1977), (1986). These structures, in turn, occupy a central role in the enactments in transference and recovery of memory as derived from the free-associational process. Thus, Freud posited universal tendencies that were more or less influenced by actuality. Clearly there was not a one-to-one correspondence between stimulus and response, past and present, memory and recall. What we analyze is current experience in terms of the past. We describe the anachronistic intrusions of structured past experiences on current problems, and we point to the prestructured behavior as the basis of current attitudes, behaviors, and conflicts. We study the symbolic representations and transformations of intentions, wishes, and drive components as they conflictedly enter and color surface behavior under the sway of mental agencies. As Anna Freud (1936) noted, we never see the drives in their pure form; we only see their derivatives as filtered through the ego. Later she added that we do not study events, but repercussion of events on the mind.

Insofar as we are doomed by the empirical limitations of our senses to observe surface behavior, it is certainly plausible and possible to derive any variety of theory that would account for the various experiences and interactions; but in order to maintain a coherent and usable theory, we have to posit a small number of deeper memorial organizations that are transformed and amply describe the substructures of surface behaviors. This model links us to other twentieth-century schools of structural thought (Shapiro, 1988). Ego psychology depends upon the experiential past to account for that which is idiosyncratic and unique in the meaning of behavior, as well as for the universals. The distinction used in anthropology between the ideographic and nomothetic clearly coheres with this idea (Barratt, 1990). Spence (1986) also calls for moving from the specific (idiographic) to the general (nomothetic) in his argument that we must present our data in a manner that is logical and not rhetorical, so that others may be "independently convinced" (p. 20). At a conference on remembering, he offered: "Subtle transformations in the 'repeated' memory may allow for the emergence of new material" (p. 320), and later, "Memory [in computers] is unchanging… and uninfluenced by use. That clearly is not the way human memory is organized" (p. 321). At that same conference, Fivush (1988) stated, regarding autobiographical memories: "[It] is not simply memories of previously experienced events: it is memory of the self engaging in these activities" (p. 277). Moreover, object-relations theory is highly dependent upon how the past is re-rendered by the mind in accordance with the interactions between wishes arising during development of infants' interacting with their parents. Even Spence, and others too, within and outside of psychoanalysis, show continuing interest in the past. Nonetheless, by arguing from the extremes of any position, we can tease apart the themes that add to our knowledge and discard those notions that prevent progress or create confusion.

Curiously, while some ferment still exists in academic psychology regarding memory studies, the last 15 or 20 years of psychoanalysis has seen a major shift in focus away from these prior considerations of how we remember. Instead of continuous reworking of the theory of the mind, we currently seem to be focusing upon technical issues about the process of understanding patients. This shift has been instructive and in many ways revitalizing, because we had become too involved in small-minded metapsychological issues. These recent technical concerns have led to analysts' becoming interested in interactional and process variables that include the countertransference-transference continuum (Jacobs, 1986); analyst-patient fit (Kantrowitz et al., 1989); and recasting of the meaning of neutrality formerly seen as an inappropriate imposition of positivistic science (Shapiro, 1984); (Hoffer, 1985). This is the unique vantage point of the analyst who observes with rapt empathic attention, and, finally, explorations of the way in which hermeneutic or interpretive procedures apply to analysis, as they do to texts cover our journal pages (see Spence, 1982), (1986); (Schafer, 1985). The general shift in attention is to the narratives that patients tell in the here-and-now. The encouragement to listen in order to perceive the current psychic reality is expressed in Schwaber's (1983) rendering of the road to discovery. Gray's (1992) close appraisal of the surface is an ego-psychological adaptation to this view. The analyst's actions also have become the object of scrutiny, because they influence the patient's perceptions (Jacobs, 1986). In fairness to the fullness of their positions, Schafer, Schwaber, Gray, and Jacobs are not simply hermeneutic in their view, as they acknowledge some capacity to discover the past in the present, but their emphasis is on placing greater import on the here-and-now. In contrast, we can point to Kohut's (1977) view of how the breaks in empathy in the here-and-now reveal an almost untransformed past interaction representing a reverse tendency, rendering the present as the past unchanged. This represents a reverse trend from the hermeneutic premise. Otherwise, there seems to be an ambient despair in the psychoanalytic community concerning our capacity to capture the past. Indeed, Masson's *Assault on Truth*(1984) and *Final Analysis*(1990), though largely ignored by "official psychoanalysis," seem to have driven some even more resistantly to hermeneutic barricades. There was some small response in a panel of the American Psychoanalytic Association in 1985 and certain book reviews as well, but otherwise, most analysts have turned away from consideration of his argumentative assault.

The strong form of the hermeneutic argument asserts there is no possibility of verification of past experience because the analyst is stuck in the present with his patient and does not probe into the environment or have access to external documentation about *what happened*. The data are filtered through 20 to 40 years of experience. Freud's archeological metaphor of the pot sherd and the reconstructions around it are dismissed as pertaining to analogies to historical truth which bear little congruence to narrative truth (Spence, 1982). Even as this stance is espoused by some, psychoanalysis is further prodded and challenged by philosophers of science such as Grünbaum (1985). Because we call psychoanalysis a science, we are challenged to demonstrate the possibility of verification from within. The battle cry has become "internal probity fails!" Hermeneutic scholars are not ruffled by such assaults, since they lay no claim to verifiability; they admit only to multiple readings of texts. They dismiss science in this instance with growl words such as *scientism* and *positivism*. Kohutians return to the nineteenth-century refuge of *Geisteswissenschaft* and empathy, as a way to beg off the challenge of how to describe the appropriate scientific vantage of analysis.

Thus far, I have laid out the existing arguments as I see them, and reiterated that if we accept the hermeneutic view unexamined, we certainly will also have to accept that we no longer suffer from reminiscences, but rather from narratives, and that we are at risk because the narratives seem so arbitrary since they obey *gestalt*ist-like rules of closure and parsimony, which only create coherent stories designed to persuade, as if there were no memory, no reminiscence, no traumas, no actual past, no primary maternal bosom or cradle experience, no rage at siblings, no childhood and no polymorphous perverse infantile paradise to rediscover. Concepts such as transference lose their meaning since this idea has no referential significance without accepting that something is transferred, falsely connected, displaced, misapplied to a current circumstance, that belongs to attitudes and stances toward earlier objects and memories. These are the metaphors of current reference. Moreover, the attribution of polymorphous perverse infantile sexuality invoked to explain perversion, neurosis, and foreplay (Freud, 1905) has little significance in helping us to understand the diverse practices available for man's sexual activity or, for that matter, to the ubiquitous repugnance toward some of these activities. In addition, the developmental and genetic notions of psychoanalysis should probably pass in the wind as useless, archaic formulations fit for the history shelves as dusty curiosities from an earlier time. While we explore these ideas intramurally, explorers in other sciences are making much of memory and reminiscence in causal proposals. Some psychoanalytic thinkers (Edelson, 1985) also are trying to salvage causal propositions for psychoanalysts. Let me catalogue but a few of the nonpsychoanalytic trends that run counter to the antimemory tendencies indicated:

Psychiatry has recently revived post-traumatic stress disorder as an observable entity deriving from verified stressors in the real world. The idea of stress psychology is so central to our modern thought because there are psychophysiological biologically based responses to such states, and there is epidemiological evidence that stress is associated with falling ill. Terr (1991) shows prospectively that observed trauma in childhood leads to play which is easily recognized years later as representational of the traumatic events. She even anecdotally records external evidence of an early sexual trauma from the preverbal period being represented in later life. Her frame of reference is clearly psychoanalytic. Pynoos and others (Nader et al., 1990) have managed to show a dose-response curve with respect to traumatic effect. Children who were closer to the traumatic event of a sniper peppering a schoolyard with bullets, killing some peers, experienced guilt and other post-traumatic effects. Friendship with the children killed added to strain for those who were not at school. They too experienced guilt. Similarly, Holocaust survivors attest to the role of memory in later suffering (Moskovitz, 1985). How can we not attend to these discoveries, especially since it was a prehermeneutic psychoanalytic model that has given rise to the propositions that led to the studies.

Developmental psychologists (M. J. Ward et al., 1990, unpublished); (Bretherton et al., 1990) learned that the strange-situation paradigm measuring security of attachment employed between twelve and eighteen months could be well predicted by taking careful histories from the mother even before the children were born. The agreement has been so good prospectively that developmental psychologists now look retrospectively at adult women subjects' structured narratives relating to their early experience with their mothers, and use the derived results of this careful inquiry to measure the early security of attachment (Main et al., 1985). This is a further extension of Bowlby's (1969) idea that we deal with our children in terms of "working models" of mother- infant interaction, and that these models can be verified in life. Thus, again we are treated to a hypothesis that it may be sufficient to work with or examine a psychological content rather than an external behavior because they are so well correlated.

Primate deprivation research (Suomi et al., 1972), similarly, attests to the effect of early life experience on later behavior. Lack of mothering in young chimps does not have the same effect as in geese following the ethologist, Konrad Z. Lorenz, because he was seen first. Rather, we see effects at a distance over time, with a shift from the specific domain of insult. Isolated or poorly mothered male chimps are later not able to perform mounting postures when sexual contact is prompted by female chimps in estrous. Indeed, we would have no immunology, molecular biology, or genetics, but for concepts analogous to memory as organized in biological systems. In fact, we are stamped by most insistent systems of memory, lock-and-key, by the arrangements of nuclear peptides in DNA molecules. Moreover, Kandel and his co-workers (1979) have shown specific permanent biochemical changes in the nerve endings of sea slugs by virtue of introduction of actual external stimuli.

All of these propositions lead to causal statements that can be studied scientifically, while at the same time, we back off at the accusations of "no probity from within" and embed ourselves in questions of technique and a misapplied version of deconstructionism. I believe that the recent indulgence in studying technique stems in part from disappointment with our ability to elaborate propositions that would be useful in the scientific realm. We seem to be shrinking from our responsibilities rather than accepting them as challenges.

My particular rationale for considering this area arises from prior studies of the abiding effect of language on human experience, and the proposal that we must understand the formative role of language in both theory-building and interpretation. If we do so we may track, predict, and apprehend the symbolic exchange between patient and analyst in a manner that may even provide a better understanding of how the mind works. How that exchange permits inclusion of the past as an essential element in current behavior remains as crucial to us as it was to Freud. What the analyst does when he designates or interprets has been very much in the minds of analysts as a factor that fosters change during treatment. I used a language framework when I suggested that an interpretation is an act of naming (Shapiro, 1970). The essential notion is that unconscious fantasies are placed in the realm of ego control by turning them into language. We *discover* by naming, and at the same time, we mimic a developmental process that teases apart wishes from the past and their derivatives in current form, when we designate the enemy as an unconscious conflictual pattern. It also helps us to understand the presumed displacements to current issues from earlier objects and earlier events.

I toyed with the notion that naming may be creating, but would like to disavow that now, although it is an idea that has been taken up by others more seriously in recent years. For example, Schafer (1977) has written that every interpretation is a new creation, since what is being interpreted and said may never have been said in words: "...interpretation creates new meanings or new actions" (p. 419). Spence (1982) takes a rather bold contrary step by suggesting that the process of verbalization distorts experience by being expressed. This seems to me to foster an antirational notion that experience is unrepresentable. These assertions permit us to avoid the problem of probity, as Grünbaum (1985) suggests. Namely, we increasingly emphasize the intrapsychic, the method and technique of extracting ideas, and show decreasing interest in determining that what we do

41

bears any relation to the effect of past events on the mind's later representations. Grossman and Stewart (1976) wrote about how we can go wrong in the interpretive process if we treat our formulations as "theoretical clichés" (p. 210). They entreat that interpretations must permit patients to use language as references to experience— they note, "It [interpretation of penis envy] is incorrect as a clinical interpretation because it forces a theoretical impersonal form onto the material" (p. 210). They encourage, instead, a personalized referential system to raise verbal proposals to conviction. This is but one instance of language distorting, but it is surely ill-thought usage and careless jargon that leads to distortion. Having teased apart some of these matters, let us look to Freud for a moment with respect to his position on how the mind integrates memories.

I propose that, from the outset, Freud understood and believed in narrative formation as a feature of memory, but not at the expense of actuality. As early as 1899, in his paper on "Screen Memories," he proposed that there were two species of memory. He quoted a paper by the Henris (1897) that indicated that vivid memories were not simply the recovery of facts of the historical past, but they were constructed and reconstructed repeatedly during life in order to signify a composite of events that had become meaningful to the individual. The Henris' discovery that there are continuous and isolated early memories parallels other contemporary ideas as well. For example, William James stated: "All human thinking is essentially of two kinds—reasoning on the one hand, and narrative, descriptive, contemplative thinking on the other—that is to say only what every reader's experience will corroborate" (quoted by Bruner, 1986). Freud cited Jessen (1855) in *The Interpretation of Dreams*: "Total forgetfulness is not serious; but partial forgetfulness is treacherous. For if we then proceed to give an account of what we have forgotten, we are liable to fill in from our imagination the incoherent and disjointed fragments furnished by memory... We unwillingly become creative artists" (Freud, 1900, p. 47n). These fragments within analysis have special significance. Freud used the metaphor of the sham that lies near the gold, in order to indicate that what we remember in screen memories, for example, are only signifiers of something "much deeper," more meaningful, and potentially much more painful. Indeed, the need to hide arises because of the anticipated pain of direct expression. And he discussed these as "works of fiction" which made one wonder about their genuineness. He ends his 1899 tract with the idea that we have memories *about*, not *from* childhood.

Toward the end of his life, Freud (1937) approached the issue of reconstruction. He indicated that the analyst as a reconstructor is only using small bits of data in order to build a story around which a patient organizes experience of the world. Thus, from the beginning of his career to the end, he shared much with the "psychological constructivists." He did not believe wholeheartedly in the truth of events as remembered, or in their simple isomorphic representation of the past. Nor did he continue to espouse actual trauma as the sole etiology of hysteria. Kris (1962) in his classic paper on "The Recovery of Childhood Memories," notes, "the model of hysteria had lost its paramount importance [p. 55]... We are misled if we believe that we are, except in rare instances, able to find 'the events' of the afternoon on the staircase where the seduction happened" (p. 73). Arlow (1969) writes, "This constant intermingling of fantasy and perception helps make it clear why memory is so unreliable, especially memories from childhood" (p. 37). Blum (1980) writes, "Analysts would no longer be seduced by memories" (p. 40). At the academic Conference on Autobiographical Memory cited earlier,

Neisser (Neisser and Winograd, 1988) spoke about the conference as it would be remembered later.

> The events I have been considering are (or were) all real. They are not figments of my imagination, or yours; they are not hypothetical constructs or intervening variables; they are not codes or mental representations or schemata or scripts. In describing them, I am referring to something that actually happened. Of course, my description is not the only one possible; different people may see the same situation quite differently.

> ...we perceive and remember events at many levels of analysis. We remember conferences, talks, and sentences; lasting personal relationships, special evenings, and pregnant moments; graduate school years, particular seminars, memorable remarks. The organization of autobiographical memory evidently parallels the hierarchical organization of the remembered events themselves [p. 363].

And yet, Spence and others consider Freud and his followers to have been in error arguing that they used narrative truth as though it were historical truth. Why this particular misreading of Freud and mainstream ego psychologists by those who suggest that the only truth is in a reading? Perhaps some are belaboring the earliest hysteria model of recovered events blindly. I think that insofar as they do, they also are likely to use the concept-object as though it were a person, and to concretize the psychoanalytic process as though the dyad of analyst and analysand do not work together in the inquiry. Certainly, Masson has damned us for not listening enough for the truth of events as reported—that in turn would be akin to a mindless return to the psychology of sensation, as though perception were not a complex organizing enterprise.

It is a failing in our critiques of each other that we pick the worst of our theories and use them as the norm, turning them into whipping boys for our own, sometime new, ideas. I tend toward the same error, for I think this pendular sway to the here-and-now and the real interaction have been oversold as the significant determinants of behavior. This warrants as strong an argument as can be mustered to alert the reader to the other pole. It does, however, provide a defensive response that I address as a strawman. If I can turn attention to the strongest form of the hermeneutic position, I can better address its flaws. I must also apologize to those who argue more nuanced and less militant positions. I would like to offer that remembering, repeating, and working through are still the central signposts of our work and in need of renewal and reminder.

Loewald (1986) suggests epigraphically, "the patient instead of having a past *is* his past." He also invokes stored interactions without stored objects; this has a ring of truth. It has face validity. The question for us as analysts is not whether the past is there, but how the analyst works with what is here in order to discover how the symbolic process over time organizes the earlier experiences. What experiences attain valence, and how do we represent our findings to the patient in such manner that he achieves conviction? We assume that the patient represents his past to the analyst in every interaction with the analyst. We could not work if we did not believe this.

It is the use of language and an understanding of that form of symbolic representation of actions that permit us to tease apart *what* in the presentation relates to the past and *how* it is to be integrated in the present. In short, it is naïve to expect that the past will rerepresent itself simply—that there has been no experiential mediation between event and theme. As the analyst turns into words that which may never have been spoken, some (Schafer, 1977); (Stern, 1983) suggest that this is a creative moment. They disavow that this is a moment of discovery or a *description* of that which is now understood. If what the analyst says does not *coincide* with something that is already there to be *described*, then we might as well throw away our claim that we describe anything with our words—we become poets of the couch. The meaning of a symbol is not only embedded in the symbol, but in the symbol maker, and involves understanding how the symbol is used. The vehicle of presentation, however, may be in an enactment in the transference or in what recent philosophers of language describe as *performatives*(Austin, 1962) or speech acts (Searle, 1969). These in turn are related to what the new cognitive psychologists designate as procedural memories instead of declarative memories (Clyman, 1991). We not only remember in words, do things with words—we perform acts and create interactions that have an effect beyond the meaning of what we have to say. There is an intention that gives force to the acts as well as the words. The intention may be to seduce or to convince, but it may also be to inform, and informing encompasses describing. These are types of naming.

Even prior to these newer formal conceptions, the developmental psychological Carl Buehler suggested that the appeal comes to supersede the expressive function of language. Loewenstein (1956), referring to psychoanalysis, wrote that ultimately the appeal gives way to the propositional function as a mature form of informing. It is the job of the analyst to discover the rules of how memories are embedded in the discourse. As such, remembering is structured by categorical verbal usage, by classes of interactions, by words and by performatives. They are turned from idiosyncratic personal systems into generalized verbal descriptions (from ideographic to nomothetic propositions—from etic to emic forms).

Each time we listen we also look for redundant themes. Thematic categories become more important than surface particulars. In play therapy, the child patient "tells" us using cars, using crayons, using clay. The same story is expressed in different communicative vehicles, but they pertain to the same category of reference. They signify something that demands expression that is there beyond the vehicle of representation. Similarly, classes of interaction apply to repetitious remembered habitual past interactions with a person. The patient in a resistant phase, who uses every excuse not to come, will also use every excuse not to say, or every excuse to be obtuse or chatter on, indifferent to the communicative function of words. The passive patient may leave all the work for the analyst—may not make any formulations himself, may obey the rule of free association as though there were no observing ego, and does not change in the least.

Remembering in words is just one species of remembering. Even Freud reminds us of that. The words used, while they have a common code designation, also have an idiosyncratic significance as they refer to more personal experiences and usage. I have noted that among the various words for excrement, some are stronger as elicitors of affects such as shock or disgust, just as baby words used for feces could bring a blush to anyone's cheeks. Just think of your affective response as you say aloud publicly: excrement, stool, shit, poop, doodoo.

And then finally, among the performatives, there is the forcefulness of words as actions. The meaning of the word is not only in what the word itself means, but in the context of expression, where words do things. The bride saying *I do* "performs an act of union (Austin, 1962). A patient saying "I had the thought that" is not only isolating thought from himself, but performing an act for the analyst suggesting that he is embarrassed to lay claim to those thoughts. "I see red" may describe an observation, but, "Each time he speaks I see red" evokes a new meaning because of the new verbal context.

The context of an analysis is unique, but it is also in a continuum with other dialogues from the past. It is a two-person circumstance, with special features that permits the individual not to focus so much on the responsiveness of the analyst. It is a dialogue in which patients can project the inquiry and the interaction onto the analyst. Freud (1915) suggested that the rhetorical force of the development of love is the context in which interpretations are accepted. He recognized that this is seductive to truth. Those feelings—and their illocutionary force—can distort the degree to which the patient accepts what the analyst says. But if that is all there is, and no rational remembering is elicited, it seems to me that an analysis would ultimately falter and be hobbled, because it would remain too distant from the influences of the patient's past experiences, and the patient's assent would serve only as surrender to a powerful guru. Freud said, when the young woman threw her arms around his neck, he could not assume he had an "irresistible personal attraction." Surely, we do not intend to be so seductive. Surely our training is designed to diminish some of the narcissism that revels only in admiration. Surely the pain involved in the analytic procedure must have some hope of greater truth than an unrequited love affair with a shrink. Moreover, we are aware of those regressive pulls and are cautious to bring our patients back to reality. Freud gave up hypnosis on those grounds. Screen memories certainly are an example of distorted memories that constitute constructed narratives. With great conviction, the patient retells the remembered, often vivid, story and then proceeds to learn by elemental association that what he thought was true is only true in the sense that the memory is constructed to represent an unconscious fantasy. The patient says, "Aha," "That fits," "That makes sense." The memory begins to lose its poignancy as specified, and even the patient begins to lose his conviction that it all happened the way in which he had thought it happened. In order to disavow there has to be a reciprocal alternative avowal that has been discovered for reason's sake.

The conflation of rigid categories is reordered, and disparate associations fall into new places that make better sense to the observing ego. Some of these ideas could be illuminated by case material so that the context of discovery could be discussed and the process of how the recovery of memories would become explicit as we examine the idiom of presentation. Psychoanalysis has added a motivational hitch to simple storage models. Although we tacitly use the same episodic, semantic, or procedural declarative niches of academic psychology, we believe that patients rearrange nature in accord with motives, just as perception depends on prior experience. Memory, again, is not simply like sensation, i.e., passive reception—a camera, a tape recorder.

This is a case that was partially exploited in another presentation (Shapiro, 1974). I shall use it to explore the significance of the patient's representations and interactions in order to determine the effect of past on present: it seems much like other cases, but it provides a clue to a transferential experience that helped illuminate a *false memory* and aided the patient to access a bit of historic storage that was isolated and possibly repressed, and then presented with current distortions. Notice I write false memory, as though I know the true memory. This knowledge derives from the improbability of the stated memory. The case also reveals that the analyst is always working with the stuff of the past. If not, our work would be of another sort.

A man in his late twenties sought treatment because of difficulties in settling down in a relationship, chronic depression, and low self-esteem. He had recently broken a relationship with a woman that had lasted for some years, because he could not commit himself to marriage. He reported a vivid memory from early childhood a number of times. He was standing in the back yard with three or four boys and one girl, designated as Cindy, who was a "bad girl." They were all urinating over a fence, and Cindy beat the boys in the distance of her stream. This reported contest was not doubted as to the possibility of its occurrence. It was a memory indeed, a vivid memory as far as our patient was concerned. It was attributed to the fourth year of his life. Perhaps, not surprisingly to an analytic audience, this man had an abiding anxiety about impotence; he reported, as well, multiple dreams and fantasies of phallic women. The latter, too, we recognize as constructs, since hermaphroditism is a rare occurrence and rarely observed by four-year-olds. We are always making judgments about the truth of statements. Thus, we are always testing our patients' reports for truth against known standards.

Some years into the analysis, the patient related a fantasy. I had told him that I was about to go away for a brief period of time. Knowing that I was affiliated with a university, he created a mental situation in which he could undo his feelings of dependency and inequality and growing gratitude. He had the fantasy that I was to go to a hospital as a consultant, and that I was to be a discussant at a Grand Rounds, which experience he knew about from an early hospitalization. He would help me. He associated to an event designated as a memory. When he was twelve years old, he was in a hospital for observation, and ultimately was subjected to surgery. He was wheeled before a group for presentation. He was frightened. No one examined him, but he remembered a cold and ugly atmosphere;

he felt humiliated by the exposure to the onlookers—a group of physicians. He then reported a current image of his girlfriend, squatting on a tile bathroom floor, partially clothed. The tile reminded him of children on the ward in the hospital where he was a patient. He then recalled a girl squatting on a bedpan, but rejected that as uncertain; but there was a burned girl at the far end of the ward whose image became vivid. She had a large curved tin thing over her body, like a tent that prevented covers from touching her burned legs. He quickly had the idea, this time an intrusive fantasy, that she was promiscuous, "She was a wild type—one that you could play doctor with." He remembered always being frightened to do that when invited as a boy. The girl under the tent asked if he would like to see her burns, and she lifted the covers as he peered. He remembered seeing her genitals instead, and only incidentally noted the burns. He felt both revolted and curious. He quickly associated to being reprimanded by the nurse because he was sitting at the edge of the bed of another little girl who had had an appendectomy. He then shifted to the present and thought that his new girlfriend was like all those other dirty little girls. It was a terrible way to describe her, but he realized there was excitement brewing even in the midst of his anxiety, as he remembered and thought anew of the girl who would urinate with the boys. This led back to remembering the "pissing contest" at four that had been isolated from its roots of formation years before.

Later on, we were able to confront the issue of the unlikelihood of that memory. For the first time, he could entertain the notion that it was a constructed mental image that embodied and expressed his fear of women. His frequent current impotence was due to anxiety about fantasied castration called up by images of controlling, forceful, and assertive women which derive from even earlier views of his mother and aunt.

Let us return to this brief sequence of analytic work and look for the *memory work* in these representations. Certainly the memory of the little girl beating the boys in a "pissing contest" is incongruous, given what we know about the nature of the anatomical differences between the sexes and the capacity for projecting a stream.

The analytic query is why this man needs such a construct. What is its use in the context of his life and in the need to report it to me with such blind faith? The answer may be found, I believe, in the impact of real experience on the immature mind, and in the telescoping of time sequences under the sway of developing mental complexes that utilize new experience in the service of old, well-fused cognitive emotional constellations. This patient's anxieties are redundantly stated in the fact that he has to make up for his sense of defect in his recurrent dreams of phallic women. Or the false memory then could alleviate the anxiety he felt in entertaining the notion that women are not like men, and when they become categorized as man-like in their assertiveness, they become frightening. I shall not belabor the contributory relationship to his parents, because these data are redundant with the rhetorical need he had to convince me of the dangers he experienced. Historical truth lies in the replay of his experience of an actuality that is restructured to personal purpose. *The external observer may not have seen it as he did. But the external viewer also could not have heard the truth about his experienced world as the analyst did.*

In the current situation of the analysis, he was very eager to come with me to exhibit himself. He looked at accompanying me to the meeting as an opportunity to be my equal. He would show that he was "okay" or better, he and I would be okay together or even that I needed him, and not he, me. The passive-dependent arm of the idea was reversed in the fantasy. He also made up for his apprehension about loss by coming with me. The fantasy further stated he had no warrant to fear being alone and abandoned as I went off. He also might deal with the anger he felt toward me in leaving him by showing me how necessary he was for my performance. Curiously enough, again it is in exhibiting his prowess and his centrality to my being that we see a parallel structure in the complementary pair—woman and phallus, analyst and patient, man and woman, independent hermaphrodite.

We must remember also that there were a number of historically accurate elements in his presentation that somehow reinforced the possibility of the variety of memories he presented. It is unlikely that he concocted the burn tent—it is too close to the reality of devices used in hospitals. It is unlikely that he did not go to the hospital, especially since he bore a scar from the surgery performed. It is likely that he also was presented at Rounds, since his was an unusual case. None of those are important in and of themselves, as historically accurate facts, but they are important insofar as he then incorporated them into a unified narrative that is presented for interpretation of what is being represented.

The transferential moment of my departure, moreover, was no random issue in the recovery of the past. It was a cue to the unconscious; it prodded memory. Mind you, I use the word "represented," not "created." Here Freud has given future generations of analysts a leg up on prior notions about what memory *does* record. Memory records the affectively laden information in codes that analysts must decipher by applying the knowledge gained about transformation of unconscious derivatives in interaction with ego defenses for adaptive purposes. Analysts use words to link the past to the present. They use words also to change enactments into categorical understandings that provide the patient with a verbal grasp of how he uses the past in the present to achieve miscarried aims—how the patient anachronistically replays events that have signifying effects on his current life. This, too, is the stuff of transference. The analysand is in a laboratory of life in his or her relationship with the analyst. If it is simply a creation of the transference relationship that is to be described, and it has no relation to the past, or better, if the past has no role in its creation, then what are we analyzing, except the here- and-now? Again, we suffer from reminiscences, and these are not arbitrary creations of the here-and-now designed to create coherence. Edelson (1985) remarks that hermeneutics is characterized by subjectivity, the pursuit of meaning, complexity, and uniqueness. Scientific inquiry, on the other hand, is characterized by objectivity, causal notions, abstraction, and generalization. I believe that the search for truth in representation of the past is not equal to the continuous or repeated rereading of a text that is the hermeneutic objective, because an analysis is not a static event to be interpreted and reinterpreted or deconstructed. An analysis employs a means by which a patient can reiterate the significant constellations of his psychological organization in symbolic representations that the analyst then discovers and puts into words, so that they can be used in order to understand the motives for current behavior and later applied to redundant reaction patterns.

Narrative appeal and persuasion have been used to support constructivist elements in memory, but leave out the obvious referential significance of how the past impinges on the present. There is a parsimony in remembering that permits constructs such as Luborsky's (1984) core conflictual relationship constellations, or Kris' (1956) personal myth. These are the deep structures that dictate behavior and thought in the individual, and these are the elements to be uncovered in the analysis. They prestructure behavior. They have causal impact as well, because these elements are drawn from meaningful past impingements that fuel current behavior.

We know from the social psychologists that nobody "tells it like it happened." It is only in the telling that we discover something about the referential system of the teller. Were it not that he experiences events in a unique and repetitive way, there would not be a need for psychoanalysis. We would be closer to a behaviorist's construct than a human being. What we take hold of is the telling and the retelling. The medium of expression does not matter. It is the redundancy of the base referred to, the fantasy defended against, that is represented in many guises.

In my patient, a little girl who can pee further than the boy, dreams about phallic women, anxiety in looking under the tent, problems with impotence, concern about good girls and bad girls, all point insistently to a thoroughgoing problem representing an anxiety that was stimulated when he did not know any better about the safety of his valued sexual organ. Freud (1937) said, in his paper on *Constructions*, "It might have happened." His archeological models, that some take such pleasure in criticizing, involve the idea that what is reconstructed from that sham or sherd must have an imaginative element to it, but what is new in that? That has been bread-and-butter psychoanalysis since 1899.

The need for narrative persuasion comes from a force that is related to the disturbed equilibrium created by memory. We are straining to remember the thing that made us feel so good or so bad. It is like having something on the tips of our tongues. There is indeed a causal link, as well as a meaningful link, between past experiences and current behavior—but we have not been able to determine prospectively which link makes a difference. Finally, if we can translate some of those causal links into hypotheses to be tested, psychoanalysis would have a place among the sciences rather than become a strawman for those who seek probity or a polysemantic set of readings that varies with the reader or the reader's context.

I hold that there are more and less compelling interpretations, and that the more compelling ones have effect, because they accurately represent in words the way the past was incorporated in the mind. They capture the wishes deriving from childhood that have been recast in the present. Meaningful systems have to be linked to motivational systems if psychoanalysis is to work. Our concepts are embedded not so much in historical truths, and here I agree with Spence (1982), but in the impact of the past upon current narratives. Our stories are not made up for the analyst in the immediate sense; they are made up for the patient, so that he can have a view of his life that feels reasonable and be helped to grasp his experience. Analysts help patients to discover those truths through the understanding of the symbolic transformations that accrue. If being together is all there is, and analysis of the here-and-now relationship is the only aim, why do we need the analyst? I do not mean that we should again hide behind neutrality—that would be regressive—but I do mean that we should provide the rules by which we transform experience in varying media through which such truths can be discovered.

Freud stimulated a century of intellectual furor around the subjective accretions of remembering. He was first among peers in establishing some scientific bases for notions that only poets had expressed before him. We should not relegate his discoveries to another act of literary criticism before we seriously test and examine the virtues he has provided in systematizing knowledge about *the how of remembering.*

Moreover, every act of representation distorts; so does every line on a graph describing the relation of variable X to Y. Each line is a compromise that obeys the rules of *a priori* analytic mathematical relations, but only approximates nature. Every description in words is once removed from the immediacy of experience. We must remember that words have a referential intersubjective nonmystical purpose. What they signify is embedded in a common human code. If every description of the mental terrain obeys the laws of our scientific generalizations, which include Oedipal conflict, unconscious fantasy, defense, transference, then we are operating within a scientific set of constructs with generalizable lawsand predictive value, which increases our understanding of how the past, as stored, interacts with the present. This is nomothetic; this is discovery of what is there; this is subject to lawful categorization.

Can we say what happened? No! Can we say how what happened was internalized and recreated in the present? Yes, if we use the analytic method to undo the various forms of disavowing repression and motivated forgetting of which we all are guilty.

As F. Scott Fitzgerald (1925) wrote in the last lines of *The Great Gatsby*, "So we beat on, boats against the current, borne back ceaselessly into the past."

REFERENCES

Arlow, J.A. (1969). Fantasy, memory, and reality testing. *Psychoanal. Q.* 38:28–51.

Austin, J.L. (1962). *How to Do Things With Words.* New York: Oxford Univ. Press.

Barratt, B.D. (1990). Reawakening the revolution of psychoanalytic method: notes on the human subject, semiosis, and desire. *Psychoanal. Contemp. Thought* 13 139–163.

Blum, H.P. (1980). Reconstruction in adult psychoanalysis. *Int. J. Psychoanal.* 61:39–52.

Bowlby, J. (1969). *Attachment and Loss: I. Attachment.* New York: Basic Books.

Bretherton, I., Ridgeway, D. & Cassidy, J. (1990). Assessing internal working models of the attachment relationship. In *Attachment in the Preschool Years* ed. M. T. Greenberg, D. Cichetti & E. M. Cummings. Chicago: Univ. Chicago Press, pp. 273–310.

Breuer, J. & Freud, S. (1895). Studies on hysteria. *Standard Edition* 2.

Bruner, J. (1986). *Actual Minds, Possible Worlds* Cambridge, MA: Harvard Univ. Press.

Clyman, R.B. (1991). *The Procedural Organization of Emotions: A Contribution From Cognitive Science to the Psychoanalytic Theory of Therapeutic Action.* Madison, CT: Int. Univ. Press.

Edelson, M. (1985). The hermeneutic turn and the single case study in psychoanalysis,. *Psychoanal. Contemp. Thought* 8 567–614.

Erdelyi, M.H. (1990). Repression, reconstruction, and defense: history and integration of the psychoanalytic and experimental frameworks. In *Repression and Dissociation* ed. J. L. Singer. Chicago, IL: Univ. Chicago Press.

Fitzgerald, F.S. (1925). *The Great Gatsby.* New York: Scribner's.

Fivush, R. (1988). The functions of event memory: some comments on Nelson and Barsalou. In *Remembering Reconsidered: Ecological and Traditional Approaches to the Study of Memory* ed. U. Neisser & E. Winograd. New York: Cambridge Univ. Press, pp. 277–282.

Freud, A. (1936). *The Ego and the Mechanisms of Defense. Writings 2.* New York: Int. Univ. Press, 1966.

Freud, S. (1899). Screen memories. *Standard Edition* 3.

——— (1900). The interpretation of dreams. S *Standard Edition* 4 & 5.

——— (1905). Three essays on the theory of sexuality. *S.E.* 7.

——— (1915). Observations on transference love. *S.E.* 12.

——— (1920). Beyond the pleasure principle. *S.E.* 18.

——— (1925). An autobiographical study. *S.E.* 20.

——— (1937). Constructions in analysis. *S.E.* 23.

Gray, P. (1992). Memory as resistance, and the telling of a dream. *J. Am. Psychoanal. Assoc.* 40:307–326.

Grossman, W.I. & Stewart, W.A. (1976). Penis envy: From childhood wish to developmental metaphor. *J. Am. Psychoanal. Assoc.* 24(Suppl.):193–212.

Grünbaum, A. (1985). *The Foundations of Psychoanalysis.* Berkeley, CA: Univ. California Press.

Henri, V. & Henri, C. (1897). Enquête sur les premiers souvenirs de l'enfance. *Année Psychol.* 3 184.

HOFFER, A. (1985). Toward a definition of psychoanalytic neutrality. *J. Am. Psychoanal. Assoc.* 33:771–795.

JACOBS, T.J. (1986). On countertransference enactments. *Psychoanal. Q.* 34:289–606.

JESSEN, P. (1855). Versuch einer wissenschaftichen. *Begrundung der Psychologie* Berlin.

KANDEL, E. (1979). Psychotherapy and the single synapse. *New Eng. J. Med.* 301 1028–1037

Kantrowitz, J.L.; Katz, A.L.; Greenman, D.A.; Morris, H.; Paolitto, F.; Sashin, J. & Solomon, L. (1989). The patient-analyst match and the outcome of psychoanalysis. *J. Am. Psychoanal. Assoc.* 37:893–920.

Kohut, H. (1977). *The Restoration of the Self.* New York: Int. Univ. Press.

KRIS, E. (1956). The personal myth: a problem in psychoanalytic technique. *J. Am. Psychoanal. Assoc.* 4:653–681.

——— (1962). The recovery of childhood memories in psychoanalysis. *Psychoanal. Study Child* 9:54–88.

Loewald, H. W. (1986). Transference-countertransference. *J. Am. Psychoanal. Assoc.* 34:275–287.

Loewenstein, R.M. (1956). Some remarks on the role of speech in psychoanalytic technique. *Int. J. Psychoanal.* 37:460–468.

Luborsky, L. (1984). *Principles of Psychoanalytic Psychotherapy: A Manual for Supportive Expressive Treatment.* New York: Basic Books.

Main, M., Kaplan, N. & Cassidy, J. (1985). Security in infancy, childhood, and adulthood: a move to the level of representation. In *Growing Points in Attachment Theory and Research* ed. I. Bretherton & E. Waters. Chicago: Univ. Chicago Press, pp. 66–106.

MASSON, J.M. (1984). *The Assault on Truth: Freud's Suppression of the Seduction Theory.* New York: Penguin, 1985.

Masson, J. M. (1990). *The Final Analysis: The Making and Unmaking of a Psychoanalys.t* New York: Addison-Wesley.

Moskovitz, S. (1985). Longitudinal follow up of child survivors of the Holocaust. *J. Amer. Acad. Child Psychiat.* 24 401–407.

Nader, K.; Pynoos, R.; Fairbanks, L. & Frederick, C. (1990). Children's PTSD reactions one year after a sniper attack at their school. *Amer. J. Psychiat* 147 1526–1530.

Neisser, U. & Winograd, E. (1988). *Remembering Reconsidered: Ecological and Traditional Approaches to the Study of Memory* New York: Cambridge Univ. Press.

Schafer, R. (1977). The interpretation of transferences and the conditions for loving. *J. Am. Psychoanal. Assoc.* 25:335–362.

———— (1985). The interpretation of psychic reality, developmental influences, and unconscious communication *J. Am. Psychoanal. Assoc.* 33:537–554.

———— 1988 Discussion of panel presentations on psychic structure. *J. Am. Psychoanal. Assoc.* 36(Suppl.):295–311.

Schwaber, E.A. (1983). Psychoanalytic listening and psychic reality. *Int. J. Psychoanal..* 10:379–392.

Searle, J.R. (1969). *Speech Acts: An Essay on Philosophy of Language* New York: Cambridge Univ. Press.

Shapiro, T. (1970). Interpretation and naming. *J. Am. Psychoanal. Assoc.* 18:399–421.

———— (1974). Development and distortions of empathy. *Psychoanal. Q.* 43:4–25.

———— (1977). Varieties of Oedipal distortions in severe character pathologies: developmental and theoretical considerations. *Psychoanal. Q.* 46:559–579.

———— (1984). On neutrality. *J. Am. Psychoanal. Assoc.* 32:269–282.

———— (1986). Nuclear conflict and the nuclear self. *Psychoanal. Inq.* 6 349–365.

———— (1987). Language structure and psychoanalysis. *J. Am. Psychoanal. Assoc.* 36:339–358.

———— (1988). Language structure and psychoanalysis. *J. Am. Psychoanal. Assoc.* 36(Suppl.):339–358

Spence, D P. (1982). Narrative Truth and Historical Truth New York: Norton.

———— (1986). When interpretation masquerades as explanation. *J. Am. Psychoanal. Assoc.* 34:3–22.

———— (1987). *The Freudian Metaphor.* New York: Norton.

———— (1988). *Passive remembering In Remembering Reconsidered: Ecological and Traditional Approaches to the Study of Memory.* ed. U. Neisser & E. Winograd. New York: Cambridge Univ. Press, pp. 311–325.

Stern, D.B., (1983). Unformulated experience: from familiar chaos to creative disorder. *Contemp. Psychoanal.* 19:71–99.

Suomi, S., Harlow, H.F. & McKinney, W.T. (1972). Monkey psychiatrists. *Amer. J. Psychiat* 128 927–932.

Terr, L.C. (1991). Childhood traumas: an outline and overview. *Amer. J. Psychiat.* 148 10–2.0.

The Representational World and The Linguistic Idiom

(1999). *In Psychoanalysis on the Move: The Work of Joseph Sandler,* (eds. P. Fonagy, A. Cooper, R.S., Wallerstein). New York: Routledge / The Institute of Psychoanalysis, London, pp. 105–117.

Abstract:

Joseph Sandler has contributed immensely to our understanding of the representational world, bringing together the views of the object-relational and ego-psychological viewpoints. In this essay, I will seek to expand that vision to include what we know about the rules of translation, by which we formulate the representational world into language or personal idiom. Since our desired contacts with our patients are through words, we should see how words enable and facilitate movement away from senseless repetitions and enactments of the past; and whether the mental constellations can be translated into meaningful new statements or interpretations. A case example will serve as a vehicle to describe the translation from action to language and the move toward change.

Joseph Sandler's larger contribution to psychoanalysis cannot be summarized in one brief piece, but his specific interest in the representational world has been a persistent theme of his work. In his 1988 Plenary Address to the American Psychoanalytical Association (Sandler, J., 1990) he distinguished his point of view as following a consistent thread that addresses the way patients present themselves and how their inner worlds dictate their behavior. His unique modification of Kleinian theory, and adaptation of ego psychology provides us with an amalgam of the important ways in which people represent their experiences. This body of work forces us to see the role of memory storage of experience on action and interaction, as well as the effect of significant past interactions on intrapsychic life.

He writes (Sandler, J., 1990, p. 866) that there are four areas concerning the relationship of memory and thought to conscious and unconscious fantasies that relate to self- and object-representations:

1. the wish for interaction with an object;
2. concern for the way wishes are fulfilled with guiding drives of instinctual wishes, safety, reassurance, affirmation, narcissistic gratification and the wish to do away with pain or anxiety;
3. seeking actualization i.e., as Freud suggested, to make perception reperception and finally,
4. transference as the closest actualization of a wish for a relationship in seeking to make the analyst conform to a wish-fulfilling role. Sandler (1990) further writes, that the patient tries to actualize, and the analyst tries to interpret.

I would like to offer a complementary set of observations derived from my interest in and work with language regarding the interpretative process that could well be grafted onto Sandler's scheme. I believe there is intellectual and practical virtue in having a clear description of the process of interpretation from the standpoint of linguistics, in order to state better and thereby understand the relationship of the verbal process to unconscious fantasy. Before doing this, however, let me note that Sandler indicated that he had been guilty of some misrepresentation "in not distinguishing between the experiential content of the mental representation—the perceptual and ideational content—and the structural organization behind that content, an organization that lies outside the realm of conscious or unconscious experience" (1990, p. 869).

Sandler and Joffe (1966) did offer an addendum allowing for the sharp distinction between the experiential and the nonexperiential realms. They wrote "the realm of subjective experience (in German, *Erlebnis*, but not *Erfahrung*) refers to the experience of the phenomenal content of wishes, impulses, memories, fantasies, sensation, percepts, feelings and the like. All we know, we know only through subjective phenomenal representation. Later on, he commented on the notion that it is not just the child's perception of an interaction that is internalized, but these fantasy images are also "unconsciously" manipulated by the ego by means of the ego-function of fantasy, thereby modifying the experience in a highly idiosyncratic manner. (Sandler and Nagera, 1963, p. 871).

These proposals offer the groundwork for further understanding of how the interpretative process helps to bring the patient into relationship with his own fantasies, and also to bring the fantasies into consciousness under the control of the ego, rather than permitting them to dictate the patient's behavior without conscious appraisal, reappraisal, and judgment about the wisdom of such action and interaction.

The linguistic frame of reference to which I refer is initially elaborated in the paper "Interpretation and Naming" where I wrote (Shapiro, T., 1970) "The interpretation of an unconscious fantasy is an event during the course of an analysis which may be viewed as naming. Varying phenomena, motivational, verbal situational, interpersonal, are synthesized by the analyst into a more or less concise sentence or complex name. This designation can now be considered by patient and analyst as a common lexical property and can be tested for its congruence with the patient's experience in the past, present and future." (p. 399)

At a later point, (Shapiro, T., 1988) I added, "Insofar as the analytic task and the aim of theory are advanced by the interpretation of unconscious fantasy, we must know how such interpretation is possible, and how it comes about. It is in this light that our interest in symbol formation, the linguistic mode of expression and the mechanisms underlying these processes might be considered." (p. 82) In short, I would like to introduce an addendum to Sandler's interest in mental representation in the form of a discussion that taps our understanding of linguistic representation that stands alongside other forms of representation. The patient represents his compromise formations to the analyst around object relational constellations of wishes in at least two forms: by actualization in words and narratives whose deeper meaning is barely understood by both patient and analyst or in enactments in the transference. These elements can be viewed from the standpoint of a number of rules of transformation derived from language theory and semiotics. (Shapiro, T., 1979) By such a view, we can approach a closer description of the mode of interaction of the interpretative process in words and better describe the analytic relationship. The analytic situation includes the controlled actualization of object- and subject-related wishes, demonstrates how they are defended, and how they become visible in the flow of associations and choice of stories told, as well as those expressed in transference enactments. Knowing these constellations and how the analyst uses words to interpret these developing actualizations is central to furthering our aim of comprehending the therapeutic process.

In order to address these issues, let us first ask, "What is an interpretation?" My earlier comments suggest that it is a *translation into a verbal medium* of that which has been represented in another form. In that sense, the vehicle of representation is altered by the analyst in the service of creating a *useable verbal statement* that can be shared in consciousness and *re-referred to repeatedly* by analyst and patient in the search for the shortest, most useful, description that can be employed as a mediational paradigm representing the various manifestations and multiple appearances of these interactions. Thus, a single phrase is used as a cipher representing multiple events, enactments, and narratives, as well as serving multiple functions. This cypher or phrase, therefore, can aptly be designated as a polysemantic auditory verbal image and, therefore, can be explored from the standpoint of how symbols organize experience. I suggest it may refer to Sandler's nonexperiential realm, insofar as it can be translated into words.

Mahoney (1987) notes that there are three forms of translation, intra-linguistic, inter- linguistic, and semiotic. In the first, we describe a word or an event in other terms than in the same code. A dictionary definition is a simple example of intra-linguistic translation. When we ask, "What is a bachelor?" we might answer, "an unmarried male" Note, however, that the word *spinster*, an unmarried female, has a different array of connotations and a broader array of affective responses, making the translation of particular words particularly eventful and demonstrating that words are not simply labels. Parenthetically, it is similarly not possible to make only one form of an interpretation or suggest that other forms are equal.

Words have affective valence as well as a designative signifying function. Inter-linguistic translation would simply be the translation from one language to another. However, easy as this may seem, it, too, is more complex. For example, in translating a noun, there is often a change in nuance and connotation between languages. Words may have a common semantic, e.g., moon in English is translated into *La Lune* in French. Nonetheless, each has different connotative significance. Moon, having to do with measurement or month, the French choice reflects a bias toward brightness and light. Both are attributes of the referent but lead us to different mental images if we become aware of our network of associations. (We can well note the intrapsychoanalytic controversies concerning cathexis and *Besetzung or the Ego and das Ich.*) The latter problem has made some, to wit, Whorf & Sapir (1962) suggest that there is no possibility of true inter-linguistic translation on a one-to-one basis if one takes into account connotative factors. Indeed, they offer that each language provides its own world view of reality. I would add that affective additions derived from group and personal use are also relevant.

The third, or semiotic translation, involves a translation from one vehicle of representation to another. The relationship of the sign to the symbol can be looked at as arbitrary in common lexical tokens, such as words, but the relationship of the sign to its referent also may be explained better by contiguity or simile, as in metonymy and metaphor. We speak of "the Crown" when we mean the Queen, we speak of "10 Downing Street," when we mean the Prime Minister.

In the metaphoric or simile relationship, the sign is chosen by token of a relationship by form. "Rosy-fingered-dawn" for Homer is a clear representation of what a sunrise appeared to be then and, not surprisingly, serves us even now. We can appreciate the metaphor even today over the centuries, suggesting that sunrises have not changed much during historical times. An interesting variation on this theme comes in the way references encode different referents. There is some question as to how the letter representing the "B" sounded in ancient Greek, since there has been some phonic drift from B to V as is found in other language codes. Fortunately, there is a sequence in one of Aristophanes' plays where the bleat of a sheep is represented—it surely is not *Vaa Vaa*—so the phonic shape had to agree with the sound for B as we use it in modern English. Linguistic drift provides another example of shift in meaning and representation. Shakespearean English approximates modern lexical meanings, but does not do so uniformly.

Psychoanalytic translations correspond most closely to the area of symbolic representation that is semiotic. In the relationship of the patient to the analyst, especially in the transference, we frequently see an enactment of a wished-for relationship to an object. We detect this from redundant descriptions by the patient of relationships with others, either in the present (synchronically) or from the past (diachronically). Such redundant and concordant stories, expressed in various vehicles, aid us in our search for a paradigmatic statement that would describe the current interaction. Indeed, more rigorous, empirically defined concepts such as core critical relationship themes (CCRTs), (Luborsky, L. and Luborsky, E., 1993) correspond nicely to Sandler's (1990) clinical concept of *role-responsiveness*. The latter is a more general clinical way of stating the characteristic stance in relation to interactions between patient and analyst. As Sandler

(1990) notes: "In the analytic situation, the patient unpacks the object aspects of his mental furniture, so to speak, and tries to position this furniture in ways that make it seem as if it belongs and is appropriate." (p. 878). This metaphor renders what has transpired interpersonally into words, permitting us to grasp the experiential aspects of a patient and conveys the experience in a vehicle that goes beyond a simple communion attaining the level of communication. Indeed, a carefully crafted relational syntax offers a precise linguistic model of what has occurred, which may be accepted or refuted on the basis of any distinctive feature, such as who is the subject or object, or how active or passive the verb is that represents the interaction.

What are the tacit frames of reference we use, whether we call ourselves object relationalists or classical structural ego theorists? What metastructure do we employ to account for the forms in which we cast interpretations, so that they achieve status as a communal property in language? I will elaborate how linguistic explanations provide us with three ways to analyze the manner in which we represent core stories in language. These overlapping areas include syntax, semantics, and pragmatics. (See Shapiro, T., 1979).

Syntax refers to the organization of phrases and sentences to express the relational aspects of subject and object, passivity and activity, and their verbal strength and force as imperatives. Insofar as the organization of syntax rests upon case grammar, it is a perfect vehicle to represent agent, action, object and indirect object. Insofar as this structure can be pinned down, the self/object oscillations that are described by Sandler may be seen to have a syntactic format. The forms are then played out with a shift in *who* is the *agent* and *whom* is the *passive* or *active object* in relation to the action sought, the verb. The patient becomes empowered by the language used, by knowing that he unwittingly is falling into one or another of these role designators, and that they were beyond his conscious grasp before they were verbalized. (Teller, V. & Dahl, H., 1993; Schaffer, R., 1976; Shapiro, T., 1988)

Semantics refers to the sign relationship of meaning and signification. What do what you are doing and saying stand for?

What is the relationship of the referent to the reference? However, here we must elaborate that we are pointing beyond the simplest denotative form of a statement. We are more interested in how the image the patient presents, or the story told, refers to an unconscious fantasy or a preconceived standing format that has not been articulated. Moreover, how does that format and its representation become a synchronic statement derived from formats of past organizations that remain relatively rigid within the individual's mental life? They may even have been encoded in early procedural memories and unconscious fantasies, and up to now have been inexpressible (Clyman R, 1992; Shapiro T, 1992).

Finally, pragmatics refers to the sector of linguistics that refers to communication and implied intention that cannot be accounted for solely through semantics and syntaxis. Such an analysis requires observation of language in use and can be determined only in the context of a human relationship. It is deciphered in the metalinguistic contextual analysis of a statement as expressed in the interactions between two people who have additional knowledge of each other, such as role expectations and social conventions and intentions.

An individual entering a room where an elder sits, hearing "It is warm in here," does not take that as a declarative sentence alone to describe the temperature of ambient air, but as an *action request* to open the window and offer relief or to turn on the air conditioner. In this sense, language in use is a vehicle whose aim is to get things done. The semantics alone or the structure of the sentence do not betray the intended wish, and certainly not the unconscious wish.

In a psychoanalysis, the prolonged interaction between the patient and the analyst provides numerous opportunities for redundant expression of what we consider to be a common small set of ideas, in varying vehicles and at various times designed to get something done or to recreate an old pattern. It is through the redundant recognition and re-recognition of these *common themes* that the analyst is able to interpret with some certainty the productions of the patient and the re-enactments of the patient in the analysis that derive from earlier interactions in the family. Sandler's representational world is rendered manageable by the analyst's interpretative words.

A case presentation referred to elsewhere (Shapiro, T., 1977) for different purposes will be used to illustrate the varying aspects of the interpretative process from a psychoanalytic linguistic standpoint. This exercise will be used to demonstrate the patient's various vehicles of expression that the analyst used to arrive at a verbal characterization of the patient's behavior for common scrutiny in the analysis.

CASE EXAMPLE

A young professional in his early twenties entered analysis complaining about difficulties functioning in many areas of life.

He was married but avoided intercourse with his wife, masturbating instead to fantasies of oral genital contact with young girls, alternating with dreams of seduction by older women. He also would provoke violent arguments with his wife instead of providing her with the solace of a caring or even sexually satisfying marriage.

Even as he felt righteous about his behavior, he also felt he was an imposter and his self-esteem lagged. He frequently changed facts impulsively to correspond with his fantasy in order to achieve some praise. These mixed motives led to the experience of shame and apprehension about discovery.

During his early adolescence, he was discovered and reprimanded for rubbing his body against the buttocks of a sleeping girl at a party. During the initial phases of the analysis he worried greatly about whether the analyst liked him. He continually sought approval, while he fantasized that the analyst would take advantage of him and seduce him, with growing anxiety that he would be passively victimized in the way in which he had victimized the girl in adolescence. This was the first representation of his identification with women. Somewhat later in the analytic work, he began to talk about his wife's older cousin. He spoke of her with great affection, revealing very soon that his wife was merely a vehicle by which he could become close to this older woman.

After confessing these ideas, he went away from the analyst on vacation and was increasingly sexually active with his wife. This, however, stopped again once we resumed treatment. During this next phase, he frequently dozed on the couch. His waking comments, however, concerned sexual exploits and the esteem that these exploits afforded him when he told his friends. Indeed, this wish for admiration by friends expanded into increasing ambition and derivative wishes that the boys admire his prowess at many enterprises. On the other hand, ambition made him anxious, because his "avaricious mother" would necessarily exact her share of the results. The latter characterization of his mother was in sharp contrast to the giving that he felt his wife's cousin provided.

As the analyst interpreted the passive wishes to be sexually intruded on while sleeping, the comments were met with pseudo-stupidity reflected in lack of understanding and naïveté. Even with such denial, this interpretation led to his expanded revelation that during early latency, that he "manipulated a girl" his own age, as she "played dumb."

There was growing evidence, as well, that his passivity was enhanced as a strong defense against castration anxiety. These interpretations were given further force by a dream interpretation.

In one dream he described being in a tub with a small frog that grew very large. The animal's skin was associated to a skin condition that he suffered and was related to his penis. Indeed, the skin condition was on his groin and genitals which he felt marked him as a masturbator. As an adolescent, he had, indeed, masturbated in the tub. This guilty revelation also turned him from an aggressive stance into a pitiable condition because he was to be considered a mere child in a tub with a tub toy.

Once these areas were interpreted with respect to their defensive nature, he began more frankly to expose his sexual wishes towards his wife's cousin in the analysis. She possessed a series of traits which he contrasted strongly to his depriving mother toward whom he felt only rage and suspicion. The analyst too was now viewed as a depriving mother.

The analyst interpreted that he had symbolically married his own Oedipal daughter. His wife was his sister and he was the triumphant partner of a mature woman who was exactly the opposite of his biological mother. His psychologically absent father became even more absent from his verbalization. The interpretation of his symbolic plight was re-represented in a condensed form in a dream: He was behind a woman molesting her. She was wearing "little girl's pants" which reminded him of his wife's underclothing, but she had the breasts of an older woman. This event was visualized in a large open area, where mother and grandmother were looking down at him while cooking his favorite food.

The analyst's interpretation addressed the exhibitionistic elements evidenced in this dream, as shown in the wish to be admired and loved. The anxieties about castration as represented in the preferred approach to the woman from behind were also aired. In the wake of these presentations, the patient's impulsiveness decreased, he became more attentive to his work, and he ceased to masturbate.

In another dream, he was flying about the city as everyone watched. As we proceeded, these phallic narcissistic exhibitionistic acts diminished as well. His mother's tendency to give him food at her expense, but not respect his adulthood, then became prominent, revealing his wish to take without having to show that he wanted. He always feared death. These emerging themes were also represented in the organizing fantasy and experience during adolescence that he tried to seduce a sleeping young woman, that is, to take without being noticed and to thereby deny his need as well as his castration anxiety.

Even as he continued to do well, the patient began to complain to the analyst, accusing him of playing with himself behind the couch. This reversal reinforced the patient's idea that the analyst would become excited by the patient as he slept, giving way to anxiety that he would be forced into fellatio in order to feed him the analyst's strength orally.

At one juncture, during the analysis, his wish to display inadequacy and pseudo-stupidity became most prominent in an enactment. The analyst had had a carpet cleaned, and when the patient entered the room he looked at the paper on the floor and asked, as though an innocent child, "Where shall I walk, on the carpet or the paper?

DISCUSSION

An analysis unfolds even as a drama does. However, neither the analyst nor the patient know the script explicitly. They are more like a new audience than the author, director, or actors.

The analyst comes prepared with some predetermined formulae that set the broad outlines of the parameters of the human script and the patient has a dim awareness of his or her tendencies to act repetitively in certain ways. Nonetheless, it takes the development of the unique relationship known as a psychoanalysis to make the script's variations explicit. As the themes become apparent, the analyst gives structure to the shadow narrative (Makari G. and Shapiro T., 1993) by verbalizing the interactions and providing a shorthand description of the significance of the associative links in words in terms of wish and defense. This is an interpretation.

The case presented provides a variety of verbalizations, story lines, enactments, and visualizations in dreams that point to a narrow range of unconscious fantasies redundantly presented in surface forms for those who are trained to see beyond the obvious.

In its briefest verbal form, the young man here described suffered from severe castration anxiety and fear of begin overwhelmed by his mother, whom he viewed as controlling and infantilizing. Moreover, he did not have the protection of his father, who was seen as weak and irrelevant. Thus he identified with the passive sleeping younger woman and could achieve sexual arousal and satisfaction only by stealing sexual fulfillment from a girl/woman from behind. He longingly sought a caring and passionately praising mother who would extol his playing at manhood, but because of the dangers of such assertiveness, had to deny his ambition in feigned weakness, pseudo-stupidity, illness, and infantilism. His narcissistic fragility is ever apparent in his repeated need for affirmation hiding his aggression and rage.

This is too formulaic to help our patient because it sounds pat, and yet such description does encapsulate the trends of the case for a most generalized verbal psychoanalytic description. It does not work as a representation for the patient, because he will recognize himself only in the general outlines and not in the specifics of the content (the *Erlebnis*). Here the concise form in words overwhelms the content. This is further confounded by the level of verbal description which is cast in metalanguage. Thus, language, when applied to the wrong context, can confound communication as well as facilitate it.

Viewed from a linguistic vantage point, we thus must consider the language of interpretation not only as a general message, but also as specific words and grammatical formats used and their appropriateness to the interaction between analyst and patient.

Do they touch the patient, are they specific enough, can they be referred to profitably again? Often, we use the patient's words and preferred references to designate interaction, or we use repetitive phrases that are familiar or laden with affect to make our interventions familiar and less intellectual.

The syntax of the relationship of subject to object is clear but oscillating. The patient wants the analyst's praise and affection initially, but is fearful that he will not get it if he reveals his secret wishes. He feels like an imposter, even to the point of changing facts and becoming one perhaps thereby inviting punishment though he consciously wants praise, but also protects his narcissistic self-image.

The first revelation is made about an adolescent seduction while the woman slept. The syntax of agent-action-object remained the same as the analysis proceeded, but the object and agent changed and had to be interpreted as such. He who seduces from behind now wishes to be seduced from behind. These relationships are further exploited and expressed later in the analysis in visual form in dreams. At first he is a child in a tub with a disease as represented by a warty frog, and then he is a masterful exhibitionistic sexual acrobat admired from the grandstand by his mother who cooks for him as well.

These shifting opposites are given life by many object-relations theorists and by ego psychologists (J. Arlow, 1977) in the well-known tendency to turn active to passive and vice versa. The defensiveness of both alternatives is a contribution of psychoanalysis. The minimalist syntactic description gives a description of agency in action, helping us to be alert to hearing who is doing what to whom and to interpret in words the direction of wishes.

The semantic portion of the equation is most closely related to psychoanalytic symbol formation. Even as Lacan (1956) referred to the play of the signifier, Freud (1899) referred to overdetermination and Waelder (1936) to multiple function. Linguistics refers to polysemy, i.e., many meanings or a rich array of meanings. In this instance the meaning of the theme of seduction while asleep and applause for such achievement apparently went back to latency-stage sexual play as indicated in the case history. If that is not indeed a historical fact, it is nonetheless a fact of this man's mental life, and therefore meaningful and salient now.

Generalized Oedipal ambitions were not abandoned: they were transformed into more acceptable forms that would permit this man to function in some adaptive capacities as a man, a husband, a son. None of these were accomplished very successfully, because the meanings of the experiences were subject to personal reinterpretation in the form of unconscious fantasies that only permitted sexual arousal if the object was immature, a girl who slept, approached from behind so that he could not see that she was penis-less and he could steal satisfaction.

These are no longer formulaic requirements; they are presented as variations on a specific semantic referent. The vehicles of representation change even as the roles of the patient and analyst change, but there is a unique referent that takes a number of forms derived from his past memories.

We learn about the adolescent seduction first, as the initial revelation that he feared would interfere with the analytic relationship. We learned about the latency event even later, but we also have the juxtaposed confession of lust for the older cousin, the impotence and avoidance of coital contact with his wife, and the expressed belief that the analyst was getting excited. All these pronouncements converge on the listener, forcing him to make a concise verbal statement that encompasses the varied experiences.

The pragmatic area of language in use is perhaps the most exciting as it links the representations to transference enactments in what Sandler calls role responsiveness.

The analyst's actions or even inactions are subjected to personal idiosyncratic interpretations by the patient within the context of his unique idiom. Meanings are no longer simply denotative or connotative; they become personally idiosyncratic or they are recast in terms of the patient's irrational need to see things in his own way and in his need to influence the analyst to adopt a specific view of him. The pseudo-stupidity exhibited in the query about where to walk on a newly shampooed rug was an easy reference to the analyst that the query was preceded by a forbidden aggressively sexual fantasy. The belief that the analyst would act with the patient as he himself described that he acted with two young girls was predetermined by the patient's narrative pull to his own carefully created, though unconscious, story line.

Thus when we listen to what patients say, we simultaneously must attend to what they do, and how they assign roles to us derived from their personal history.

This description of the text of the analysis is rather dry and formal, but does force us to focus on the elements of symbolic play that confront us in an analysis. Such analysis is not only applicable to our work, of course, but to any dialogue. We have not yet taken the fullest advantage of this approach for our work.

Joseph Sandler has alerted us and riveted our attention to the highly significant role of mental representation in psychological life. I would like to say that we need a further explication of how we become aware of these unities and how we encode them for verbalization, instruction and dialogue.

I might add that until they are verbalized within the context of the analysis, they remain entities to be wrestled with within the patient's own mind. When cast in appropriate words, they are communicated and become a common property to be reviewed and argued about, to be considered and modified and re-reviewed to achieve a better fit.

There is no guarantee, however, that the verbal cast will create the change that is desired. For the patient in the throes of positive transference may accept too readily, just as the negative transferential state may yield further negativism.

Nonetheless, the feat of stating that which had been clothed in polysemantic forms in various vehicles (dream, narrative, enactment) can, once interpreted, be used in the service of understanding and change. The representational world is now a public issue in concise form, ready for discourse, disagreement, and dialogue.

REFERENCES

Arlow, J. (1977). Affects and the psychoanalytic situation. *Int. J. Psychoanalysis* 58:158–170.

Clyman, R. (1992).The Procedural Organization of Emotions.In *Affect: Psychoanalytic Perspectives,* ed.by T.Shapiro and R.N.Emde. New York: Int.Univ.Press.

Freud, S. (1899).Screen Memories. *S.E.,* Vol. 3, p.301.

Lacan, J. (1956).*The Language of the Self: the Function of Language in Psychoanalysis* (translated by A.Wilden).Baltimore: The John Hopkins Press.

Luborsky, L.& Luborsky, E. (1993).The Era of Measures of Transference the CCRT and Other Measures.In supplement: *J.American Psychoanalytic Assoc.* 41(suppl.): 329–351).

Mahoney, P. (1987). *Psychoanalysis and Discourse.*London: Tavistock. Makari, G. & Shapiro, T. (1993).Psychoanalytic Listening: Language and Unconscious. *J. American Psychoanalytic Assoc.* (4):991–1020.

Sandler, J.(1990).On Internal Object Relations. *J. American Psychoanalytic Assoc.* 38:859–880.

——— Joffe, W.G.(1966).On Sublimation.In *From Safety to Superego,* ed.J.Sandler.New York: Guilford Press, 1987, pp.191– 207.

——— Nagera, H.(1963).The Metapsychology of Fantasy.In *From Safety to Superego,* ed.by J.Sandler.Guilford Press, 1987, pp.90– 120.

Schaffer, R. (1976).A New Language for Psychoanalysis. New Haven: Yale University Press

Shapiro, T. (1970).Interpretation and Naming. *J. American Psychoanalytic Assoc.* 18:399–421.

——— (1977). Oedipal Distortions in Severe Character Pathologies: Developmental and Theoretical Considerations.*Psychoanalytic Ouarterly.*66: 559–579.

——— (1979).*Clinical Psycholinguistics.*New York: Plenum Press.

——— (1988).Language Structure and Psychoanalysis.In Supplement: *J.of the American Psychoanalytic Assoc.*Vol.36. Madison, CT: Int'l. Univ. Press.

———(1992). Words and Feelings in the Psychoanalytic Dialogue. In *Affect: Psychoanalytic Perspectives,* ed.by T.Shapiro and R.N. Emde. New York: Int.Univ.Press.

Teller, V.& Dahl, H. (1993).What Psychoanalysis Needs Is More Empirical Researchers. *J. American Psychoanalytic Assoc.* (Suppl.): 31–49.

Waelder (1936).The Principle of Multiple Function.*The Psychoanalytic Ouarterly* 5:45–62.

Whorf, B.L. (1962).*Language, Thought and Reality.*Cambridge: MIT Press.

Naming the Unnameable

(2005). *Psychoanalytic Inquiry* 25(4):506–515.

An analogy is drawn between the naming of preverbal mental constellations and the intrusion on aboriginal fixed beliefs and rituals. In order to interpret the unnamed complexes, we must venture past many personal taboos and time our interventions, taking care to secure a workable alliance. A review of current practices in psychoanalysis shows many breaches in the older requirement of neutrality in the name of empathy, alliance, and intersubjectivity. Nonetheless, the verbalization of unconscious patterned behaviors must be rendered in words and mentalized, if patients are to proceed in life with fewer restraints.

Naming the unconscious fantasies designates the patient's psychic reality. The factual basis of psychic reality as memories of the past remains uncertain.

In many religious groups, and in certain African and Pacific societies until recently untouched by Western civilization, there is a taboo about naming God, uttering someone's name, or having a photograph that represents someone's image. This is a puzzling practice unless we understand that a name is more than a label and has added value because it entails all the symbolic power of the god or the person, and is full of affective valence and mystery. Demystifying the name for inhabitants of these societies or religious groups takes a good deal of work, and even a change of view, which undoes years of prior individual experience and training in the culture of origin. The unnameable is the repository of the secret power of the life itself; its panoply of powers underlie existence, but also restrain the community from certain actions and commit them to promises made in the name of the culture which include such things as blood revenge, Satanic possession, ritual prayer, talisman, sanctity of family, cult secrets, and a host of other expectable and respectable societal rules.

Freud (1901) sought to demystify the usual, the banal, the commonplace in his late-19th-early-20th-century world by helping us to understand the unconscious underpinnings of the beliefs, dreams, parapraxes, and day-to-day neuroses that made up the ego-syntonic routines of humdrum quotidian existence. He entered the personal arena of patients, however, only when they hurt or were just plain out of step and seemed not to fit. Initially, they were thought to have neurological diseases. He alluded, for example, to the similarity of the rituals of compulsions and religious practice, again bringing psychopathology into the realm of the banal. In his various analyses, he discovered that so-called civilized humankind was afflicted by taboos similar to the constraints of the other societies I mention. They were bound to practices that they thought of as necessary to their existence, which he was able to analyze and name (Shapiro, 1979). And, in naming them, Freud sought to free the sufferers from the constraints of their anachronistic bonds, which supported action and reaction patterns that may have been appropriate to childhood when dependent, and when in a relationship to parents who as adults were no longer the lords of the manor in which the person lived and grew up. He worked his magic verbally and by slowly habilitating patients to name the unconscious constellations that he thought supported the foolish and constraining actions that had become their lives. The psychoneuroses Freud (1895) assaulted were rampant and epidemic.

There then were issues to be dealt with about which Freud never satisfactorily came to rest: Did the repressed have to be conscious, or are there primal repressions that exert an afterpressure, drawing the new experiences into old conservative and even biologically based mind-sets? Was a construction (Freud, 1937) about the past really what had happened, or was it a construction requiring a qualifier stating that you act as if x had happened? Are there preOedipal residua that shine through in adult behavior as action patterns, as if a series of bad habits learned through many interactions with mother emerged from the sheer force of early conditioning? All these and many other solutions have been part of the history of our modern approaches to interpreting—or, as I have written about it, naming that which has eluded the patient's conscious apprehension of the world (Shapiro, 1976).

Freud's initial belief was that making the unconscious conscious would do it all; then followed the quantum of affect to be discharged in catharsis; then the idea of deciphering the actions of patients as resistances and turning the patterns of action into words; and finally the transference interpretations that were mutative. His ideas about change received their penultimate form in his last metaphor: Like the Zuider Zee where the sea was reclaimed as land, the Ego would drain the Id and become usable to increase the scope of action of the fortunate patient (Freud, 1940). Later theorists have offered variant forms of these old saws in new concepts such as *corrective emotional experience* and *transmuting internalization* (Kohut 1977) where the new relationship with the analyst permits the self to heal and become *cohesive*, where the special relationship with the analyst permits an *inter-subjective* (Greenberg, 1995) apprehension of the other's inner self, where the *mentalization*(Fonagy, 1999) of the *enactments* between patient and analyst becomes the stuff of change, or where the *now moments* (Stern et al., 1998) between analyst and patient replicate the best of times with mother so they can now move along without uttering the name of the unnameable.

All these approaches have been proffered to address the fixity of our action patterns and repetitive maladroitness with life: The repetition compulsion was invoked to account for our moral masochism, to help us face over and over again the helplessness we felt when traumatized, to create a new experience that will disprove that people are "no damn good" and "unreliable, abusive cads." The victim in us wants to be on top, but if to be on top means to kill our fathers, then let's take on the mantle of victimization again and back off. Notice that whatever theory we hold about change—some require confrontation with the devil in words and others involve the therapeutic relationship and cradling and holding or whatever other device convinces the person called patient—they have to change behavior and belief to feel better. Patients have to change their beliefs, their actions, and their tendency to slip back into old ways. Even as we take hold and redirect our lives, the tides that pull us to the past must be overcome. As the last lines of *The Great Gatsby* boldly state, "So we beat on boats against the current borne back ceaselessly into the past" (Fitzgerald, 1925).

The power of the past is invoked in almost every construal I have mentioned, but as a means of change some demand words and others do not. Sweeney, in Eliot's (1930) poem, cries out, "I've got to use words when I talk to you!" My response is, "Yes!" I believe that psychoanalysis is a talking cure, and no matter how we twist and turn and complain about the austerity and indeterminacy of words and the need to cradle and comfort and "hold" in many instances, in the end we are a profession of word-users. In addition, we use our words to influence, and we time our phrases so that what is said can be listened to; we do not make tacit or inauthentic promises that create an illusion of fulfillment of longed-for wishes, or a magical reunion with God. The latter is the most egregious of our potentials for malpractice.

As for the boundaries of our professional obligations as analysts, many of us seek to help others, and many treatments do many different things. We should, however, constrain our zeal to help. There has been a rash of recent papers that offer pragmatic justifications for breaching old rules that many think are obsolete, but nonetheless require scrutiny as to their intent and may continue to be used as guides rather than rules. "I do not mind revealing myself," the average modern analyst says. Analysts, in fact, are advised to do so, and then the slippery slope of mutual confession and transference-countertransference constellations takes hold in enactments, and treatment can be destroyed by no conscious intent but by the mutual seductiveness entailed in the intimacy of the therapy. I believe that there is a lot that is not understood as we proceed and we do hit impasses, but we should first try to determine what is going on in order to clear the way toward understanding. This, I believe, involves words as a means of bridging the gap between two subjective participants (Shapiro, 2002).

The recent focus on the patient's narrative is a happy turn, because it requires a retelling of that which was not told, as a map of the territory that has been explored. It should include the traps and declivities where the patient may again fall and also serve the patient as a reusable guide to future action as the path of life is resumed. There is much said about coconstruction of such maps, which for some mimics the mother-child coconstruction of the childhood narrative, creating the illusion that what is said is a social construct without designative power (Greenberg, 1995). However, as I see it, the designation is that of a description of the repetitive tendencies of patients to trip into old potholes even when they have new knowledge. The latter issue has taken life in the well-worn notion that insight may be present, but the patient cannot use it. It is the usual idea of knowing, but the knowing is not enabling. Our analytic parents used to cite the difference between intellectual insight and emotional insight to distinguish the two. Others called on Waelder's (1930) notion of multiple function, requiring the repetitive working through by the patient so that he can become acquainted with the various dimensions of symptomatic acts—that is, their relation to guilt, their reality justifications, their compromise role, and so forth. It was Nietzsche who reminded us that every word we utter is an interpretation, and, insofar as that is true, every word we utter has to be timed and thought about in terms of what the speech-act theorists call the illocutionary force of the utterance (Searle, 1969).

Illocutionary force may be a new version of Freud's earlier idea that speech is trial action. The newer form grew out of the work of Austin, an English philosopher and linguist, who reminded us that words not only point to things and ideas (i.e., mean), they also perform acts. He called them performatives. When we say "I do" at a wedding, for example, we promise. These performatives were expanded by Searle (1969), the Berkeley philosopher, into a theory of speech acts that show that if we did not know the context of the usage, we could not understand the pragmatic meaning of the utterance. It would not be possible to grasp the ritual of the analytic arrangement for a Martian who in its experience on Earth had become accustomed to people's greeting face-to- face and saying, "How are you?" The visitor to Earth would have to have become acquainted with the specific intracultural, ritualized feature of the analytic situation. The extension of finding meaning in the arrangement and the intention or illocutionary force of an exchange opens the door for considering the array of gestural and mimetic components of discourse as fair game for interpretation as well (Makari and Shapiro, 1993).

There are those who believe strongly in the possibility of interpreting the preverbal past and coming close to the mark of an actual happening. Some few examples come to mind. Terr (1988), who studies trauma, reported on a young woman who as a child had been abusively used in pornographic movies, describing a sexual practice which was so idiosyncratic that its origins could not be discerned. At some point in the therapy, the porn films in which she was a participant were found and reviewed, showing the same postural gestures that were her route to arousal as an adult enacted in her not-remembered past. Levine (1990) has reported on a number of cases in which he could surmise a past event which was then proven as a factual happening. These types of *post hoc* findings and verifications of the preverbal or early verbal past are few in the literature. Freud in the beginning of his career in a paper on "Screen Memories" (1899) and then later in "Constructions in Analysis" (1937) was very careful to say these memories were from the past and about the past, but not of the past. His caution was warranted, because his entire edifice was based on the idea of the power of psychic reality in constructing organizing fantasies that direct action at a distance that have value as afterpressures, *Nachträglichkeit*, or, as the French say, *après coup*.

The significant issues that have arisen from what has infelicitously been called the "false-memory movement" have come to haunt us, because there is an issue of the effect of suggestion again on the land. Doubt has been replaced with certainty; and there is a split among us in regard to patients' beliefs in their memories or in the analyst's wish to prove his theory. Ferenczi (1949), of course, fought that battle with Freud in his suggestion that patients will tell of the horrors experienced only if they have an accepting audience and that traumatized patients can only trust if the recipient of the confession is tolerant and willing to join the conversation. There is, unfortunately, no way to become a detective or private agent in the discovery of verity. Rather, we accompany patients in their quest, and we examine their convictions for their defensive value and for the way in which the psychic organization profits from the beliefs and how the patient's adaptation depends on such beliefs. Like the aboriginal's unwillingness to tell us the name of his god, he has the comfort of the internalized teaching of his community as a protection to proceed as usual so long as it is confined to the world in which he lives and he does not venture beyond the borders.

Turning briefly to the theorists of childhood in our quest for the possible origins of mental registration of action patterns that are socially detectable later, we must start with Freud (1926) himself, whose "Inhibitions, Symptoms, and Anxiety" was written in part as a refutation of Rank's notion of birth anxiety. Freud was too wily a developmentalist to believe that the human infant was able to register a long-lasting pattern for behavior at the first instances of life. The cerebral cortex was not so ready to be a source of instantaneous imprinting that lasted without the possibility of modification, which

90

marked the developmental danger signals that he posited. Anna Freud (1936) also suggested that it was not the events of life that mattered, but the repercussion of events on the mind that analysts dealt with. She called the first six months of life the period of the need-satisfying object; that is, the object was vague and anaclitic, as her father had noted. More recent observers seem to provide some warrant that over the first 18 months a pattern of mother-infant interactions becomes fixed that has a lasting impact on our social tendencies. Stern (1998) especially has taken Bowlby's internal working-model idea one step further in his belief that there is a coconstruction of the motherhood constellation... a new version of Winnicott's (1960) assertion, "There is no such thing as an infant."

The implicit memory system holds the "now moments"in place over time, so that the subsequent experiences do not supersede the earliest pattern. These patterns continue to be sought in subsequent human experience, as though dormant and reactivated with each new relationship, perhaps someday awaiting declarative translation. Such views are distinctly linear and do not obey the alternative developmental view of hierarchic reorganization, in which the past is superseded until a relatively fixed pattern of interaction is congealed into an organizing fantasy, as in the Freudian Oedipal constellation. Those who take the nuclear constellation position say, as does Anna Freud (1936), that we can see that preOedipal past only dimly through the thick veil of the Oedipal constellation. What can we say about the schools that believe, as the self-psychologists do, that we must await the hurt that we inevitably will effect, and the insult that the narcissistically damaged patient will feel, so that a new modification can be effected in a transmuting internalization? There are many among us who do name the unnameable in the search for the patient's core beliefs, so that the pragmatic effect of the relationship can take the patient a step further in life trajectory on the basis of the alliance alone. An Italian saying, roughly translated, is, "Even if not true, it is indeed well-conceived." Good intentions may go awry, however.

The following vignette describes a naming of the past in a manner that offers a better ground to even consider how to proceed. It entails a linguistic trope that makes me feel better because I do not commit myself to the belief that it is necessarily true. It carries the proviso of a conditional clause that says to the patient, "Does it fit you?" Is this an approximation of your wish that you cannot ask for, because it seems unsuitable to your current status and would not satisfy the restraints of the current relationship and not be seductive. It is the "as-if" clause, or the metaphorical "You seem to be saying" preamble. We all do it, and whenever I have been a reader of a paper on reconstruction, the best intentioned among us use it. It refutes the certainty and yet it fits the affective climate of inquiry and curiosity; it puts words on an unuttered constellation that we can observe in gesture, sequence of ideas, and the like. It has illocutionary force.

I once saw a 10-year-old girl who longed desperately for a better quality of contact and feeling of love from her mother who was mighty busy and tended to be unseemly angry. As the child spoke and could not find the words for what she wanted, she was running her hand slowly and gently inside her fleece-lined coat sleeve. It was not difficult to see the soothing effect it had on her agitation. I suggested she acted as if she wanted her mother to soothingly and softly hold her even as she was gently comforting her own arm. She brightened and seemed to become more fluent, complaining of the deprivation she felt from her busy mother both presently and in the past [Shapiro, 1977].

In another instance, I was confronted with a woman who was in an endless struggle regarding who needed more, her husband or her. I was finally able to metaphorically say that she acted "as if" she were angrily competing with her twin brother like newborn birds open-mouthed in a nest as to who would be fed first.

Yet another patient provided an opportunity to grasp at an artifact in my office as a reference for an interpretation. The photo of Freud is an incidental part of the decoration about the room. This patient never accepted interpretation or help of any sort. Instead he remained austerely self-sufficient and uncompromising in his "do it myself " attitude. He also did not join his father's lucrative business as his only son but remained fixated on his pursuit of writing, experiencing disappointment upon disappointment. One day I learned that his father's name was Sigmund and then the link could be made to my own intellectual father. It was as if he could not take from this Sigmund or and father representation or follower of the father. The icon was mistaken for the person (Shapiro, 1977). I raise the latter examples as a means of showing that language enables a wonderful flexibility of reference insofar as it does not simply denote but allows a hypothetical contrary-to-fact possibility for referencing the real. It is an approximation similar to the iconic and the symbolic. The patient can now reject, modify, or accept what has been offered in words and the negativity may abate with aid of the 'as-if' maneuver. This permits a different illocutionary force to begin the new iterative process of therapy.

When we interpret, if we do, we make a statement about something we have witnessed derived from the patient's behavior and verbalizations. We designate an empirically based coherent datum. This is what I mean by an analytic fact. I make no claim, however, that what I say actually happened in the past. Rather, I am telling it as I see it from the vantage point of the patient's unconscious fantasy, or, better yet, the inner unspoken psychic reality that can now make its way into consciousness by the miracle of words. The form of the interpretation can then be manipulated by the patient in the service of breaking the former magical bond of the unsaid and increase his flexibility to act in accord with a newly recognized reality.

REFERENCES

Eliot, T. S. (1930), Sweeny Agonistes. In: *Collected Poems*. New York: Harcourt Brace.

Ferenczi, S. (1949). Confusion of the tongues between the adults and the child (language of tenderness and of passion). *Int. J. Psycho-Anal.*, 30: 225-230.

Fitzgerald, F.S. (1925). *The Great Gatsby*. New York: Scribners.

Fonagy, P. (1999). Memory and therapeutic action. *Int. J. Psycho-Anal.*, 80: 215–223.

Freud, A. (1936). *The Ego and the Mechanisms of Defense*. New York: International Universities Press.

Freud, S. (1895). Studies in hysteria. *Standard Edition* 2: 1–309. London: Hogarth Press, 1955.

——— (1899). Screen memories. *Standard Edition* 3: 303–322. London: Hogarth Press, 1962.

——— (1901). Psychopathology of everyday life. *Standard Edition*, 6: 1–290. London: Hogarth Press, 1960.

——— (1926). Inhibitions, symptoms, and anxiety. *Standard Edition* 20: 87–175. London: Hogarth Press, 1959.

——— (1937). Constructions in analysis. *Standard Edition* 23: 255–269. London: Hogarth Press, 1964.

————— (1940). Outline of psychoanalysis. *Standard Edition* 23: 144–207. London: Hogarth Press, 1964.

————— (1940). Outline of psychoanalysis. *Standard Edition* 23: 144–207. London: Hogarth Press, 1964.

Greenberg, J. (1995). Psychoanalytic technique and the interactive matrix. *Psychoanal. Q.*, 64: 1–22.

Kohut, H. (1977). *The Restoration of the Self.* New York: International Universities Press.

Levine, H.B. (1990).

Makari, G. & Shapiro, T. (1993). Psychoanalytic listening: Language and unconscious communication. *J. Amer. Psychoanal. Assn.*, 41: 991–1019.

Searle, J. R. (1969). *Speech Acts: An Essay on the Philosophy of Language.* : Cambridge University Press.

Shapiro, T. (1970). Interpretation and naming. *J. Amer. Psychoanal. Assn.*, 18: 399–421.

————— (1977). Oedipal distortions in severe character pathologies: Developmental and theoretical considerations. *Psychoanal. Q.*, 46: 559–579.

————— (1979). *Clinical Psycholinguistics.* New York: Plenum Press.

————— (2002). From monologue to dialogue. *J. Amer. Psychoanal. Assn.*, 50: 199–220.

Stern, D., Sander, L. & Nahum, J. (1998). Non-interpretative mechanisms in psychoanalytic therapy. *Int. J. Psycho-Anal.*, 79: 903–921.

Terr, L. (1988). What happens to early memories of trauma. *J. Amer. Acad. Child Psychiat.*, 27: 96–104.

Waelder, R. (1930). *The Principle of Multiple Function.* ed. S. A. Guttman. New York: International Universities Press, 1976, pp. 68–83.

Winnicott, D.W. (1960). The theory of the parent-infant relationship. In: *The Maturational Processes and the Facilitating Environment.* New York: International Universities Press, 1965, pp. 37–55.

Now Moments in Psychotherapy and Psychoanalysis and Baby Watching

(2018). *Psychoanalytic Inquiry* 38:120–129.

Now moments and moments of meeting are concepts derived from careful observation of mother-infant interaction using a theoretical frame that employs implicit knowing and nondeterminate sloppy processing. This dyadically derived construct has been transported and applied to the therapeutic dyad by Daniel Stern and his colleagues at the Boston Change Process Study Group (BCPSG) as a means to understand the something more that complements classically modeled psychoanalytic interpretation in promoting change. Tracking the origin, development and application of this idea opens the concept to scrutiny and will permit testing of its explanatory power, its flaws, and offer direction for future study.

It is not by chance that some psychoanalysts in the United States during the 1960s and '70s took to baby-watching and immersed themselves in new technology and methodology of infant-mother observation. The seeds were sowed by Freud himself when he posited polymorphous perverse infantile sexuality and drove his theory backward in time toward infancy by making fixations and regressions into the anlage of symptom formation. He was a developmentalist by proxy, so much so that when filling out the key points of view that psychoanalysis comprises, Rappaport included development as an essential viewpoint among the others.

Within the psychoanalytic world, Anna Freud and Melanie Klein explored the psyches of children within the broad strokes of the method, using play as a substitute for free association. At approximately the same time, clinical theorists wrote seriously about an early undifferentiated phase, Mahler (1963) about an early autistic phase, Anna Freud (1960) about a stage of need-satisfying object, and so on. All of these models regarding the early months and their meaning to later psychology were left as theoretical constructs yet to be substantiated. The new baby-watchers expanded empirical knowledge of how early interaction with mother (I use mother as shorthand for caretaker) shaped behavior and was internalized as mental complexes that led to behavioral consequences in later life. As psychoanalysts, Stern among others, were interested in how these early observations and internalizations affected adult human interaction and the therapeutic encounter itself. One might suggest that these investigators provided an unbeckoned empirical arm to object relations theory. On the side of biological research, they provided the behavioral data that could be used to account for epigenetic changes and variability in gene expression.

In addition to, and prior to, Stern's pioneering efforts, other analysts took off into empirical studies of infancy and mothering using the techniques of modern observational science. The most distinguished and enduring of these were Rene Spitz and John Bowlby. They actually watched children of early age. Spitz (1946) and colleagues watched babies in extreme circumstances in institutions and discovered that infants need mothers not only to offer physical care, as Freud posited in his anaclitic, evolutionarily derived model, but to provide consistent loving and affectively charged environments. Bowlby (1953, 1969) studied and described the effects of war and family separation on children and built attachment theory, and with it a huge edifice of research that carries on. Since his death, coworkers and disciples such as Ainsworth et al. (1978). and later Sroufe (1999) were all devoted to establishing an empirical description of the consequences of security of attachment as a determinant of later outcomes. Many of these students concentrated on 12- to 24-month-old toddlers, leaving infancy to others. However, they did not study infant- mother dyads closely or as systematically as Stern did.

These mid-century baby watchers spawned huge legacies of developmental psychological interest and research that also included some selected psychoanalysts who took as their life work the study of infants and their mothers (Sander, 1975). Dan Stern was one of the most creative and persistent of this new breed. Also prominent in the group were Robert Emde, Louis Sander, Edward Tronick, and others who have contributed to our knowledge, left students to carry on, and developed models to work with and revise in accord with new data. I write this piece partly from the inside, because I had the opportunity to work closely with Sander, Emde, and Stern in various settings and even share published works with each. However, this article also draws on my view from the outside, as a clinical psychoanalyst and clinical investigator working with developmentally afflicted children and, only sometimes, with normal children, rather than with the normal developmental process as it occurs in average expectable environments.

The analysts *cum* baby watchers, as noted, were influenced by Freud's retrospective reconstructions of the experienced preverbal beginnings of intrapsychic development, leading to the later representations of these processes during therapy. Stern's (2004) foray into what he has called the "now moments" derives from his early-life observations carried forward into the dyadic interactions during psychoanalytic therapy. He gathered together like-minded colleagues to inaugurate the Boston Change Process Study Group (BCPSG; which, by the way, included Louis Sander and Edward Tronick, among others). and is foundational to his book, *The Present Moment* (Stern, 2004). The group took as its task the expansion of observations during infancy to further understand the influence of past patterns on interrelationships such as the psychoanalytic dyad, as well as interactions in everyday life. Hence, the full title of his book is *The Present Moment in Psychotherapy and Everyday Life*. The project has a scope that includes the idea that all interactions are derivatives of the earliest maternal influences. Just to remind the reader, John Bowlby's (1953) first popular presentation to the public of his ideas was titled *Child Care and the Growth of Love*. During the late nineties and early millennium, the BCPSG (Stern et al., 1998) grasped the opportunity to apply the early data and constructs regarding interaction, and devoted their efforts to seeking the something more that facilitates change during therapy. The "something more" refers to that which is necessary to complement interpretation in order that change takes place.

The conditions that permit change during psychoanalysis also were a prominent concern in Freud's day, and resulted in his discovery of transference and countertransference. The importance of these phenomena are central to our current models of change and have been the hallmarks of post ego psychological theory permitting the addition of concepts such as inter-subjectivity, two-person psychology, and non-interpretive factors that foster change. The same issues in treatment that had driven the introduction of these terms in psychoanalysis had earlier driven some, including Mahler, Pine, and Bergmann (1976) among others, to consider the therapeutic process as an analogue to the vicissitudes of mother-infant interactions during development. More recently, some theorists have turned to attachment literature, ascribing the roots of serious ruptures in adult relationships and treatment to disordered attachment. Primitive defensive operations that show up again in mature life are viewed as new versions of earlier interactional challenges. Kernberg (1967) has considered disordered attachment as a contributing root of the chaotic emotional experience in borderline personality disorder.

Kohut's (1984) self-psychology also grew out of what he saw as deficient therapeutic interactions in narcissistic patients, requiring the introduction of a developmental line referencing the Self. Stern was, for many years, a co-teacher with members of the Kohut circle, applying his baby-watching data to clinical understanding. He was pleased to apply infancy data provided from dyadic mother-infant observations. He and the Kohutian clinicians believed they could be used to explain narcissistic self-development. Stern, in his book *The Present Moment* (Stern, 2004) carefully elaborated his ideas about the past's operating in the present, as well as the roots of capacity for intimacy. He draws on what the developmental psychologist Jerome Bruner (1990) referred to as "acts of meaning" or "decisive moments" as high points of readiness for interaction during treatment. There may be some overlap between this idea and what others had called the *therapeutic alliance*, the *benign positive transference*, and other terms that inadequately explain the significant prods to change. These interactional facilitators work against the stubborn inertia of the defensive rigidity of personality and the unyielding cohesion of maladaptive organizations. These initial notes represent my reading of the essential historical context surrounding the intellectual and clinical themes that overlap with moments of meeting (MOM). I proceed to explore how Dan Stern applied his careful study of mother-infant interaction to the therapeutic situation and also offer a running critical commentary.

Studies of infant-mother behavior

Stern's (1971) microanalyses of mother-infant encounters in split-screen recordings enabled him to recognize the emergent experiences of the dyad as an increasingly patterned set of rituals that includes nativist inbuilt infantile capacities, enhanced by experienced maternal care and leading to what he called a limited set of co-created interactions around quotidian encounters, such as feeding and play and other maternal ministrations. His careful observations led Stern to the conclusion that much of what the infant brings evolutionarily is patterned by regular and consistent maternal effort; and the reciprocal love and pleasure that emerges from caring, as Bowlby predicted, is implicitly the basis of positive object relations and behavioral patterns. Simple early interactions such as sequences of vocalization and infant referencing and seeking responses and attunement, become part of a baby's expectations and take on appeal functions that later include calling and expressions of desire. Cocreation of games and covocalization that lead to pleasure and the posited experience of love are part of the mix.

In a similar vein, irregular and noncontingent surprise can lead to disruption of bonds based on built-up expectation. Tronick (1989) has offered the still-face intrusion in the dyad as a test situation, in which the mother either turns away or becomes less animated, assuming a blank face, and the child seems at a loss, turns away, or cries, and the interaction is disrupted. Stern learned from this and other similar encounters that there emerges a special dyadic encounter that is the MOM during which time the mutuality in the pair is at an affective apogee and reciprocity is maximal.

These MOMs partly derive from idea of acts of meaning (Bruner, 1990) that Stern adopted as decisive (Stern, 2004). Indeed, he averred that both parties in the dyad come to intuit the other's intentions and next move. This observation can be seen as another version of the linguistic pragmatic assertion that language in conversation is more than a referential word exchange; it is full of mutual intention requiring perception of inferred meaning. In a similar vein, Searle (1969) and other speech-act linguists have noted that a mere semantic parsing of words is insufficient for understanding and message comprehension, unless it is complemented by the pragmatic inclusion of intentionality. Thus, Stern has offered, in these early descriptions, a reference to the peak affective and cognitive arousal that becomes internalized in concrete infantile communion. In other volumes (Stern, 1985), regarding the developmental path of selfhood, he noted that in the earliest version of core-self communion is superseded by a later verbal Self, and life is never again the same for the child—as it was in infancy. There is a gap in affective immediacy by achieving language that we may mourn and long for as we try to match immediate experience with memory. I have always looked at that construction as an expression of Stern's romanticism and even mysticism, which is a counterpoint to his staunch empirical stance. It can seem to be a revenant from Freud's postulated preverbal memories that called for constructions from the past. He, too, wanted, so much, to offer a science of the mind, but at times gave way to speculative romantic musings. One such event is his speculation that the oceanic experience represents the infant at the breast. Similarly, the vital conflict of Eros and Thanatos presented in his later years is cut of similar romantic cloth.

Stern, a close friend of the choreographer, Jerome Robbins, was also very taken by the temporal contexts of dyadic movement and sought coactive rhythms and coordination of synchrony as roots of interactive and intersubjective capacities to figuratively mind-read. These mind-body states are precursors to developmental accomplishments of the second and third years of life, where attunement and social referencing become the scaffolding of healthy communication and mutual satisfaction. These landmarks are built on sequential registration of moments of high-intensity mutuality that, in his view, increase the possibility of new representations internalized and generalized (Stern, 1985), or composited experiential schema that may be determinate of later templates of interactive sensitivity. He noted, "These temporal contours of stimulus play upon and within our nervous system and are transposed into contours of feelings in us. It is these contoured feelings that I am calling vitality affects" (Stern, 2004, p. 64)

The implication of these phenomenological findings is that they permit us to reach from behavior to psyche and brain for the establishment of lifelong expectations that later determine the most favorable conditions for learning. Congenial synchronized meetings with high affective charge, seen as reproductions of such moments permit maximum receptivity. The moments themselves are an abstraction, called MOM. They have precursors and temporal, cognitive progressions expressed in dyads. Most important, they represent the best opportunity to experience the significance of an interaction, whether pre- or post- verbal. The general message is that they offer high alertness and promote learning. There are neurodevelopmental studies to support the idea that learning is facilitated in specific contexts.

However, not every experience leading to a MOM goes smoothly. Stern proffered the sloppiness of the process. How such moments evolve in real time with real couples seems not to be as orderly as one might imagine. It is here that Stern suggested an open and dynamic system of indeterminacy as the mechanism of self-organizing dyads. These forays into microanalytic techniques during infancy derived from dyadic observation led Stern and the BCPSG to employ a dynamic-systems model and the new-age language of open systems that serves their program and fits their data from therapies. In open systems, there is uncertainty and fuzziness. We should not be fooled by the homely words, just as we should not be fooled by Winnicott's (1965) homely vocabulary, good enough mothering, no such thing as a baby. They are complex systems by virtue of their dynamic changing and unpredictable paths. The model is said to be sloppy because it is interactive, and, as such, is also deemed creative with both parties serving as cocreators. It is in this manner that Stern has rendered a process in motion as one that drives toward no particular end or goal, but one that requires patience and dialogue in pursuit of what turns out to be a more cohesive expectation of future encounters.

Open systems reference a self-organizing dyad that derives from each participant. It is transactional and emergent. The process itself is referred to as "moving along." I interject that rivers also roll along, with each change of tide seeming indeterminate, but even large fluid systems such as rivers and oceans have their predictability. Tides are high or low. Winds affect the direction of flow, as does topology. This rub will have to be addressed as we unravel the process in terms of theoretical determinacy and its relationship to dynamic systems and their analysis. This is not an objection to the idea, but rather an optimistic offering that may take us to a more complete description that could be encoded in some prediction, once all the variables are identified. I am reminded of the oral and observational traditions in prehistoric music and dance that had to await the development of a means of graphic notation to preserve their forms without tedious repetition and concrete presentation. During the recent past within psychoanalysis, kinesiologists and Judith Kestenberg (1967) introduced dance notation to describe the nonverbal motoric and gestural sequences in treatment, but the idea did not have momentum at the time and did not catch on as an object of interest.

These musings, again, are drawn from the baby-watching basis of the model. Stern referred to implicit emotional knowing as a process between mother and infant that draws on pre-symbolic nonword emotional contact (Varela et al., 1993). I presume these are the roots of a more general theme known as intersubjectivity, which has caught on inthe psychoanalytic world and, in my estimate, mired us in even more uncertainty, even as it is introduced as an attempt to escape the mechanistic language of Ego Psychology. It is appealing and draws us to inferences that go way beyond the professed empirical attention that the baby-watchers use as data in their mapping of interaction. Stern described "process of inferring intentions through parsing of actions as central to how the brain works and how we understand others" (Stern, 1985). He used the term "fuzzy internalization" in a similar vein. The application of these twenty-first century ideas draws us in as scientific, but awaits data for a good fit to model.

I now turn to another trend in the literature concerning the relevance of infant observation to later behavioral organization. In service of this task, I turn to the work of another baby-watcher born of the same psychoanalytic muse, Peter Wolff (1996). He revised his position on the relevance of baby-watching and joined those of the hermeneutic camp in asserting that because psychoanalysis is interested in meanings, and meanings are registered and are revised during development, prospective empirical observation cannot be counted on for causal outcomes. "Psychoanalytic theories should concern themselves with the phenomena subsumed under the concept of unconscious ideas, hidden motives, and repression, and they should specify a method or methods for exploring the polysemous meanings of irrational fantasies, dreams, and actions that are presumed to be motivated by unconscious ideas"(Wolff, 1996, p. 370).

He continues saying "the goals of the talking cure are understanding of the psychological present in terms of the forgotten personal past by confronting patients with their unconscious desires rather than to explain the psychological present in terms of events in the past" (Wolff, 1996, p. 370).

I wrote a response to Wolffs proposal that eliminates any need to study infancy (Shapiro, 1996). I employed a Freudian proposal that is echoed by the developmental psychologist Heinz Werner (1943) positing hierarchic reorganization during development. This theory posits that each new stage is characterized by a new organization that supersedes prior structures of mind and creates new complexes and mental tendencies that are more than the sum of prior parts. Such a construct is also represented in Freud's idea that the Oedipus is the nuclear conflict and buries prior stages. As Anna Freud (1937) further stated, the prior stages are dimly divined through the veil of new ego structures. Thus, we see constantly revised fantasies, let's say from oral and anal phases, as restructured epigenetically complex schemata. In addition, development is ongoing, covering prior remnants with the silt of recent experience. The past, as it happened, is but dimly represented in the past as experienced and repackaged in the mature mind. Freud (1937) noted that constrictions are merely memories from the past, not of the past (also see Donald Spence, 1982).

Nonetheless, scientists often provide explanation by analogy and perhaps the constant harking-back is a way of analogizing that offers some promise of understanding about unusual phenomena seen in adult behavior. The mother-infant dyadic model may be seen as such an explanatory model. It fits well to the analyst-patient dyad. In a similar vein, Winnicott's (1965) No such thing as a baby and transitional space have been used by intersubjectivists as a model for field theories; and the idea of play has been adapted as the work the dyads employ to achieve change. Sloppy encounters and the distressing wanderings along the path to understanding and the achievement of MOM may similarly apply to such analogous sequences. Finally, in this arena they surely are not simple re-enactments of the dyadic past that have not traveled through the modifying paths and underbrush of experiential tribulation.

The interpretation made by the analyst may also be seen as a growing coconstruction from the vantage point of "Where is the information coming from in the first place?" The patient is the sole source. Indeed, one of the traps of that fact is the power of the transference to skew what is told, how it is told, and what sort of conviction the patient is ready for. Is the denial defensive?—and a myriad of other possible interactional sourced distortions intervene. Unfortunately, I reveal my conviction that the patient comes to therapy saddled by a meaning system that is structured by unconscious fantasies that are indeed derived from childhood distortions. These live on and lead to maladaptive interactions and persistent symptoms that are representations of compromise formations derived from conflicts.

This model is somewhat at odds with the model of the BCPSG or, at best, is complementary, because they are by their own admission not trying to undo the idea of unconscious repressed meanings, but to determine if the something more in the therapeutic interaction can be found in procedural memories from infancy that underlie human interaction throughout the lifespan.

Reconsidering the clinical theory from the standpoint of change

The BCPSG has seriously placed its bets on an open-system model that offers implicit relational knowing and sloppy encounters. The dyadic cocreation is the central theme that permits understanding of this model that promotes change that does not replace interpretive efforts, but represents the something more. It complements other processes. They are enamored of this interactionally grounded idea as a parallel to Freud's devotion to retrospectively based theories regarding the march of the drives and their derivatives of early bodily representations as the source of unconscious fantasy constellations. Bruner's (1990) acts of meaning are clearly a recent version of the incorporation of early interaction into meaningful systems that serve as the whole constellation of current meaning. I am not sure that the BCPSG means to go that far. Rather, they seem to be seeking the nonverbal procedural memories as independent factors alongside of more organized and coded fantasies, which define the units of meaning.

My reading suggests that the BCPSG are interested in procedural encounters from the past that they assert can be revisited in the present in enactments rather than in formed fantasies that have been restructured into coded units of meaning (i.e., unconscious fantasy). This is truly a complementary theory that does not cut across meaning, but remains phenomenological and close to the surface. It is behavioral and apprehended by what the anthropologists call thick description. I have no quarrel with these musings, but ask, "How much of the variance of the change achieved in therapy is accounted for by this model that is uniquely descriptive and references data derived from observation of dyadic parent-child interactions?" The continuous thrust of the baby-watchers' ideas about fuzzy and sloppy beginnings leads to another favorite of our recent psychoanalytic buzz-words—the development of intersubjectivity as a means to the end of understanding.

Proposals such as intersubjectivity are invoked with some obeisance to our scientific posture that learning from observing a system in motion will give the clues to how we acquire and share meaning and how analytic work is possible and, most important, how we build up and support what we say in interpretation. It indicates that the object of the interpretation is a cocreation of the verbal interactions we call interpretations, thereby adding to the conviction of their relevance. These proposals say nothing of their truth or referential value and use for future application, scaffolding a possible change of behavior. It is said that the aim of the interpretive effort is to loosen the maladaptive, binding, rigidly held beliefs that make for neurotic behaviors. The latter is, indeed, the intent of the interpretive process, and the patient must be able work with the analyst's utterance as though it was true enough to take hold as an enlightenment that moves him emotionally. The common experiences of being understood do sometimes end in a burst of emotion, tears or joy, etc. On the other hand, if the patient is caught in a defensive struggle to justify his behavior, there may be continuing doubt or negative transferential confounds that permit neither relief nor change. I thus agree that the interpretive process may be sloppy, insofar as we are straddling a barrier of defense and wish to know that the analyst must tactfully breach and lay the groundwork in the therapeutic alliance, which is indeed a process of coconstruction and procedurally sloppy, but not immediately apprehended in consciousness.

In the Motherhood Constellation, Stern (1995) describes work with dyads with one nonverbal partner, the baby, as warranting a therapeutic choice of portal-of-entry into the system. Behavioral or intrapsychic choices are possible (because the infant is silent, its mental life must be visited and posited from the behavior of both it and its mother's talk). Bertrand Cramer, a Geneva psychoanalyst who was trained in the United States, and others who do psychoanalytically oriented dyadic therapy, analyze the dyad using and referencing the mother's spoken and enacted fantasies (Cramer & Stern, 1988). Others have the therapist speak for the baby (see Lieberman et al., 2005) Yet others watch closely and do a debriefing after the interactions with mother as cowatcher of her behavior in retrospect on a tape (Beebe and Lachman, 2002). It can be seen that none of this deals with or represents a coded meaning system or a plan that employs plumbing meaning and the repercussion of events on the mind. The latter is Anna Freud's (1960) suggestion of what separates psychoanalysis from behaviorism, and also calls the earliest nondifferentiated six months the period of the need- satisfying object, omitting any reference to growing interactive patterning and awaiting future cognitive organization.

Bonnie Litowitz (2002) addresses the matter of meaning from the standpoint of the role of language in her discussion of the BCPSG, noting, as classical analytic authors have, that the soul (read mind) is not in the pineal, as Descartes suggested, and that the mind is not in the brain *per se*, but that the mental apparatus is an organization seriously constrained by meaning units and cast in a language. Although impossible to envision a mind without a brain, the mechanism and construction are surely epigenetic and not purely isomorphic with what we now know of brain circuitry derived from fMRI and other studies—at least not yet. As the child learns and ascribes salient meaning and affective valence to experience, that meaning does change and expectations are altered as development proceeds and experience dictates. Real events are incorporated sequentially as memories, fantasies, and complexes that are encoded by language. Moreover, the progressive changes are dictated by the new cognitive capacities of the child to recognize, name, and assign salience to the psychologically new objects referencing the people in his/her world.

The maternal infant dyad becomes triadic as the mother's adult partner or sibs can be reorganized as competition for love, etc. These are the mental templates that dictate a range of constellations that prestructure interactions. They are met head-on in later life and in the transference. Enactments may be driven by preverbal and procedural memory, but I believe the ones we deal with in psychoanalysis are more likely due to what Joseph Sandler (1987) called role-responsiveness—the tendency to project onto the object the expectations gleaned from early interactions, as in transference. In addition, sometimes the preverbal unformed memory traces can be put into words via naming (Shapiro, 1970) and future reflective revision. Thus, in real-life therapeutic interchanges, we seek to verbalize for the sake of ease of reference and reflective function, and the expectation that the patient may broaden his/her range of response. Such encounters increase the degree of freedom for new possible actions freeing the patient from the binding symptomatic world views that constrain the neurotic mind.

Transporting the baby-watchers' now moments and sloppy fuzzy encounters into later life interactions does have some appeal, but it is hardly the fullest description that, perforce, must include a more complex cognitive-emotional mind. This is so despite Bion's poetic dream of meeting the patient without desire and memory. We meet the patient with the hope of trust, offering understanding and an opportunity to convey the idea of being read accurately. The end is not cocreativity alone, but getting it right! It entails understanding what the patient is about and what unconscious fantasies are driving rigid unexamined solutions. It means discovering what compromise formations are protecting the patient from imagined horrors and anxiety that are the result of anachronistic impingement of the past memories still full of poignancy in the present. This model is bound by formed fantasies, not by inchoate parallel procedural memories that need enactment to be recognized.

One avenue that does seem relevant to the path prescribed in MOM is that the working interpretation will be more effective only when there has been a MOM, i.e., the trust is highest permitting conviction about interpretation at those moments. Spoken in another jargon, the interpretation takes hold when the positive transference is the prevailing relational climate and/or the therapeutic alliance is secure. From an Eriksonian (1946) vantage point, basic trust has been established and revisited.

The value of the models employing verbal interpretation is that they are cast in the language we use to collectively encode meaning and do not depend on an irrevocable past dyadic schema that seeks replication in the current relationship as an unexpected guest. In such a system, the current developing patient-doctor interaction mimics a preverbal past that, as yet, has been unsaid. It is thus very unhandy and cannot be recruited in the process. By contrast, a verbal representation may be inexact, but close enough to a mark to allow salience and revisable for further reflection.

The latter idea, of course, may be why so many have wanted to look hard at the noninterpretive something else that will account for change when interpretation, alone, fails. Within the past 75 years, theorists have reached for other models to deal with a broader swath of patients. The roster includes Leo Stone's (1954) reference to a widening scope, Kohut's Self theory, derived from treating narcissists, and the later analytic third (Ogden, 1994). Oher field theories, intersubjectivity, and two-person psychology all representthe backdrop of a greater extreme of pathology. Mimicking nineteenth-century Freud, they direct their theories toward early interactive dyadic internalization of maladaptive patterns and the consequent expectations of human contact that causes pain, strain, and anxiety . These patients have a lability and easy arousal that seems eruptive and destructive to positive human contact, which is said to mimic the early object relationship that distorts the dyadic pair and lives on as pathologic relationships, that may or may not be related to traditional views of intra-psychic unconscious fantasies.

Patients who do not respond to traditional psychoanalytic techniques and who are said to have ego deficits may need different approaches. The therapist must be on guard not to drive them away, as they expect. They must be ready to tolerate the extremes of emotion that make these poorly modulated patients feel crazy and make others back off. Theories that employ data from early childhood dyadic interaction and implicit emotional knowing seem best directed to them and the cohort that Kernberg (1967) called borderline and psychotic personality organizations. The therapists in those encounters must gingerly engage the patient, ever vigilant of their role as emotional modulator and cautious that a revenant of the past may easily emerge in memory and that the patient may be playing the role-responsive game, prompting an emergent enactment that was not intended by the therapist. The so-called holding environment must precede interpretation.

In the more neurotically organized patient, the open-system dyadic interaction may be played out in sloppy encounters too, but the path toward interpretation is less devious and less impeded by extreme emotional derailment, because the therapist can trust the patient's observing ego not to be swamped by the participating ego, and the countertransference of the therapist does not seek collusion with the patient's tendency to act out. I have experienced many a patient with whom we have had to slowly coconstruct the interpretation in a transference that is fraught with distortion. Similar coconstruction takes place in patients whose past sources of current interactive rigidity derived from the past are only slowly revealed. This is a process that may be a part of the now moment process described. It is characterized by questions and clarifications and observations of redundancy and recognition of parallels within the therapy to events in a patient's life. Some like to think of this, as the BCPSG does, as cocreated. I am not sure, because I prefer to think of it as a gradual slow discovery of how the past dictates and patterns experienced in the here-and-now.

The next example shows such a pursuit. Following a tentative query or rough-hewn interpretive probe, the patient often responds with new history, or a triggered memory, or a partial correction that makes the verbalization more tolerable, more complete, or closer to the mark. This next comment often clinches a rounded revision of the initial interpretation, permitting a more acceptable idea that the patient can use to make his/her narrative cohere and permit moving on. The path described is acceptable to me as a psychoanalytically sound MOM built up by coconstruction. The process is in the pragmatics of the verbal interaction and the modulation of affects, permitting a better-coded description of the patient's experience. It makes sense! It is a "hurrah" because it means something. It is not new, it is only newly stated and suitable to ward off miscarried irrational beliefs built up by a child's mind and reenacted in adult formats to be analyzed in reflective functioning.

Thus, MOMs and fuzzy process become acceptable as analogies to interactions derived from infancy. They either serve as parallel processes to interpretation in more severely ill patients, whose behavior does not permit interpretation of unconscious fantasies. On the other hand, maybe MOMs represent the pretransferential matrix that permits interpretative paraphrases of procedural memories which are trusted as salient. The biggest query concerns how much of the something else is needed for change. Indeed, where do such constructs fit into reflective function? How does interpretation sow the seeds that permit new horizons and offer greater latitude for functioning in patients—and does the affective relaxation permit more MOMs?

In a different vein, I am not sure how that idea, MOM, gives us strategic advantage or a better means to conduct our work toward better outcomes. This takes us to the domain traditionally known as the balance between relational issues (therapeutic relationship) and transference in promoting change. As Greenson (1965) suggested, some people in treatment, at specific times, require more of one than the other. The heightening of positively balanced excitement at the peak of the MOM may indeed promote trust and conviction in healing, and alignment that advances change. The baby-watchers, such as Stern, are experts in viewing such alterations in affect and attention and switches *in situ*. Therapists with adult, meaning-seeking, patients work in more modular units of time and larger units of signification, such as narratives, that may not be detectable in micro-analysis. A crude analogy concerns scanning a slide with a microscope for relational observations in cellular patterns as opposed to an oil-immersion view of intracellular structure.

In fact, if psychoanalysis is a process that seeks meaning that is defensively protected and embedded in anxious worry. The units of time are indeed long as discovery is sought. The quickly labile, and rapidly projecting and splitting, borderline patient may be more subject to rapid-affect escalations that can be witnessed in one session; but the languid neurotic takes time both to trust and to reveal meaningful unconscious fantasies. In a small group experiment that I conducted, I provided process notes of one session. The group achieved more reliable and congruent judgments regarding process and meaning if they were presented in a series of three or more sessions than in data from only a single session.

All these arguments should be viewed against what I consider to be a more important background note that should give us pause. The developmental model proposing hierarchic reorganization is a serious glitch for any theory that posits full representation of past interaction in a progressively reorganizing person. Humans are ever-maturing organisms, especially so because they are progressively psychosocially reorganized around the achievement of a code, language. A truly developmentalist explanation requires change in the schemata, the templates of meaning, with some stabilization at various maturational landmarks. They are continuously in flux during early childhood, with resulting temporal succession and increasing complexity; the flux does not seem to abate until maturity, and even then new developmental structures may ensue within a lived life. I suggest that even procedural memories are subject to such revision.

Yet, as I end this tribute to Dan Stern's scholarship, enthusiasm, and creativity, I admit there are moments in life that involve others that seem reminiscent of a time and valence that had less accumulated cognitive baggage and compounded structure. Perhaps these moments that feel so pure and unencumbered still harken back to an ideal, high-valence emotional tie we attribute to the mother-infant pair as they engage in MOM. Stern's work puts therapists in mind of that early interactive time and alerts us to a dim past of high excitement and discovery in the arms of a safe, loving caretaker. It has the ring of a fantasy sought after but difficult to remember in its fullest dimensions.

REFERENCES

Ainsworth, M.D.S., Blehar, M.C., Waters, E., & Wall, W. (1978). Patterns of Attachment. Hillside, NJ: Erlbaum.

Beebe, B., & F. Lachman. (2002). Infant Research and Adult Treatment: Coconstructing Interactions. Hillside, NJ: The Analytic Press.

Bowlby, J. (1953). Attachment and Loss Vol 1. New York: Basic Books.

——— (1969). Child Care and the Growth of Love. London: Penguin Books.

Bruner, J.S. (1990). Acts of Meaning. New York: Basic Books.

Cramer, B., & Stern, D.N. (1988). Evaluation of changes in mother-infant brief psychotherapy. Infant Mental Health J., 9: 20–45.

Erikson, E.H. (1946). Ego development and historical change. Psychoanal. Study of Child, 2: 359–396. Freud, A. (1937). The Ego and the Mechanisms of Defense. New York: International University Press.

——— (1960). Discussion of John Bowlby's paper. Psychoanal. Study of Child, 15: 53–62.

Freud, S. (1937). Constructions in Analysis. Standard Edition, 23: 255–276. London: Hogarth Press. 1953.

Greenson, R. (1965). The working alliance and the transference. Psychoanal. Quart., 34: 155–181.

Kernberg, O. (1967). Borderline personality organization. J. Amer. Psychoanal. Assn., 15: 641–685.

Kestenberg, J.S. (1967). The role of movement patterns in development. Psychoanal. Quart., 36: 356–409.

Kohut, H. (1984). How Does Analysis Cure? Chicago: University of Chicago Press.

Lieberman, A., E. Padron, P. van Horn, & W. Harris. (2005). Angels in the nursery. Infant Mental Health J., 25: 504–520.

Litowitz, B. (2002). When something more is less: Commentary. J. Amer. Psychoanal. Assn., 5: 751–759.

Mahler, M. (1963). Thoughts about development and individuation. Psychoanal. Study of Child, 18: 307–324.

Pine, F. & A. Bergmann. (1976). The Psychological Birth of the Human Infant. New York: Basic Books.

Ogden, T. (1994). The analytic third. Internat. J. Psycho–Anal., 75: 3–19.

Sander, L. (1975). Infant and caretaking environment: Investigation and conceptualization of adaptive behavior in a system of increasing complexity. In: Explorations in Child Psychiatry, ed. E. J. Anthony. New York: Plenum, pp. 29–166.

Sandler, J. (1987). Projection, Identification, Projective Identification. New York: International University Press.

Searle, J. R. (1969). Speech Acts. An Essay on the Philosophy of Language. New York: Cambridge University Press.

Shapiro, T. (1970). Interpretation and naming. J. Amer. Psychoanal. Assn., 18: 399–421.

——— (1996). Commentary on Peter Wolff paper. J. Amer. Psychoanal. Assn., 44: 446-453.

Spence, D. (1982). Narrative truth and theoretical truth. Psychoanal. Quart., 51: 43–69.

Spitz, R. (1946). Hospitalism, a follow-up report. Psychoanal. Study of Child, 2: 113–117.

Sroufe, A. (1999). Implications of attachment theory for developmental psychopathology. Develop. and Psychopath., 11: 1–13.

Stern, D. (1971). A microanalysis of mother-infant interaction. Amer. Acad. Child Psych., 10: 501–517.

——— (1985). The Interpersonal World of the Infant. New York: Basic Books.

——— (1995). The Motherhood Constellation. New York: Basic Books.

——— (2004). The Present Moment in Psychotherapy and Everyday Life. New York: W. W. Norton & Co.

——— Sander, L., Nahum, J.P., Harrison, A.M., Lyons-Ruth, K. Morgan, A.C,. Bruschweiler-Stern. N. & Tronick, E.Z., (1998). Non-interpretive mechanisms in psychoanalytic therapy: The something-more than interpretation. Internat. J. Psycho-Anal., 79: 903–921.

Stone, L. (1954). The widening scope for indications of psychoanalysis. J. Amer. Psychoanal. Assn., 2: 567-594.

Tronick, E. (1989). Emotions and emotional communication in infants. Amer. Psychol., 44: 112–119.

Varela, F.J., Thompson, E., & Rosch, E., (1993). The Embedded Mind. Cognitive Science and the Human Experience. Cambridge, MA: MIT Press.

Werner, H. (1943). Comparative Psychology of Mental Development. New York: International University Press.

Winnicott, D. (1965). The Maturational Process and the Facilitating Environment. New York: International University Press.

Wolff, P. (1996). The irrelevance of infant observations for psychoanalysis. J. Amer. Psychoanal. Assn., 44: 369–392.

PART II.

INTERPRETING AND FEELING (CHANGING LANDSCAPE OF UNDERSTANDING)

The subheading of this section refers to the changing landscape of understanding that I used in the last editorial, "A View from the Bridge," at the end of my tenure as editor of *JAPA* (1983–1992). In another later review (2011) of the psychoanalytic movements that occupied the psychoanalytic community during my tenure as editor, I refer to "Psychoanalysis in the U.S.—Recovered Memories and New Experiences of a Former Editor" That paper covers similar ground to the former reference, including some later observations in a text that celebrates 100 years of American psychoanalysis.

The very fact that I may uses two topographical metaphors to refer to the same idea is, in itself, a remarkable feature of our human symbolic system, language. Indeed, each paper in this section concerns the dynamic interplay among signs and symbols, as well as idiosyncratic and personal references that children use during individual maturation. The additional flexibility of using symbols to reference our cultural past historically, and then again to say something current, is a great advantage to efficiency and parsimony in communication. These condensations over time and within the personal psyche are a remarkable feat of the imaginative and the common-sense perceptual worlds that are integrated in the mind (notice the spatial metaphor that employs the word *in*).

The shifting focus within the psychoanalytic community from the initial interest in depth psychology and the unconscious to the ego (that references adaptations to reality and the changing issues of object relations at the dictates of the reality principle) is the story of the psychoanalytic vocabulary and its changing syntax. These changes empower Freud's notion that maturation requires renunciation of pleasure for civilization to progress. Within the psychoanalytic movement, we have ventured from interpreting derivatives of drives and their repression to highlighting the need for defense and the role of internalized constraints, leading to compromise and symptom formation. The latter, of course, evokes my gratitude to Charles Brenner and Jacob Arlow, who were significant influences in my understanding of the psychoanalytic process. The continuing query and doubt regarding the curative effect of depth interpretation has led to interest in therapeutic mediators other than interpretation, such as relational roles. Timing, tact and the emergence of significant interpersonal aspects of a therapeutic relationship placed the role of therapeutic alliance and transference and countertransference at center stage at clinic time.

Psychoanalytic developmentalists such as Mahler and Erikson led us from depth outward to the primacy of the ego. The role of narcissism awaited Kohut, who abandoned conflict theory for the Self as a new hypothetical structure including self -esteem and self-objects—an area foretold by the Kleinians and neo-Kleinians that was argued brilliantly in America by Roy Shafer and Otto Kernberg. Lingering in the hallway of change, object-relational theory caught hold south of the border and especially in the treatment of Borderlines. These movements were soon augmented or replaced by relationist and intersubjectivist points of view, each reaching back to understand how the infantile past is registered and repeated in the therapeutic relationship. Depth psychology was retired by many, as experience with models minus metapsychology stepped boldly forward. This section picks up on the various modules of classical theory that had to be revisited in order to understand our patients. I also choose to revive a regressive new look at old theory, specifically the topographic model, because it was isometric with modern linguistic models of deep structure espoused by Chomsky. In short, I was suspected of discarding the past models without further scrutiny regarding a need for complementary system to be used in understanding our patients.

My first paper was deeply ensconced in the interpretive-depth model, integrating language theory. It highlights interpretation as an aspect of naming. Naming has a long history in developmental theory, as the toddler begins to learn that naming things and persons leads to mastery and that the capacity to use words to reference the now, as well as future and past, is useful for fitting into the broadened world of childhood. Naming can anticipate and secure affects into pleasurable actions, while symptoms dissolve in the daylight of understanding. The need to revive the topographic theory was a surprise in a climate where structural theory was shining at its brightest. Indeed, Brenner and Arlow were at work with Occam's Razor, slicing away excess conceptual baggage such as the pcs (?), while ignoring the powerful tool provided by topography to reference the word-and-thing representation. These entities helped to mesh the role of referencing and transforming symbols into deeper structures. The simultaneous appearance on the intellectual horizon of Chomsky's linguistics brought his generative grammar closer to psychoanalytic referential theory. Each had surface and depth dimensions and transformative mechanisms to account for surface variability. Both models shared structural paths to understanding.

The issues stated above are addressed in the paper "Sign, Symbol, and Structural Theory" that was written as part of a *Festschrift* in honor of Jack Arlow. Piaget's criteria for the label *Structuralism* required the following elements: 1.Wholeness;2.Transformations; 3.Generativity . The paper explores how psychoanalytic structuralism overlaps with the new linguistic generative grammar introduced by Chomsky.

The two papers on empathy and words and feelings are an examination and critique of Kohut's idea of understanding through empathy and its posited necessary role in the interpretive arena. The introduction of the primacy of feeling during analysis is worth raising, insofar as feelings are at the root of the whole spectrum of positive and negative valence and poignance during the analytic process. That very issue may be reconsidered, as I state in the paper on "Words and Feelings" by using a new schema for word definition that allows for an essential new dimension of affective tone that should be included when designating the features of a word's meaning. The associated emotional valence to word meaning carries *gravitas* in interpretation. And in practice such valence is much desired, adding profundity to the words we use.

In the service of applying the new knowledge of linguistic behavior and theory to technique, George Makari and I coauthored a "guide" (1993) that describes an approach to listening based on language theory. It is directed toward semiotic understanding of the way in which patients speak, think and act and revealthe symbolic underpinnings of unconscious fantasy in treatment sessions. We approached patients' language using surface data of speech and accompanying communicative channels such as gesture, mimetics and prosody to discover the meaning of the behavior and stories told. Affect-ridden constellations have a continuing influence on scripts that effect human interaction as they are exposed during treatment. My work received a boost when I was asked to teach a semester-long course at the NY Psychoanalytic Institute on language and psychoanalysis to third-year candidates.

"The Unconscious still Occupies Us" is a tribute paper in honor of my Child-Analytic supervisor, Marianne Kris, whose lively appreciation of children and the analytic process were contagious.

It is a detailed consultation with a 5-year old, in which drawings and a non-verbal encounter with a young child blossoms into fuller verbal understanding during a brief two-session, therapeutic consultation. It is a dense example of deep meaning and multiple function embedded in a child's story, pieced together from drawings and progressive elaboration of her personal interpretation of recent events that leads to a deep structural understanding of her fright and plight. It can be looked at as a polysemantic and transferential triumphant encounter that led to relief of symptoms and revives our idea that depth interpretation is alive and well, and even necessary, in this larger world of intersubjectivity and interpersonal surface interpretation. It also is an indirect tribute to Winnicott, who introduced me to the idea of a Therapeutic Consultation and the Squiggle Game. This and the following section are complementary insofar as they stress the continuing role of representation and meaning and may be studied in sequence.

Interpretation and Naming

(1970). *Journal of the American Psychoanalytic Association* 18:399–421.

The interpretation of an "unconscious fantasy" is an event during the course of an analysis which may be viewed as *naming*. Varying phenomena—motor, verbal, situational, interpersonal—are synthesized by the analyst into a more or less concise sentence or complex name. This designation can now be considered by patient and analyst as a common lexical property and can be tested for its congruence with the patient's experience in the past, present, and future. Thus, the *words* are matched to the *things* and *events* of experience, as a first step prior to working through. It is a shorthand verbal note referring to a concept which was formerly expressed only at other levels of behavior. It pinpoints errant experience in a vehicle which can now be manipulated as a shared conceptual property.

Psychoanalysts have long insisted that the analytic situation is a "process" during which the analyst is allied to the analysand's observing ego in an attempt to clarify the "meaning" of the analysand's behavior (Menninger, 1958); (Kris, 1956); (Loewenstein, 1951). Fenichel (1941) commented that during this process, "The correct guessing and naming of the unconscious meanings of a neurotic symptom can sometimes cause its disappearance" (p. 43). He further suggested that the next therapeutic innovation in the history of technique was the analysis of resistance. That naming, of and by itself, was not sufficient to cause analytic cure was later taken up by Loewenstein, who used a linguistic frame of reference to clarify the importance of verbalization in the analytic process (1951), (1956).

Drawing upon Kris' earlier comments about the synthesizing effect of interpretation as an aid to recognition and recall, and finally to integration, Loewenstein (1956) commented that "language performs the function of a kind of scaffolding that permits conscious thought to be built inside... he [the analyst] lends the words... which will meet the patient's thoughts and emotions half-way" (p. 465).

Kris (1950) said that the final integration of the verbal statement changes the patient's attitude from that of "I know" to "I believe." In Lewin's terms, there is a re-establishment of the infantile omniscience (1939). Despite these studies Beres (1962) wrote that "the content of the unconscious fantasy, its relation to verbalization and imagery, remains unexplored" (p. 325).

Recently Balkányi (1964), Rosen (1966), and Edelheit (1969) directed our attention to the importance of linguistics to psychoanalysis.

With this brief background in view, it seems justified to look at the interpretation of an unconscious fantasy as a verbal event, which is therefore subject to linguistic formulations which lie outside of our particular psychoanalytic science. To my view, the notion of an interpretation as a designative event should enable us to synthesize disparate data that have been collected on the interpretive process. Moreover, the problems which accrue from inexact interpretations or, if I may, *misnaming,* can also be understood in these terms (Glover, 1955).

Thus far, I have suggested that there are descriptive and dynamic reasons for this approach. There are, in addition, genetic data concerning the early mother-infant interaction in the social process of learning how to name things that could be useful to psychoanalysts. The naming process is an early feature of object relations, as well as a first step in language development (A. Katan, 1961). Clarification of these events can provide us with useful explanations which underlie behavior seen in the course of certain transference reactions.

Linguistic Theories of Naming

Although originally preoccupied with a neurophysiology of mentation, Freud's earliest thoughts on psychology were well stated in his treatise *On Aphasia* (1891), which antedates his psychoanalytic writings. The very efficacy of the psychoanalytic method rests upon a linguistic postulate that thought is trial action, and that verbal residues bind small amounts of cathectic energy (Freud, 1900). He also wrote extensively on the theme of the relationship of words to things, which is the central problem of the theory of reference. The early topographical theory provided a theory of reference, whereas the structural theory does not. Freud placed the verbal representations and images in the system "preconscious." However, in his *Outline of Psychoanalysis,* Freud (1940) stated that the connections of unconscious residues with memory traces of speech are not a necessary requisite for the preconscious condition. Beres (1962) later turned his attention to the fate of the verbal content in the situation of descriptive unconsciousness, while Hartmann (1952) discussed the fate of the cathexes of these verbal residues. Rosen (1966) suggested "that the conventional shared meaning of words... depend[s]... upon concepts or referential categories... rather than upon images" (p. 641). Thus, using the Ogden-Richards formulation (1923), he considered the naming process as a triangle, referring not only to thing presentation and word presentation, but also to concept presentation (see Fig. 1).

As psychoanalysts, we would be most interested in how speech influences behavior. It has long been acknowledged by stimulus-response behaviorists and Pavlovian experimentalists that verbal suggestions can interrupt even reasonably fixed conditioned responses (Watson, 1919); (Luria, 1960). The traditional mind-body problem is obviated by these thinkers by their not asking the question: how does the mind influence the body? Instead they view the influence of language in terms of neurophysiological adaptation or simple response systems.

However, many philosophers and psychologists have not been satisfied with the black- box and neurophysiological explanations of the organization of behavior (C. I. Lewis, 1949); (Werner and Kaplan, 1963). Werner and Kaplan (1963) stated that hypotheses based on the idea that words and things elicit similar reactors do not adequately distinguish between reacting and knowing. It is here, in the act of knowing, that naming and mental representation emerge as mediators of behavioral response. "Representation is... an emergent activity not reducible to the overlap of responses" (p. 24). This was demonstrated by two conditions: one is the lapse-of-meaning experiments when a symbol, because of loss of its connection to thing presentations, changes into a mere sign; and secondly, the instance of magical speech, where the symbol loses its representational function because of *fusion* with its referent to become an object in itself (see Fig. 1). In the latter instance, for example, we experience awe at the name of God rather than His manifestations.

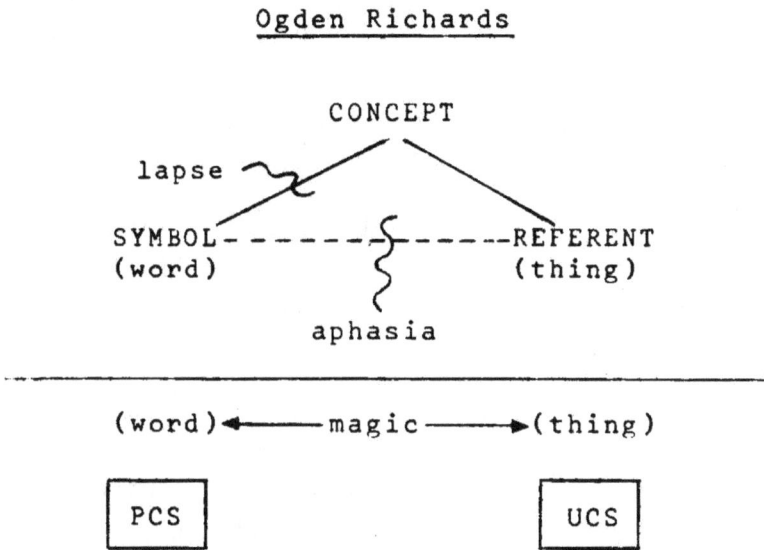

Figure 1. Ogden Richards

The nature of the connections between the things, their labels, and the concepts they refer to can be understood through a study of development. Werner and Kaplan (1963) parallel Piaget's ontogenetic work in noting that "objects are given form, structure and meaning through inner dynamic schematizing activity" (p. 18). Through development, man progresses from a period of *things of action* where sensory impressions are bound globally with motor impressions to a later stage of *things of contemplation*. Only the latter can be manipulated in their own right in the service of representation (Werner, 1926). How efficient to have a map to plan a trip "in our thoughts" rather than having to traverse the territory (Sapir, 1921).

During development, a mother's words become an intimate functional complement to the child's visual, tactile sensory experience of things. That concepts emerge in the course of this growing body of experience is a built-in feature of the human mental apparatus. *The tendency of the central nervous system to integrate is paralleled on the level of psychology by the tendency to synthesize and categorize and to make hierarchic organizations in accordance with meaning.*

While the *words* or phonetic patterns that a child learns may remain unaltered throughout life, the connotated referent is typically modified by the accidents of experience (Vygotsky, 1934); (Ullman, 1962). Because of his concern with idiosyncratic and personal meaning, it is to this area that the analyst turns his attention (Rosen, 1961). For this purpose we must first describe two models for semantic understanding. I have already discussed the first or *referential* model. The second is the *contextual model,* wherein the meaning of a word is related more to its use in language than to its independent existence as a unit of meaning (Wittgenstein, 1922).[1] While group usage changes the meaning of words historically within a language community (diachronic change), as analysts we are more interested in ontogenetic changes within the life of an individual. Observers of children have described the global use of words as gross referential categories in early childhood, progressing to the more specific

---

1   For example, a word such as *door* has a simple referent which is unambiguous. The word *strike,* however, can only be understood in context: 1. The umpire called a strike; 2. The union called a strike; 3. I strike a match. For those interested in the philosophical background of these ideas, Kant's arguments about *a priori* synthetic judgment are relevant.

differentiated use of words in later life (Stern, 1928); (M. M. Lewis, 1936); (Leopold, 1939–1949). Transitional forms from a baby word to an adult word are common. For example, the word *boom* has a reference not only to the sound as an onomatopoeic expression, but also to the efficient cause of the sound, namely, to the hammer that makes it. The ultimate reference, hammer, may go through a stage of depiction in which it is called a "boom-hammer." There is a transfer of meaning from the earlier forms to the later.

Werner and Kaplan account for this transfer of meaning by suggesting that mental schematizing takes place in a dynamic matrix. Words are apprehended and integrated in age-specific mental structures which remain more or less pliable throughout life. Motor, vocal, auditory, and visual experiences can be transferred and associated one to the other, e.g., in pointing, speaking, and reading. In the beginning, words serve as signals or elicitors or inhibitors of action. Later, schematization takes place, which helps develop anticipation and symbol function. The latter binds energies in the construction of a representational reality rather than the immediate discharge in response to a specific event at hand.

"In reference by pointing the object remains stuck in the concrete situation, in reference by symbolization the characteristic features of the object (its connotations) are lifted out, so to speak, and are realized in another material medium (an auditory, visual, gestural, etc.)" (Werner and Kaplan, 1963p. 43).[2]

---

2   It should be indicated that a name is linguistically somewhat different from a sentence. "Naming was treated primarily with respect to the development of the depictive or designatory function... With the shift to an analysis of sentence-formation we moved to a new function quite distinct from the designative function... we made a distinction between 'names,' the function of which is solely designatory, and 'words' which have a syntagmatic function, that is, whose referents are located within a network of syntactic-grammatical categories" (Werner and

The further notion that speech is only one instrumentality of language allows that ideas and thoughts can be expressed in behavioral media other than verbal (de Saussure, 1916). It is from this basic principle of *organization of thought in terms of meaning* that the psychoanalytic principle of rendering the unconscious conscious takes its origins. The essential thesis of this presentation, then, is that an interpretation of an unconscious fantasy is the restatement in speech of language expressions formerly indicated by more cumbersome, idiosyncratic vehicles.

Naming and Psychoanalysis

During the process of psychoanalysis, a number of possible interventions have been described under such categories as confrontations, clarifications, and interpretations. For the purpose of this discussion, I shall consider only the interpretation of an unconscious fantasy.

As Fenichel (1941) stated, there are three reasons why a patient accepts an interpretation: (1) he recognizes it as true; (2) it is a rationalization in the transference; (3) it is an identification with the analyst. If it is indeed true that interpretation in its initial phases is naming, what is the referent to which the analyst's words refer?

Kaplan, p. 384). Although this extension of function from designative to syntagmatic is well taken, it seems that even the latter is merely an extension of the designative function. At any rate, we will simplify our discussion by using the concept *names* as the smallest unit that carries *referential* significance in usage. Morphemes and phonemes, smaller linguistic units, are unnecessary for our purposes. If we limit our discussion to the designation of an unconscious fantasy, we need not consider the functional relationships necessarily relevant in other classes of interpretation, e.g., dynamic statements of ego-id tension or interpretation of defense and resistance.

Leo Stone (1961) said it is a "transformation of what the patient has shown into something manifestly different, albeit latent or implicit in what was shown" (p. 26f.). In short, it is the classification of experience into a verbal message, which now exists as an auditory trace carrying the efficiency of speech over action.

The enchanting possibility that interpretation is a synthesis as well as an analysis is brought to light by G. H. Mead (1956). "Language does not simply symbolize a situation or object which is already there in advance; it makes possible the existence or appearance of that situation or object, for it is part of the mechanism whereby it... is created" (p. 180). It is in this light that classification into names represents only the first step in the analytic process. The "knowing process" demands a firm synthetic link not only between what is said and what is experienced at other levels (in the transference or in life, or with genetic roots), but this linkage leads to new mental schemata which may be the scaffolding of what has been called insight.

This brings to our attention the second step after *naming*, that of *seeking congruence* between that which is named and that which has been experienced or reacted to in the past. Just as the *label* book learned in a specific context is generalized to include the *concept* book, the next time an object fitting the criteria is met, so the interpretation must enhance recall (Kris, 1956); (Brown, 1958). Finally, the new name and its variations in experience must be integrated into the *system of belief* of the individual. Then he may proceed in his future activities with a degree of cognitive control which will permit him to change his behavior in the future.[3]

---

3   Varying explanations of the unconscious meaning of accepting an interpretation have been given. Kris (1956) related the acceptance of an interpretation to receiving the paternal phallus, and Lewin (1950) indicated the oral receptivity of the patient at rest. Interpretations have also been viewed as gifts on an anal level. While the

The process of *classification in words* begins with the patient's experience with the analyst, but goes on to influence cognitive structures. As Fenichel (1941) wisely commented, interpretations work through one of five avenues: what has been interpreted had formerly been *isolated;* the patient's *attention is drawn* to his own activity which he formerly viewed as passive; he *comprehends* that he had motives of which he did not know; *new connections* have been made in the associative process; and these new observations correct former distortions. The distinction between simple recognition and insight is cogently stated in the *Book of Job* where, when confronted with God in the whirlwind, Job stated, "I have heard of you by the hearing of the ear, but now I see you by the seeing of the eye."

Since our interest in interpretation must finally focus on insight and behavioral changes, we may use a patient's initial response to an interpretation as a handy observable index to its cognitive and emotional value. In order to demonstrate that the linguistic view of interpretation has heuristic value, consider the following experiences that every analyst has undoubtedly had with patients on the couch:

1. The patient claims *not to understand* the interpretation, although he can repeat the words of the analyst.
2. The patient takes what the analyst says at face value and says that *reminds him of x, y or z,* or modifies the interpretation by saying that it is almost so and adds to it.
3. The analyst may notice a *relief of tension* in the patient, though no new analytic work in regard to uncovering and understanding is accomplished.

---

interpretation of these phenomena seems to broaden the consciousness, they sometimes do not lead to dynamic changes in the ego where adaptive behavior and flexibility are enhanced.

4. The analyst may notice a *relief of tension* with a consequent better relationship with the analyst, such that former negative affects seem to be dissolved. There is a *better working alliance* and better object relations.

5. The patient may *deny the interpretation,* either calmly or with increased affect.

6. The patient may take whatever the analyst says and attempt to use it as an *explain-all* (panchreston).

Consideration of the six phenomena mentioned will provide a clinical touchstone to test the use of looking at interpretation as an example of naming.

A Linguistic Model of the Mental Apparatus as a Means of Understanding Six Responses

From its beginnings the focus of psychoanalytic theorizing has been on intrapsychic processes. Despite this fact, Freud (1924a), (1924b) found it necessary to consider problems of the ego in relation to outer reality. Moreover, since the method depends upon the periodic intrusion of the analyst, he also had to consider the ways of influencing and understanding behavior by verbal exchange (1912–1914). The latter feature prompted later theorists to reframe the method to account for the communicational aspects of the psychoanalytic arrangement (Sullivan, 1953); (Fromm-Reichmann and Halle, 1949). The split between those who continued with classical technique and others is history by now.

Linguistic models can be applied to the intrapsychic focus of classical psychoanalysis without doing havoc to the method. In this discussion, I shall not consider the possible communicational deficits of the analyst, although it must be admitted that this is a serious omission. Figure 2 outlines the relationships of the potential phenomena seen or inferred by analysts and remolded into linguistic terms. The virtue of this system lies in the possibilities of seeing the six patient responses outlined as failures, facilitations, or short-circuits in the connections pictured. *This model is designed to focus on the area glibly passed over as the "ego function of language."* It is to be hoped that the paths outlined can aid us by pinpointing *where* in the language function a defect occurs. As such, one should not be disturbed at not seeing the usual psychoanalytic references to defense, resistance, etc. These are understood as given and enter into the reasons why changes occur in the language function. This is a schematic statement of where they occur and how many dynamic operations share a final common pathway of expression through defects in language.[4]

The words spoken by the analyst are understood by the patient because they share a common social code. They speak the same language (see Fig. 2). (There are many slips between words as intended and meaning as understood, of course, and this is accounted for by what I have labeled the "exchange barrier.") It is to this area that linguists concerned with communication have devoted their energies.

The words or names must now be associated with other aspects of the cognitive-conative system in order for "knowing" (as opposed to reacting) to occur. The words are associated with concepts that correspond to the *denotative meaning* of a word. This has the immediacy of gestural pointing. The relation between

---

4 Since explanatory hypotheses are at best constructions based on one or another model called upon to codify data, I submit the following scheme only as a temporary heuristic tool.

denotation and connotation may be two-pronged: changing usage provides a history of meanings which are clustered about a word. These remain available for social purview. It is also permissible to extend connotation to include the history of its use by an individual. In this sense, connotation may include genetic linkages that are unconsciously significant. In all these instances, concept, denotation, and connotation, there may be associational linkages which are horizontal at a single level, i.e., word-to-word-to word, or *vertical,* i.e., denotation to social-historical connotation to personal-ontogenetic connotation.

In unconscious connotational systems there are connections to affective residues which may be loosely organized in the same schemata, but not necessarily as verbal residues (see Fig. 2, Potential Affect) (Freud, 1900); (Schachtel, 1959). These latter linkages would enable the preverbal schemata to be ultimately related through the associational chain to verbal discharge as well as visceral discharge channels, as is presumed in psychosomatic illnesses.

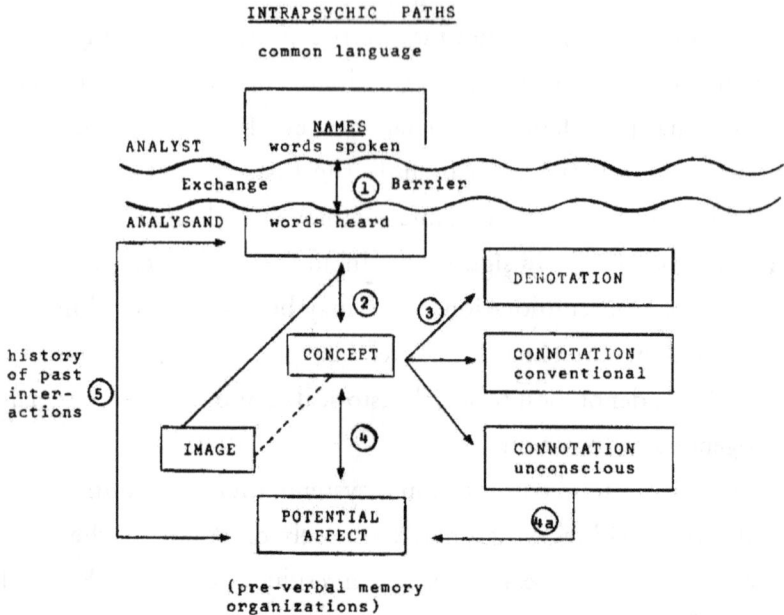

Figure 2. Intrapsychic Paths common language

This scheme is couched in linguistic terms, but includes the same postulated and observed connections which psychoanalysts have used for so long in their clinical understanding. The six paradigms can now be considered in relation to the paths described. In addition, each paradigm will also be viewed as an arrest in the development of reference and concretized by a clinical example:[5]

1. The situation where the patient can repeat the analysts's words without knowing what they mean is akin to lapse-of-meaning

---

5   By analogizing the breaks or slurs in connections to developmental stages, no equivalence is implied. Hartmann has suggested that in regression patients do not act as two- or three-year-olds do. There is an alteration in function in the face of structuralization that is established. Thus, functional alterations occur along the "faults" in the developmental lines.

experiments (break between word and concept). During these experiments, the subjects are asked to repeat a word until finally they experience a loss or diminution of its rich meaning while still feeling it is a familiar word. The connections with the concept- and thing-representations to which the words refer are lost (Jacobovits and Lambert, 1961). It is like a reversal of aphasia wherein the words are available, but they are not linked with cognitive schemata, except for the automatisms of syntax.

During the analytic process, this phenomenon occurs in certain patients who encode into words with diminished reference to concept or consideration for communicative value. They string words together for a kind of *Funktionslust*. It is akin to the stage of babbling in early infancy or of learning rhymes and catechisms by ritual mimicry at a later stage. There is a hypercathexis of the lyrical poetic function of language (Jakobson and Halle, 1956). The hearing but not understanding is often accompanied by keen sensitivity to how one says something rather than what is said. The potential for paranoid misunderstanding is evident in this type of language arrest.

A similar defect in knowing may serve a defensive purpose in the well-known pseudo naïveté of hysterics. That is to say, the functional link between what is designated and what is known may be lost in the service of a wish to keep out of awareness a potentially painful affect associated with remembering. One sees this dissociation of name and concept in the defensive isolation of obsessional neurotics as well. This link between hysteria and obsessional states because of their descriptive similarity is more likely due to factors of ego organization than factors ascribed to libidinal organization. The different levels of libidinal fixation described in each of these neurotic types are expressed through

143

a final common pathway describable in the terminology of linguistic reference.

2. The instance where the naming of an unconscious complex leads to slight verbal modifications by the patient or increased flow of associative themes is the opposite of that which we see in responses of type 1 (there is facilitation of links of word to concept and deep connotation). Here the name, the thing, and the concept referred to are well-coordinated, and congruence is immediate. This corresponds to Kris's idea (1950), (1956) that *recognition* stimulates *recall* and finally *integration*. For these reasons, the interpretation is said to be well-timed and already preconscious. The analyst's proposition "fits" what the patient feels, that is, its connections with experience and therefore its integration into a complex personal meaning schema are secured by the observer giving it a name.[6]

The particular terms in which analysts couch their interpretations are geared to estimates of "receptivity" of the patient. We know, for instance, that many analysts use anecdotal styles. Others offer direct statements. With children we use concrete terms with strong referential links to current play material. Glover advised only interpreting the transference as an attempt to appeal to the patient's immediate designative experience, as opposed to something more remote.

What is sought in interpretation is *naming* at a level which the patient can *use* (Hartmann, 1951). The linguists provide

---

6   This concept of "fit" must be related to "meanings," which are personalized syntheses generally not available to veridical demonstration. The "aha" or "light bulb" phenomenon is more akin to a truth function which is nonexperimental, non-repetitive, and highly egocentric. Its validation rests on continuing the match of experience to proposition.

a childhood example of this process. I have already alluded to the transitional forms that one sees in the naming process in childhood. The progression from "boom-boom" through "boom-hammer" to "hammer" was described. Moreover, those who have attended to the interplay between mother and child as language is taught attest to the gradual development of lexical forms. Not only does the mother speak baby-talk at first, but the parents echo the child as both parties seek congruence (M.

M. Lewis, 1936); (Brown and Bellugi, 1964). The flexibility of the parent in permitting transitional forms permits a growing sense of autonomy in the child.

This evolution of designation to more standardized, socially shared forms is akin to interpreting from the outer, more manifest derivative experiences to the more concrete or archaic representations of these experiences. During psychoanalysis, the process is often reversed, going from the *concept* to the *particular,* the *recent* to the *past*. This process not only attests to the particular state of the synthetic function of the ego (i.e., will the patient understand?), but also to the actual stages of learning to name as a means of coping with the world in a more efficient manner.

An example of broadened insight during analysis was derived from the discovery of the meaning of a childhood name which a patient used to designate his mother. This should provide a concrete example of the meaning of "analyzing from outward-in" as well as indicating the spreading effect of understanding. This patient in his mid-twenties had succeeded in extricating himself from a marriage in which he had a strong aversion to sexual contact with his wife which was associated with impotence. He complained that his wife "clutched at him" and that he felt hovered over and restrained with her.

His mother had been and still was a strong influence in his life. He never felt that any achievement was his own, but that she intrusively shared all. This feeling was so strong that at times he preferred failure to success rather than share his success with her.

Much of the latter had been interpreted in terms of the concepts outlined. Only later did he reveal a childish name he had for his mother which had two variants, "poome," "pooshe." The one stood for "poor mother," the second, "poor she." His mother had been sick frequently when the words were coined. During his discussion of his mother's sickness, he mentioned his own suffering and deprivation at this period. I interpreted the necessity for two names in that one of the poor suffering parties was himself, consequently not only poo-she (poor she), but also poo-me (poor me). This interpretation led immediately to his expanding on his own self-pity not only in the past, but in the analysis. Furthermore, he remembered that he had not called his mother "mother" until after she forbade his using the other name which she deemed babyish. He felt very strange calling her by a name which other children called their mothers. He wondered if she would know it was her little boy, since the name was not personal.

This interpretation revealed the symbiotic closeness which the childish name denoted. The patient then at a later date was able to consider the Oedipal manifestations of this early feeling in the form of his wish that his mother share his penis. This was reinforced by her constant intrusions into his privacy and successes. The latter may be considered an archaic concretization

146

of the more general concept presented earlier in the analysis and belonging to a different developmental epoch.

The associational links often will lead to expanding of consciousness, but not necessarily to new adaptations, because the affective aspects of the transference are also integral to the knowing process. Thus, although a facilitation may be evidenced at junctures 2 and 3 (see Fig. 2), between words, concepts, and connotations, this does not guarantee that the link to affect is secure.

3. Interpretation at times yields a relief of tension without any new uncovering taking place. It is a situation that evolves in patients who have specific ego structures with relevant genetic histories. In such patients there is a short-lived facilitation between words and feelings, but there is no evidence of connections to associated connotations at the same or deeper level. These are patients who beg the analyst for more activity during the course of analysis. This wish may elicit stubborn refusal on the part of the analyst, which only produces more tension. On the other hand, compliance by the analyst yields no furtherance of the analytic process, because the patient is constantly gratified. As Freud commented, we travel between Scylla and Charybdis. The case of an immature analysand provided an example of this type of nagging attitude, which was not only the replay of an unconscious wish, but a conscious repeated experience within his family. He was descriptively an obsessive nagger.

The meaning of this behavior is surely overdetermined, but it is also related to a fact of language learning. One day in the playground I noticed a child of about fourteen months (who had obviously just learned a minimal vocabulary). She was sitting in a swing as her mother casually continued a conversation with a neighbor. An airplane passed above. The child looked up at the airplane, pointed to the sky, and made a roaring sound, which was obviously her onomatopoeic designation for the airplane. She looked at her mother and again made the roaring sound. Her mother paid no heed. The child again made the roaring sound, looking at her mother. She persisted in this vocalization until the mother acknowledged her sounds and turned to her saying, "Yes, dear, that is an airplane."

This anecdote dramatically points to the dynamic matrix of mother-infant interaction in learning language. M. M. Lewis (1936) showed that mother and child gradually come to a congruence at a middle ground closer and closer to lexical speech. In a later study Brown and Bellugi (1964) showed that although children at an early level speak telegraphic syntax, their parents always answer them in an expanded syntactic form and that the interchange goes on until it is finalized by the parents' reiteration. Thus the child comes to expect that in order to end an exchange the mother must naturally repeat what has been said. In this sense the development of naming is keenly attached to the relaxation of tension through *affirmation by repetition*. Werner and Kaplan likewise introduced the relationship between learning referential speech and mother-infant differentiation (cf. "distancing"). I would suggest that in patients of the type I have been describing, the tension-relieving aspects of the analyst's talking is what is being sought and that the words are less relevant. Characteristically in these patients, however, the relief of tension is short-lived and the nagging begins again.

4. There are situations in which interpretation yields a marked tension relief with dissolution of former negative affects. Better

object relations and a working alliance ensue. This situation usually leads to favorable analytic work. As in response 3, there is a facilitation of the path to affect with gradual opening of paths to concept, finally leading to connotative associations. The cognitive links develop only later through the new work made possible by the feeling of alliance with the analyst. This situation, too, attests to the close connection between the naming process and the human matrix in which names are learned. However, in this instance the economics of tension relief without conscious understanding has priority over the cognitive steps.

One sees a similar sense of relief when we remember words which are on the tips of our tongues, that is, the linking between a verbal vehicle and a preconscious referent. When the analyst interprets an unconscious dynamism correctly, the "naming of the enemy" elicits a new sense of ability to cope. The catastrophic reactions of aphasics are likely due in part to the frustration derived from their inability to master by naming— the efficiency of thought or, better, "verbal thought" has been mentioned. The developmental link between object relations and thought organization was recognized by Abraham (1924) when he constructed a table of vicissitudes of development of libido coordinated with preambivalent, ambivalent, and postambivalent attitudes toward the object. That is to say that although many ego functions mature free of conflict (Hartmann, 1939), often the development is intimately tied to fantasy organization (Peller, 1964). A derivative behavior has connections not only with referents but with organized schemata tied to affects. Sometimes the latter are freed before the former can be utilized for "knowing."

As Freud said, a cigar is not always a phallus; and in like fashion, in child analysis, a truck is not always a penis. In order to interpret correctly one must wait to see the particular meaning at the particular time in relation to the level of the transference and context. Although at each moment in time the individual is expressing all of the multiple functions to which Waelder (1930) alluded, the level of fantasy organization which is most relevant at the time is the one which has to be named. The sense of relief the patient gets when the immediate concern is accurately designated calls into effect the second step in knowing, *seeking of congruence*, which leads to secondary correlations with more remote experiences (see Fig. 2, paths 3 and 4a). On the level of object relations it is akin to saying to the parent, "You have given me the words to designate my experience and it works for me, and therefore I feel more trust toward you and can also fit other experiences to the words."

5. Often interpretations are met only by denials or denials with an increase in negative affect. We are well enough acquainted with Freud's paper on negation (1925) to place negation in the contexts in which symbolic logicians place it: namely, that in order to represent a negation one has to present that which is being negated. Negation does not stand alone but represents a judgment about a proposition. Thus, in the course of an association a denial represents an affirmation. We sometimes use a negation as a means of demonstrating the validity of an interpretation. This has always seemed a rather spurious kind of verification, leading critics of analysis to suggest that the patient is in a coercive bind. Yet we know that often analytic data follow negations which verify what has been denied. Thus

the facilitation at path 3 is what analysts use as verification, even though the lady may not protest too much.

The patient described earlier presented a dream and raced through his associations, obviously shifting to content that bore little discoverable relationship to the manifest content of the dream. I asked for further associations to the dream, at which he balked. I then interpreted his resistance as a parallel to his feelings in marriage that the longer he stayed the more he felt trapped by what others expected of him. He denied this with little affect and proceeded on another tack. Later he slapped his head and noted that he had said "No" as he had so frequently done to his wife and mother because he could only feel free and autonomous by opposing. He felt what they or the analyst said were challenges and therefore to be denied. Another variant he often showed was: "All right, I'll do it your way." While he complied on the surface, he maintained a stubborn resistance to getting anything out of it because it was not for him, but an obedience to the other person because of guilt.

Developmentally the use of negation represents another link to the interplay between two parties who sought congruence between the symbol and its referent. Even though negativistic two-year-olds say "No," they show comprehension by their very opposition. In the analysis, negation is a continuation of the ongoing dialogue. What has been named has been heard, has been integrated, and can be used for further exploration if the opposition is lifted. That is, the word has been sufficiently related to its concept. What is lacking here, if indeed the negation does turn out to be an affirmation, is the part of the sequence which guarantees insight—*congruence seeking and belief.*

Once classification is secure, congruence and belief depend upon the recovery and elaboration of other experiences past and future (facilitation of 3, 4, 4a, in Fig. 2). In effect, Glover's admonition to interpret in the transference prevents evasion by negation, because only those things which can be pointed to with the finger are interpreted.

6. The notion of an "explain-all" has been brought to our attention by Szasz (1957). That is to say, naming may give the patient a dynamic feeling of having discovered something. This sensed discovery inhibits further activity.

One sees this in the course of the analytic process where the patient uses the interpretation in an obsessional manner and it is applied in an across-the-board manner to everything he does (facilitation of 1a and 2 with overuse of path 1). Often at a later date he finds a situation where the interpretation does not fit and then he is furious at the analyst, saying that the whole process is useless. This is often due to an initial idealization of the analyst and later wish to destroy his authority.

A patient in his late twenties was having sexual difficulties with his wife due to the encroachment of a typical madonna-prostitute split. The interpretation was offered that since he married his wife, he was unable to seek genital aims with her because she was the one who cared for and fed him like his mother. There was ample evidence for this interpretation and it led to further insight and understanding.

Later in the analysis whenever a new sexual problem arose, he would bring out the "old saw" to explain his reluctance, although new data were prominently available. At varying times the new data clearly related the wife to his sister or involved his fear of the vagina or shame regarding pregenital aims, or homosexual object choice. He would stubbornly deny any new interpretations laying the original interpretation at the analyst's doorstep. This was the "name of the animal" so how could it have another name.

Developmentally a child may use the word *dog* to describe all four-legged animals as though dog were the generic class inclusive term. An arrest at this stage may ensue if the learning is contaminated by the sadistic struggle over toileting at this crucial stage. At a later stage, the parent may help to ensconce such attitudes by saying to the child, "God made it." By decreasing the curiosity of the child by a name, he proceeds as though he had an explanation.

Linguistically, it represents an overvaluation of the word and name as information, as opposed to the word as classification. It may be akin to the fusion of concept and word as seen in magical speech—the mere pronouncement causes change. The spuriousness of this claim is gained through later experience.

SUMMARY

The interpretation of an unconscious fantasy is the first step prior to working through it. The analyst provides a shorthand verbal representation of what the patient has formally expressed in nonverbal behavior. The verbalization is viewed in the light of linguistic models of naming. The theory of reference formerly available in Freud's topographic theory is lacking in the structural theory. The linguistic model presented in this contribution is designed to describe the vicissitudes of verbal representation according to what is known about the development of reference. In this way, disparate data on the interpretative process are brought together under a single heading known as the *ego function of language.*

Six examples of patient responses are described in the light of the model. For example, there are patients who can repeat the analyst's words but have no conscious concept of what their meaning is; others have an affective response with a better working alliance, while no new associative uncovering is done. Similarly, some patients intellectually respond to interpretation with increased uncovering and remembering, but no link to the emotions is made. In addition, there are those who use the analyst's words as an explain-all, and others who negate but affirm by opening new avenues of insight. In some, their response to interpretation leads to further recall. They recognize the congruence of what has been said with the facts of life and finally integrate the interpretation into a system of belief. The latter is insight.

In all instances described the defects in verbal grasp can be viewed according to our understanding of the developmental faults in structuring language.

REFERENCES

Abraham, K. (1924). A short study of the development of the libido In: *Selected Papers on Psychoanalysis* New York: Basic Books, 1953 pp. 418–501.

Balkányi, C. (1964). On verbalization *Int. J. Psychoanal.* 45:64–74. Beres, D. (1962). The unconscious fantasy *Psychoanal. Q.* 31:309–328.

Brown, R.W. (1958). *Words and Things* New York: Free Press.

———— & Bellugi, V. (1964). Three processes in the child's acquisition of syntax In: New Directions in the Study of Language ed. E. Lennenberg. Cambridge: M.I.T. Press, pp. 131–162.

Bhler, K. (1934). *Sprachtheorie* Jena: Fischer.

Edelheit, H. (1969). Speech and psychic structure American Psychoanal. Assn. 17:381–412.

Fenichel, O. (1941). Problems of Psychoanalytic Technique New York: *Psychoanal. Q.*, Inc.

Freud, S. (1891). *On Aphasia* New York: International Universities Press, 1953.

———— (1895). Project for a scientific psychology Standard Edition 1 283–397 London: Hogarth Press, 1953.

———— (1900). The interpretation of dreams Standard Edition 4 & 5 London: Hogarth Press, 1953.

———— (1910). The antithetical meaning of primal words Standard Edition 11 153–161 London: Hogarth Press, 1957.

———— (1911). Psycho–analytic notes on an autobiographical account of a case of paranoia Standard Edition 12 3–82 London: Hogarth Press, 1958.

———— (1912–1914). Recommendations to physicians practising psycho-analysis Standard Edition 12 109–171 London: Hogarth Press, 1958.

Freud, S. (1913). The philological interest of psycho-analysis Standard Edition 13 176–178 London: Hogarth Press, 1955.

———— (1915). The unconscious Standard Edition 14 159–209 London: Hogarth Press, 1957.

———— (1924a). Neurosis and psychosis Standard Edition 19 149–153 London: Hogarth Press, 1961.

———— (1924b). Loss of reality in neurosis and psychosis Standard Edition 19 183–187 London: Hogarth Press, 1961.

———— (1925). Negation Standard Edition 19 235–239 London: Hogarth Press, 1961.

———— (1940). An outline of psycho-analysis Standard Edition 23 141–207 London: Hogarth Press, 1964

Fromm-Reichmann, F. & Halle, M. (1949). Recent Advances in Psychoanalytic Therapy New York: Hermitage Press.

Glover, E. (1955). *The Technique of Psychoanalysis* New York: International Universities Press.

Hartmann, H. (1939). *Ego Psychology and the Problem of Adaptation* New York: International Universities Press, 1958

———— (1951). Technical implications of ego psychology *Psychoanal. Q.* 20:31–43

———— (1952). The mutual influences in the development of ego and id The *Psychoanal. Study Child* 7:9–30 New York: International Universities Press.

Jakobovits, L. & Lambert, W. (1961). Semantic satiation among bilinguals J. Exp. Psychol. 67 567–582

Jakobson, R. & Halle, M. 1956 Fundamentals of Language Hague: Mouton.

Katan, A. (1961). Some thoughts about the role of verbalization in early childhood The *Psychoanal. Study Child* 16:184–188 New York: International Universities Press.

Kris, E. (1939). On inspiration *Int. J. Psychoanal.* 20:377–389.

———— (1950). On preconscious mental processes *Psychoanal. Q.* 19:540–560

———— (1956). On some vicissitudes of insight in psychoanalysis *Int. J. Psychoanal.* 37:1–11.

Leopold, W. F. (1939–1949). *Speech Development of a Bilingual Child* Evanston: Northwestern University Press.

Lewin, B.D. (1939). Some observations on knowledge, belief and the impulse to know *Int. J. Psychoanal.* 20:426–431.

——— (1950). *The Psychoanalysis of Elation* New York: Norton.

Lewis, C.I. (1949). Some logical considerations concerning the mental In: Readings in Philosophical Analysis ed. H. Feigle & W. Sellars. New York: Appleton-Century-Crofts, pp. 385–392.

Lewis, M.M. (1936). *Infant Speech* New York: Harcourt, Brace..

Loewenstein, R.M. (1951). The problem of interpretation *Psychoanal. Q.* 20:1–14.

——— 1956 Some remarks on the role of speech in psycho-analytic technique *Int. J. Psychoanal.* 37:460–468

Luria, A.R. (1960). *The Role of Speech in the Regulation of Normal and Abnormal Behavior* Bethesda: U.S. Public Health Service.

Mead, G.H. (1956). In: *The Social Psychology of G. H. Mead* ed. A. Strauss. Chicago: University of Chicago Press.

Menninger, K.A. (1958). *Theory of Psychoanalytic Technique* New York: Basic Books..

Ogden, C.K. & Richards, I. (1923). The Meaning of Meaning New York: Harcourt, Brace, 1959.

Peller, L.(1964). Language and its prestages *Bull. Phila. Psa. Assn.* 14 55-76.

Rosen, V.H. (1961). The relevance of "style" to certain aspects of defence and the synthetic function of the ego *Int. J. Psychoanal.* 42:447–457.

———(1966). Disturbances of representation and reference in ego deviations In Psychoanalysis—A General Psychology: Essays in Honor of Heinz Hartmann ed. R. M. Loewenstein, L. M. Newman, M. Schur, & A. J. Solnit. New York: International Universities Press, pp. 634–654.

Sapir, E. (1921). Language New York: Harcourt, Brace & World.

Saussure, F. de (1916). *Course in General Linguistics* New York: Philosophic Library, 1959

Schachtel, E. (1959). *Metamorphosis* New York: Basic Books. Stern, W. & Stern, C. (1928). Die Kindersprache Leipzig: Barth. Stone, L. (1961). *The Psychoanalytic Situation* New York: International Universities Press).

Sullivan, H.S. (1953). *Interpersonal Theory of Psychiatry* New York: Norton.

Szasz, T.S. (1957). The problem of psychiatric nosology *Amer. J. Psychiat.* 114 405–413.

Ullman, S. (1962). *Semantics* London: Alden Press.

Vygotsky, L.S. (1934). *Thought and Language* Cambridge: M.I.T. Press, 1962.

Waelder, R. (1930). The principle of multiple function *Psychoanal. Q.* 5:45–62 1936.

Watson, J. (1919). *Psychology from the Standpoint of a Behaviorist* Philadelphia: Lippincott.

Werner, H. (1926). *Comparative Psychology of Mental Development* New York: International Universities Press, 1940

——— & Kaplan, B. (1963). Symbol Formation New York: Wiley.

Wittgenstein, L. (1922). *Philosophical Investigations* Oxford: Oxford University Press, 1953

Empathy: A Critical Reevaluation

(1981). *Psychoanalytic Inquiry* 1(3):423–448.

In 1974, I wrote of the development and distortions of empathy. The opening sentence was, "Psychoanalytic literature abounds with references to empathy; most authors advocate its use and decry its absence" (p. 4). That statement still holds in 1981; it describes a state of our science that contrasts markedly to earlier literature, in which insight gained by interpretation was cited as the most important process to be explicated. Even though Freud mentioned empathy in his treatises on jokes (Freud, 1905) and group psychology (Freud, 1921), he never attended to it as a central instrument of analysis. Instead he espoused free-floating attention of the analyst to his associations and intuitions along with logical review of the apparently random data of analysis.[1] The nonreducible

---

1 Ferenczi (1919) best summed up the new scientific attitude toward data as follows: "On the one hand, [analytic therapy] requires of him [the doctor] the free play of association and phantasy, the full indulgence of his own unconscious; we know from Freud that only in this way is it possible to grasp intuitively the expressions of the patient's unconscious that are concealed in the manifest material of the manner of speech and behavior. On the other hand, the doctor must subject the material

central assumption that permitted such logical scrutiny was psychic determinism. Without such an assumption, associations would indeed be random.

The increasing importance of empathy over insight can be documented by the following facts: From its inception in 1932 to 1955, the *Psychoanalytic Quarterly* recorded only one citation to empathy; during the same period, there were 42 references to insight (*Cumulative Index*, 1969, 1977). By contrast, from 1967 to 1980, empathy was referenced 23 times and insight only 6. In the *Journal of the American Psychoanalytic Association*, which has been published since 1953, references to empathy and insight were roughly equal through 1969 (31:30), while the last decade showed a 41:25 preponderance of empathy over insight citations (excluding the *Supplement* where empathy: insight is 23:27) (*Cumulative Index*, 1976). What lies behind this current emphasis on empathy? The answer is to be found in a number of strains in our recent history:

1. Psychoanalysts have always attempted to analyze and understand their mode of operation by self-observation. Various authors have been interested in what Isakower called the "analyzing instrument"—its development and specialization (Balter, Lothane, and Spencer, 1980). While Isakower only recorded his thoughts *en famille*, many who were in contact with him as students recognized his efforts to grasp how the analyst appreciates the significance of psychic life from the collection

---

submitted by himself and the patient to a logical scrutiny, and in his dealings and communications may only let himself be guided exclusively by the result of this mental effort... his constant oscillation between the free play of phantasy and critical scrutiny pre-supposes a freedom and uninhibited motility of psychic excitation on the doctor's part" (p. 189).

of impressions presented by patients. Perhaps this "fictional instrument" and others like it, such as the "analytic work-ego," include empathy as one of their processes. Further trends in distinguishing the therapeutic alliance from transference phenomena, and combining an atmosphere of safety along with or in contrast to analytic neutrality, are also relevant.

2. A second and more specific determinant of our emphasis on empathy derives from increasing work with other than classical neurotics. There are those who suggest that special techniques are necessary to understand such individuals. Robert Knight, for example, as early as 1946, recommended empathy to understand a catatonic boy when all other techniques failed. Margaret Fries (1968) elaborated similar techniques in her paper on "Problems of Communication Between Therapist and Patients with Archaic Ego Functions." In a recent panel reported in the *Bulletin of the Association for Psychoanalytic Medicine* (1979), as diverse a group as Jacob Arlow, Otto Kernberg, Arnold Modell, and Aaron Karush concluded that as difficult as it is to achieve a uniform agreement on definition, all analysts utilize empathy and it is most useful in dealing with inner states remote from the analyst. Paul Ornstein (1979), in the subsequent volume of the *Bulletin,* applauded the relative uniformity of agreement and asked rhetorically, "What is the controversy all about?" (p. 96).

3. This leads to the third reason for the surge of interest in empathy. Heinz Kohut's (1977) emphasis on "tragic man" as opposed to Sigmund Freud's focus on "guilty man" has contributed to a greater entrenchment of self psychology within our science, which is said to complement the psychology of the mental apparatus. In order to accomplish the analysis of tragic man, Kohut claims empathy to be the essential tool of the

analyst. Indeed, in his later writings it is *the* tool of analysis:...
psychoanalysis is a psychology of complex mental stateswhich,
with the aid of the persevering empathic introspective
immersion of the observer into the inner life of man, gathers
its data in order to explain them [Kohut, 1977, p. 302] it is the
only one among the sciences of man that explains what it has
first understood [Kohut, 1977, p. 303].

Earlier (Kohut, 1959) he sharpened the distinction between
psychology and other sciences by suggesting that physical phenomena
are grasped by our senses, and psychological data by introspection
and empathy. Ornstein (1979), in accord with Kohut, explains that
the empathic approach differs in quality from the inferential vantage
point of natural science.

This idea of two types of apprehension for two types of science
(*Naturwissenschaft, Geisteswissenschaft*) was first elaborated by the
phenomenologist philosopher W. Dilthey. This tradition thus had
its origins prior to Kohut, but has not received much recognition
within psychoanalysis until Kohut's espousal. Within the frame
of self-psychology, Kohut further argues that scientific objectivity
can be more broadly based to include an introspective empathic
component. This claim, however, is never clearly explicated and has
required disavowals of mysticism, as though to preempt criticism.
Thus, empathy continues to be illusive with respect to procedure or
veridical measures, issues that I will address later in this essay.

A parallel to the recent willingness to employ new modes to
deal with new problems can also be found in Freud's writings.
He seemed to be in constant tension between his own wish for a
scientific vantage point for psychoanalysis, and his own humanistic
aims and cultural preparation reflecting the "Sturm and Drang" of

German Romanticism. This dichotomy can be documented in his early training in neurophysiology and wish for a scientific psychology of mental life (Freud, 1895) based on neuronal mechanisms, and the stress he placed on biological theorizing. The latter notwithstanding, his work also reveals a more openly romantic vision invoking varying *animae* within, such as libido and aggression, as drive forces creating tensions against the dictates of reality as registered in ego and superego residues, thus creating conflict. He gave way finally in his last writings to more philosophical constructs, such as Eros and Thanatos, but still valiantly hoped to maintain the scientific status of analysis—and that in a climate even more violently opposed to his revolutionary insights than we suffer today. Freud's inner struggle also is evident in the external historical scene as the prolonged polarization of models.

In his *Science and the Modern World,* Alfred North Whitehead (1925) presented an ample review of Western intellectual history to show that philosophical and scientific explanation alternates between mechanism and romanticism. Experimentation to test mechanistic hypotheses rather than introspection has long been considered more scientific. Wilhelm Wundt and other mentalists were largely discounted among the clearly scientific academic psychologists, while behaviorists and Pavlovians were included within the scientific family. The ease with which the experimental method may be taken up in these latter psychologies contrasts to the clinical mentalist emphasis of psychoanalysis.

Thus, we may not be surprised by the new movement toward empathy and immediate understanding. It is a shift toward what I choose to label a romantic vision, and may denote the continuing restlessness of a science that has for too long sought a rationalist basis.

Though always mentalist in its vantage point, psychoanalysis took on new hopes for scientific status under the banner of ego psychology and the guidance of those who agreed with Heinz Hartmann. Still others strained, even in the 1940s and 1950s, to maintain the position of psychoanalysis as a depth psychology with lesser ambitions. Parenthetically, this strong, rationalistic starting point has been bolstered in part by cognitive and developmental psychology, which has been temporarily heartening to some. Jean Piaget's and Heinz Werner's approaches to psychology are compatible in many ways with a Freudian position, even though they omit a dynamic unconscious and are dissimilar in method. At least they could be absorbed within ego psychology.

Additional problems for the scientific and rationalistic status of psychoanalysis will be cited, but not explored further. It is a method and technique carried out by unobserved dyads; even inclusion of the tape recorder for observational purposes in recent analytic experiments creates an unusual effect that cannot be discounted. Moreover, attempts by prospective developmental research to deal with the genetic point of view of psychoanalysis as a means of verifying reconstructive propositions have led to some disappointment. In my view, those analysts who became mother-infant watchers have, at best, come up with complementary rather than validating data about what classical analysts proposed (Shapiro and Stern, 1980); (Shapiro, 1981). Post-Kleinian object relations theorists have also made their mark. They have emphasized the presumed dyadic preOedipal origins of varying analytic phenomena, alerting analysts to felicitous or unhealthy mother-infant interactions. Winnicott's (1953, 1965) "holding environment" and "transitional objects" were brought to theoretical light to account for both the imaginative aspects of mental life, and to provide an explanation for impeded analyses with patients who may have been narcissistic and borderline. As a pediatrician and unique individual, he provided a humanistic vocabulary close to observation and rich in metaphor that has a compelling appeal to many, but is lacking in veridical strength.

The foregoing cited factors essentially reflect the relative failure of psychoanalysis to achieve the hoped-for status of a "science" similar to other sciences, rather than a humanistic discipline. Even the suggestion that it is a science, as astronomy and archaeology are sciences, does not comfort all, and certainly its inclusion within hermeneutics places it closer to religious exegesis than I, and many like me, would like to accept. Having been disappointed at not achieving this aim, we as psychoanalysts should not be surprised that there is impetus to assert our individual contribution and ascendancy by setting ourselves apart from science, while at the same time proclaiming our uniqueness by boasting something that other sciences do not have. Thus, I would see the emphasis on empathy as a recent *conceit* borne of disappointment.

Moreover, self-psychologists in general tend to elevate the psychoanalytic method to an art by asserting that empathy is the *sine qua non* of the psychoanalytic method. Indeed, the *only* way to plumb complex mental states according to this vision is via "vicarious introspection" or empathy. Incidental support for the view that empathy reveals a wish for extraction from science and closer alliance to art comes from the historical etymological fact that "empathy" appears in the *Oxford English Dictionary* only in its supplement, as a relative newcomer to the English language. It is a direct translation from the German *Einfühlung*, employed by Lipps to explain man's comprehension of artistic products.

Even though the new emphasis on empathy may be explained historically, I still would see our recent interest arising within

165

psychoanalysis as a new defensive conceit. It is a conceit which has its parallel in other social movements. The invention of "soul" by the Black community and the "Yiddishe kopf" by the Jewish community strike me as apt parallels. These groups reveal their sense of ostracism from a larger community as well as the wish to assert separateness in a *virtue* that is not easily shared by the rejecting community. I would regret it if psychoanalysis were to accept empathy as its tool (and the further dictum that we understand before we explain) because we would then relinquish our place among the sciences altogether. However, my regret as well as acceptance of empathy without examination of its meaning may be countertransferential, more specifically, counter-cultural-transference. That is, we on both sides of the empathic fence may be responding too hastily to relative rejection by asserting our independence. We know all too well how psychologically appealing and entrenched is the tendency to appear to win by turning the passive into the active. But such victories are to be understood as defensive, and therefore fragile; they do not result in conflict resolution.

In taking this position against the wholehearted acceptance of empathy as *our* tool, I wish purposely to sharpen our understanding of empathy in order to see if it holds up against the usual rules of discourse. In so doing, some may be alienated, but it is equally worth the risk taken by those who have accepted their allegiance to Kohut's principle. In his espousal of empathy, he metaphorically alluded to the "Emperor's new clothes" and analogized his assertion of a "new method" to that of the child's "naïve courage." If I may coin a new aphorism, "Courage is in the eye of the polemicist." Who is seen as courageous depends on whether the person is in the crowd or in the Emperor's entourage.

II

Yet, who among us would wish to be known as unempathic? Empathy, like the word "tall," shares properties that linguists call *markedness*. When we inquire about somebody's height, we do not ask if he is short, because such phrasing already prejudges the subject. However, if we ask, "How tall is he?" we equally entertain the possibilities that he may be either tall or short. I cannot conceive of anybody within our science being favorably disposed to sending a patient to an unempathic rather than an empathic therapist. In that sense, our common usage demands that empathy be revered as a precursor to understanding and interpretation. But, these common-sense-isms bring us no closer to that which we wish to achieve—an explanation of what we mean by empathy that includes something more than its assertion as the base technique or process of analysis.

Another possibility to consider is that perhaps empathy is a creative fiction of the German language, which has a propensity to agglutinate stems, prefixes and suffixes into new creations that are then falsely reified. *Einfühlung* (to feel into) has been employed not only as a cautionary counter to unempathic analysis, as Roy Schafer suggests (*Bulletin of the Association for Psychoanalytic Medicine*, 1979), but as a new organ of perception to match Theodor Reik's (1951) imaginary third ear. It is a phenomenon that can only lead to a new metapsychology of the self rather than a metapsychology of a mental apparatus. Regardless of whether we need such a new vantage point (and perhaps we do, because much of what we write about lately seems stale), we should recognize that it is indeed invoked as if it were a new organ. Kohut states:

The inner world cannot be observed with the aid of our sensory organs. Our thoughts, wishes, feelings, and fantasies cannot be seen, smelled, heard, or touched. They have no existence in physical space, and yet they are real, and we can observe them as they occur in time: through introspection in ourselves and through empathy (i.e. vicarious introspection) in others [1959 p. 459].

We may thus repeat the earlier definition in the form of an explicit statement: We designate phenomena as mental, psychic or psychological as our mode of observation includes introspection and empathy as an essential constituent [1959, p. 462].

Valid scientific research in psychoanalysis is nevertheless possible because (1) the empathic understanding of the experiences of other human beings is as basic an endowment of man as his vision, hearing, touch, taste, and smell [1977, p. 144].

Ornstein (1979) makes a clear dichotomy in his paraphrase of Kohut's complementary two layers: The first layer, *understanding psychology*, is grasped via introspection and empathy as methods to encompass meanings, motives and relationships leading to understanding. The second layer, *explaining psychology*, is grasped by inference, concept formation and theorizing. The latter seeks causal connections and evolves explanations.

Contrast this with Freud's naturalistic vision of the problems of knowing another's consciousness:

Consciousness makes each of us aware of his own states of mind; that other people too, possess a consciousness is an inference which we draw by analogy from their observable utterances and actions, in order to make this behavior of theirs intelligible to us This inference (or this identification) was formerly extended by the ego to other human beings, to animals, plants, inanimate objects, and the world at large, and proved serviceable so long as their similarity to the individual ego was overwhelmingly great [Freud, 1915 p. 169].

As stated in an earlier paper (Shapiro, 1974), Freud's assertion places us in a position as mental scientists to be concerned with *perception* of and *judgment* about the feelings and thoughts of others, but does not propose the need to construct a new organ with which to see within. In that sense, Freud keeps us well within a natural-science frame. Moreover, Gedo (1979) insists that Kohut endorses empathy as an interpersonal process that is not merely an instrument for recognition of psychological configurations, but is equally useful in treating both guilty and tragic man.

The espousal of empathy as an independent apparatus, I fear, implies a new form of animism and vitalism. This time it is not a base life force used by Bergson to instill in the human species a reasonable humanistic discontinuity within Darwinian continuities, but a property of human capacity. While we may have to accept a *gestalt*ist view that free-floating attention is directed to larger non-reducible apperceptive masses seen as wholes, I am not sure that we have to suggest a completely new function independent of other functions. Indeed, even empathy employs experience, distant and close, sensory experience and cognitive data analysis. Kohut (1977) himself makes the assumption that empathic responsiveness is increasingly possible toward those who are culturally similar in both background and situation. Such an assertion, if true, is highly dependent on the very sensory and memory inputs that are employed in natural sciences, and is logically incompatible with a view of empathy as a process apart from other modes of apprehending the surroundings.

Interestingly, such a view is in marked contrast to Harry Stack Sullivan's (1953) attempt to explain how we attend to patients such as schizophrenics with experiences different from our own, that is, his assertion that we are more similar as human beings than dissimilar as patients and therapists. It has always been somewhat troubling that Sullivan's contributions are not even mentioned by most self-psychologists. He even expressed a strong partiality for empathy and undercuts my own argument in suggesting that it may be "my kind of education" that does not permit me to see how feeling is transmitted interpersonally:

> I bridge the gap (between mother and infant; therapist and patient) simply by referring to it as a manifestation of an indefinite—that is, not yet defined—interpersonal process to which I apply the term empathy. I have had a good deal of trouble at times with people of a certain type of educational history, since they do not know whether it is transmitted by the ether waves or air waves or what not; they find it hard to accept the idea of empathy. But whether the doctrine of empathy is accepted or not, the fact remains that the tension of anxiety when present in the mothering one induces anxiety in the infant [Sullivan, 1953, p. 41].

On the other hand, a historical contrast that reveals a similar appeal to Kohut's espousal of familiarity as an empathy-enhancer comes from Charles Darwin. However, Darwin extends familiarity to affection and comes closer to Freud when he discusses the feelings of communication in love:

> The feeling of sympathy is commonly explained by assuming that, when we see or hear of suffering in another, the idea of suffering is called up so vividly in our own minds that we, ourselves, suffer. But this explanation is hardly sufficient, for it does not account for the intimate alliance between sympathy and affection. We undoubtedly sympathize far more deeply with a beloved than with an indifferent person; and the sympathy of the one gives us far more relief than that of the other. Yet assuredly we can sympathize with those for whom we feel no affection [Darwin, 1872, p. 216].

Another challenge that will have to be met by those who seek a rational understanding of empathy concerns extricating it from its designation as a *primitive* function. The thesis here is that empathy is preserved in the mature mind as though it were an inborn legacy of infancy, surviving as an apparatus that once subserved mother-infant preverbal coenaesthetic mutuality. In this vein, Olden (1958) explains that empathy has an umbilical- like function. Still others invoke Winnicott's holding environment (Modell, 1979) or suggest continuities between mature empathy and earlier mother-infant dyadic situations. These states are seen by some as the same as empathy, rather than analogous to it. Again, Freud showed his rationalism more than his followers when he looked for precursors to empathy in imitation, while identification or trial identification were considered to be later events, as more recent therapists have suggested. Loewald (1979) is illuminating in his somewhat mixed position:

If we exclude the whole realm of identification and empathy from normality, for example, we arrive at a normality that has little resemblance to actual life. Identification and empathy, where subject-object boundaries are temporarily suspended or inoperative, play a significant part in everyday interpersonal relations, not to mention the psychoanalyst's and psychotherapist's daily working life.

While its [psychoanalysis'] intent has been to penetrate unconscious mentality with the light of rational understanding it also has been and is its intent to uncover the irrational unconscious sources and forces motivating and organizing conscious and rational mental processes. In the course of these explorations, unconscious processes became accessible to rational understanding, and at the same time, rational thought itself and our rational experience of the world as an "object world" became problematic [Loewald, 1979, pp. 772-773].

Martin Hoffman (1978), an experimental developmental psychologist, places empathy on a developmental continuum. He begins with observations of reflexive action such as an infant's arousal to tears at hearing other infants cry; motor mimicry is seen next (as already noted by Freud), while conditioning and imagination follow. The possibility of thinking oneself into another's affect is demonstrable experimentally and also revealed in various physiological measures taken while an observer watches another receive ostensibly painful shocks. Both observer and subject of such experiments increase their sweating, but there is a delay in the observer, long enough for cognition and judgment to take place. Moreover, a decrease in heart rate signals attention of the observer, whereas increase in rate is shown by the subject who has received the shock. This fact of heart- rate reduction is a regular accompaniment of focused attention.

These elements of developmental progression from primitive precursor to more mature experience are also suggested by Schafer (1959), who calls the highest level of empathy *generative;* this has also been discussed by Shapiro (1974) and Beres and Arlow (1974). Kernberg (*Bulletin of the Association for Psychoanalytic Medicine,* 1979) espouses a similar view, in recommending that empathy is a precondition of interpretation, rather than understanding, as stated by Kohut.

The foregoing supports the idea that empathy is a mediated response, not simply a regression. Distance from the object observed (Shapiro, 1974) and knowledge of one's own mental state as distinct from an other's requires developmental maturity. Indeed, consider someone who is deaf and blind, and ask if he can easily establish in himself the mental state of another, no less perceive and organize the stimuli from other senses into a *gestalt* for knowing another's mind rather than one's own immediate state. A significant experience in Helen Keller's coming to understand symbolic relationships is instructive; it links man's symbolic capacities with his affects, and the interrelation among mental objects with ideas of others and personal feeling. Ms. Keller tells of the finger motions of her hands signifying letters made by Anne Sullivan. They were empty, and their relation to things were meaningless until she achieved symbolic understanding:

> One day, while I was playing with my new doll, Miss Sullivan put my big rag doll into my lap also, spelled "d-o-l-l" and tried to make me understand that "d-o-l-l" applied to both. Earlier in the day we had a tussle over the words "m-u-g" and

"w-a-t-e-r." Miss Sullivan had tried to impress it upon me that "m-u-g" is mug and that "w-a-t-e-r" is water, but I persisted in confounding the two. In despair she has dropped the subject for the time, only to renew it at the first opportunity. I became impatient of her repeated attempts, and seizing the new doll, I dashed it upon the floor. I was keenly delighted when I felt the fragments of the broken doll at my feet. Neither sorrow nor regret followed my passionate outburst. I had not loved the doll. In the still, dark world in which I lived, there was no strong sentiment or tenderness.... We walked down the path to the well-house, attracted by the fragrance of the honeysuckle with which it was covered. Someone was drawing water and my teacher placed my hand under the spout. As the cool stream gushed over one hand, she spelled into the other the word water, first slowly, then rapidly. Suddenly I felt a misty consciousness as of something forgotten—a thrill of returning thought and somehow the mystery of language was revealed to me. I knew then that "w-a-t-e-r" meant the wonderful cool something that was flowing over my hand. That living word awakened my soul, gave it light, hope, joy, set it free! There were barriers still, it is true, but barriers that could in time be swept away.... I left the well-house eager to learn. Everything had a name, and each name gave birth to a new thought. As we returned to the house, every object which I touched seemed to quiver with life. That was because I saw everything with the strange, new sight that had come to me. On entering the door, I remembered the doll I had broken. I felt my way to the hearth and picked up the pieces. I tried vainly to put them together. Then my eyes filled with tears; for I realized what I had done, and for the first time, I felt repentance and sorrow [Keller, 1913, p. 212].

This skillfully recorded event, so full of poignance and meaning, gives me courage to embark on the following line of argumentation. I will suggest that psychoanalysis is, above all, a rationalist enterprise, devoted to observations involving all the senses and employing judgments about those perceptions—without the requirement that we make of empathy an additional function that will remove us prematurely from the rest of science. Freud's aim towards scientific purposefulness was not in vain. Freudian psychology is, in the first instance, a psychology developed around clinical interpretative processes designed to generate insight, and with insight, the development of new ego organizations. Some may say that psychoanalysis is also other things, and I would agree; I also suggest that if we do not pay attention to our rationalist base, in fact the first rationalist science to include a significant theory of affects, we will find ourselves in the ranks of other artists of the mind, such as novelists. Our sense of rejection for not having fulfilled many requirements as science is no reason to defensively throw the whole show over, with an ill-conceived definition of empathy as a new guide to knowledge. Indeed, the quest for a psychology of meaning and its relation to conscious and unconscious dynamic states associated with the potential for affective expression is too important a change in psychology's object of scrutiny to segregate from science. Understanding these ideas and their disposition is, and should continue to be, the aim of psychoanalysis.

What psychoanalysts do is to analyze symbols and resistance. We have thus entered into the arena of the careful analysis of behavioral as well as ideational structure and states. The genetic point of view in analysis must also ultimately be verbalized in a veridical form. We can never know directly or for certain that our constructions are correct. Instead, we use an aspect of the current interaction as having some reflective significance, i.e., a symbolic recasting of the past. Through his tentative identifications with the patient, the analyst can come to know both sides of the dyad as projected. However, while we utilize such techniques as transient identifications and shared unconscious fantasies for understanding (Beres and Arlow, 1974) (which is probably the closest thing to a dynamic restatement of what we call empathic understanding), we also misfire; we misunderstand and may be led into the most common route of error in psychoanalysis—responding to our countertransference and unanalyzed personal needs. We then act as though we were responding to something that was elicited by our patient's behavior. Indeed, if we uncritically take every state of the analyst as being induced by the patient and analyze it as such, we will fall into error more frequently than if we keep the kind of neutrality that Anna Freud (1960) describes as a vantage point equidistant from drives, superego, reality and the defending ego.

Do not doubt for a moment that the toleration required of this demand is enormous! Freud's lack of tolerance for sociopathy and psychoses is easy to note as an example. Kohut's interest in and tolerance for the narcissistic personality is perhaps an example of his greater acceptance. Nevertheless, one might ask if what we tolerate—and yes, even "immerse ourselves in empathically" in order to know better—also satisfies something significant within each of us as therapists. The neurotic mesh between therapist and patient may be as preordained as marriages made in heaven, or equally as likely, the method may prescribe its results. As a case in point, why was libido discovered (or used as an explanation) prior to aggression,

176

rather than vice versa? Why did guilty man emerge prior to tragic man? Kohut answers on both sides of the issue: Method holds its results, and culture changes persons.

III

The sources of such errors as described have been made clear to us. We are instructed that if we are not well enough analyzed in all aspects of our functioning, our response to varying states induced by patients might not lead to correct judgments about them, even if empathically guided. Moreover, if we are preoccupied by common everyday life demands when interpretation is necessary, we may be responding to our own needs rather than to the implied needs of the patient. Too often I have seen or heard of circumstances where therapists respond to patients because of what their own analysts or supervisors did that day. For example, a young therapist in analysis for six months wondered if "everything was OK." since I had not spoken during the prior hour. In the intervening time he had the impulse to "give in" to his patient by speaking, so as to diminish his patient's suffering, as he had suffered from lack of assurance by me. I interpreted his wish to outdo me in kindness and inquired about the resolve to do as I did instead. He responded that he wanted to feel as I did as he watched new data emerge, and feel as he presumed I had felt as he virtuously waited. He then relented and admitted that he had experienced resentment and anger, and that he characteristically worked to gain my attention, not my interpretation.

Referring to his unfortunate history, I noted his sense that he was always working for his father's attention. This led to data from his early history in which he succeeded in getting his father's approval, only to be followed by long separations and a constant struggle to find out how to please him so that he would stay. One could have stopped analyzing, but what emerged was data from the past that helped in the interpretation of a dream reported two days prior. In the dream, the analysand was caught stealing and was frisked in his underwear by a storekeeper. The feeling that he had taken something that did not belong to him was a new experience. He had never thought he'd experience guilt; he always thought of himself as tragic. He had not come by his identification with me honestly; he stole it to deal with his resentment, disappointment and anger. His presumed empathy for his patient would have led to a technical intrusion that had been a response to his own need. His identification with his analyst at least permitted his behavior to be revealed and analyzed in its conflictual origins.

Another source of error concerns the unusual communicational scheme that the psychoanalytic situation produces. It tends to intensify a relationship by creating a nonvisual circumstance in which affects are built into larger dimensions that become like caricatures of real life. Such caricatures may not be easily interpreted on an empathic basis, because of their intensity or their obvious lack of appropriateness. The imagined reality that gives rise to such feelings requires studied rethinking of the person's history as remembered and alertness to symbolic reformulations.

After her return from a relatively long undiscussed absence from analysis, I interpreted that the patient, a woman, had not come because she sought to treat me as she treated her husband. The confrontation was an attempt to bring to her attention that she used sexual abstinence as a retaliation to him, and now absence from me served a similar purpose. Earlier in the marriage, her husband had spurned her when she expressed her wishes, and now she asserted her independence by infidelity to him through identification with her equally unfaithful father. The patient denied the interpretation and stated that she had been angry at me, which is why she had not come. She also implied that much more was going on within that she did not wish to share with me.

Prior to the absence, she had experienced a brief period of regression where she "felt like an infant." Moreover, she was furious at me for looking on and not responding, and no longer wanted to feel trapped. She complained that her only way of coping was not to come. She also admitted that coincident with her absence she had thought of leaving a message, but forgot. This time, unlike others, however, she knew that she was angry and purposely did not want to let me know that she would not be coming.

She complained bitterly that I did "not know her at all," that I had "no real empathy," and that I had been too "cut-and-dried." She admitted at the same time that she had chosen me because she thought that I would not "take her nonsense," would "be strong" and take care of her. She also feared the latter and resisted any implication of dependent or erotic transference. I repeated to her by way of clarification the paradox that she felt: She had acted like an infant and complained that I had seemed unempathic, yet independence was what she had wanted of me in the first place—I was to be strong, someone on whom she could lean while she indulged her own emotions without fear of seduction. This led to an elaboration of her disappointment in her husband, and the confrontation of her conflicted wishes for dependency without mature sexual participation in marriage.

She then spoke of what had transpired during her absence. She had given up a longstanding habit without aid. In that setting of absence from me in which she had relinquished something on her own, she recognized an increase in affection and sexual arousal towards her husband. He looked younger and better; they were able to talk, and her lover of the past faded from her thoughts. She even felt desirous and showed it; then when she felt his erection, she drew back thinking, "What would Dr. S. say?" She knew it was such a clearly distorted experience. In face of that, she was able to tell him that she loved him for the first time in many years; she also reported on the couch that she had a strong desire to resume her relinquished habit. Then she admitted having told her husband that she wished he did not have a penis.

Empathic listening surely permitted the analyst to appreciate the depth and sources of this patient's difficulty and pathetic regression. To have let her know about such understanding at the stage of analysis reported might have made her feel better, but I believe it also might have impeded the emergence of significant derivatives and sidetracked the analytic work. Instead, she was now able to see the two sides of her ambivalence towards me in coherent relation to her feelings towards her husband and how she selected and chose companions in her life. The wishes to be strong rather than leaning, and that the male share in her sense of inadequacy, I believe emerged because the analyst maintained a relatively neutral and analyzing stance, rather than identifying with her need and permitting seduction by her transient mood.

Another source of error and perhaps the most dangerous to the therapist is that the ready acceptance by the patient of what the analyst says leads to the analyst being fooled by his own success. Transference readiness for such acceptance becomes flattery and the "over-idealization" that Kohut writes about so cogently. Moreover, the gratification of the patient may yield a return of the gift by the analyst, making him too certain of his own perceptions. Such modes, I would submit, lead to the same mutual gratification that accrues in the child-rearing process itself, in which parents find so much pleasure in bringing up a child who is responsive (e.g., when he turns out as the parent wished him to turn out, or when he even begins to sound and look like the parent). This is not analyzing; it is child-rearing and not unpleasant confrontations.

A young man in his twenties who had been in analysis for two years began to recognize his likeness to his complaining mother. He had felt initially that he was supposed to pity her for her martyrdom, and later thought that she had "screwed him up" by augmenting his guilt. He believed that he was "a rotten son who wanted to do what he wanted to do," while he continued to feel that he was doing something wrong.

He described meeting a girl who seemed interested in him, but he hated her because she was doing to her husband what his wife had done to him. He had been and felt like a cuckold. He then protested that he did not feel contempt for the man, but that "any guy would feel contempt for him," had he known about his wife's affair. Instead, he claimed empathy for the other young man because he had "been there too." He then noted that his sense of worthlessness had come from the feeling that he never could please his parents. Now he had met somebody whom he did please.

He then made a parallel observation: He had been in class the night before, and had a good insight but could not raise his hand to report it. He felt he could have impressed the professor, that most people in his class were really stupid. He wished he could learn from the professor and become just like him, and remembered that he said similar things about a former employer. He commented on how he felt that he had to market himself all the time in order to get from the teacher what it took to improve himself. He questioned his need for teachers and bosses, and how much he yearned to be like the teacher. He then mused that he probably was as smart as that teacher anyway. He boasted that he was interesting and funny, well-liked, brilliant. On the other hand, he felt so inhibited that he couldn't even raise his hand in class; he must therefore be quite inadequate. He saw in the latter a return of his initial complaint—the identification with his mother.

Analytically, the patient repeatedly had been made aware of his success phobia, which was based on the idea that he did not want to sit at the feet of the Guru, but to wear the Guru's shoes and sit where the Guru sat. Similar attitudes had prevailed towards his father. In terms of the therapeutic process, it would have been all too easy to identify with this man's sense of despair, inhibition and inability, rather than bring to his attention his ambitious strivings, negative Oedipal attachment (his continued wish for his father's phallus), and passive identification with his mother. It would have been possible to yield to the temptation to rear him in a more empathic way than his mother had, pity his inhibition and nurse his grandiosity, rather than analyze him.

This case material can serve to make the transition from the vantage point of the therapist to that of the patient's response to interpretation.

The empathic response of the therapist may have the same effect as Glover's (1955) premature and/or exact interpretation—it may be used as an obsessional defense. One of the difficult tendencies of the interpretative process concerns diminishing the possibility of future return in deeper analysis. In fact, it is my general impression that our former devotion to depth analysis is less the aim of recent therapies. Interpretation as currently described in some hands may be couched in terms of a paraphrase of earlier-stage experiences rather than its archaic derivatives. In addition, the patient's dependency needs frequently come to the fore, providing a willingness to accept any injection of encouragement when feeling understood by the therapist. Nunberg's (1926) early and all-but-forgotten paper on the conflicting interplay of need and insight in the analytic process in producing cure is rarely read these days. Such dependencies play into therapists' needs for narcissistic flattery. The patient responds as though he were a colleague in agreement with the analyst. The ready explanation provided by the empathic definition of problems may afford the patient the general effect of what Rabkin (1977) calls an "Aunt Fanny interpretation." The interpretation is couched in nonspecific general terms so as to be noncontributory to the development of future health, no less better understanding. Such responses are useful during the induction period of an analysis perhaps, but certainly questionable in attempts to get more precision in the definition of the patient's conflicts.

IV

Rather than throw out the term empathy, I would like to suggest that we try a new definition. It might be put in line with all that we know about psychic organization, structure, and the perception of others, rather than remystify our science. Some suggest that it be renamed *sensitivity* to data (Friedman, 1980), that it be dealt with as though it were sensitivity to the patient's defensive compliance and designed to obscure his fears of greater and further exposure. That is, it would refer to an analysis of resistance derived from understanding the emotional climate of the patient's past and present life as he or she replays it in the transference.

I suggest that empathy is likely a part of the *gestalt*-building aspect of perception. One might therefore look at empathy as an attempt to build images of others which have both discursive and nondiscursive rational elements, i.e., linear sequential and spatial temporal thought forms. However, the task in the analysis should still be to deal with these configurations not so much as mystical *immediate* perceptions, but as *mediated* and able to be understood, broken down into symbolic parts and then clearly verbalized. If we cannot verbalize it, I believe we lose the analytic arena and enter the abyss of the ineffable. I contend that we have had enough of this tendency in psychoanalysis, exemplified by vague verbiage, analogies to the unknown past, or unverified human interactions with parents retrospectively perceived as monsters or weaklings.

It should be clear by now that I would find it problematic if psychoanalysis were to adopt a stance which claims that we as initiates are endowed with a capacity not definable in the terms of our own scientific understanding of symbols. Edelheit (1973) noted, in a discussion of my paper on distortions in empathy, that "a skilled and gifted person can with scrutiny of his own feelings in an encounter arrive at a close qualitative approximation of a subjective experience of another person." He cautioned, however, that he used the word "approximation" and raised the question of knowing another's mind as indicating the pitfall of circularity, i.e., in claiming to know another's mind, we may but know our own. Perhaps as Viderman, the French analyst, notes (Wilson, 1978), that is all we can know.

Instead, Edelheit decries the use of empathy as a mystical mode. He suggests that theories such as the merger model of empathy represent a sentimental reverence for a kind of primal empathic state visualized as a preverbal "Garden of Eden." He (Edelheit, 1978 also

184

notes a dialectic relationship in the development of speech and object relations that can provide a better model for the empathic process. I paraphrase him extensively because he echoes something that I myself have written, but he did it better: Empathy is not so much nonverbal as post-linguistic, since it depends on maturation of ego functions, in which language is crucially implicated. In that sense, while there is an apparent immediacy of feeling in relation to others, there is also object distance. Other writers such as Schafer (1959) also emphasize the creative aspects of such states of knowing in attempts to deal with others' feelings.

In summary, I have stated my case rather strongly in order to instill a caution designed to alert analysts. The issue is not whether empathy is a mode of apprehension, but rather whether it is analyzable as an element of our psychic organization, not something to be yielded to as an unmediated intuition.

I would submit that those who tell you about the success of their empathy are like those who invest in the stock market—they only tell you when they win! I would go as far as to suggest that the solace that we may take in our own empathic success is related to the distortion afforded by identification with a longed-for good mother who knows and understands everything. I would like to provide a counter-argument for consideration, if only as a strawman. This includes Kohut's (1959) own statement that our hesitation concerning introspection and empathy stems from the fact that they are exemplified in "catch-words such as 'mystical,' 'yoga,' 'oriental,' 'non-Western'... there still remains for us to identify the underlying reason for the prejudice against acknowledging the observational method that has given us such results" (p. 465). He then goes on to state, "Hardly anyone, however, would talk about a plant psychology. True, some enthusiastic observer of flowers might conceivably see in the turning of plants towards the sun and towards warmth something with which he can empathize... but this will be more in the sense of allegory or poetry because we cannot concede to plants... the capacity for rudimentary self-awareness" (p. 463). My only comment in closing is that Dr. Kohut's suggestion in 1959 has borne the very fruit that he predicted it would not. Many people have been advised to, and do, talk to plants. My question is, "Are they being analyzed or cajoled?" That many people feel they understand or are felt to be understood is no guarantee of such understanding.

REFERENCES

Balter, L., Lothane, Z. & Spencer, H. H. (1980). On the analyzing instrument. *Psychoanal Q.*, 49: 474–504.

Beres, D. & Arlow, J. (1974). Fantasy and identification in empathy. *Psychoanal Q.*, 43: 26–50.

Bulletin of the Association for Psychoanalytic Medicine (1979). The role of empathy in the psychoanalytic process. 18: 61–93.

Darwin, C. (1872). Expression of Emotions in Man and Animals. Chicago: University of Chicago Press, 1965.

Edelheit, H. (1973). Discussion "Development and Distortions of Empathy," by: T. Shapiro. 585th Meeting of New York Psychoanalytic Society, February 13.

Edelheit, H. (1978). On the biology of language: Darwinian/Lamarckian homology in human inheritance (with some thoughts about the Lamarckism of Freud). In: *Psychoanalysis and Language*, Vol. 3, ed. J. S. Smith. New Haven: Yale University Press, pp. 45-74.

Ferenczi, S. (1919). On the technique of psycho-analysis. In: *Further Contributions to the Theory and Technique of Psycho-analysis*. London: Hogarth Press, 1950 pp. 177–189.

Friedman, L. (1980). Kohut: A book review essay. *Psychoanal Q.*, 49: 393–422.

Fries, M.E. (1968). Problems of communication between therapist and patients with archaic ego functions. *J. Hillside Hospital*, 42: 136–160.

Freud, A. (1960). Four contributions to The Psychoanalytic Study of the Child. Four unpublished lectures presented at the Biltmore Hotel, New York City, September 15–18.

Freud, S. (1895). Project for a scientific psychology. *Standard Edition*, 1: 283–388. London: Hogarth Press, 1966.

——— (1905). Jokes and their relation to the unconscious. Standard Edition, 8. London: Hogarth Press, 1960.

——— (1915). The unconscious. *Standard Edition*, 14: 166–215. London: Hogarth Press, 1957.

——— (1921). Group psychology and the analysis of the ego. *Standard Edition*, 18: 69–143. London: Hogarth Press, 1955. Gedo, J.E. (1979). Beyond Interpretation. New York: International Universities Press.

Glover, E. (1955). The Technique of Psychoanalysis. New York: International Universities Press.

Hoffman, M.L. (1978). Toward a theory of empathic arousal and development. In: *The Development of Affect: Genesis of Behavior*. Vol. 1, ed. M. Lewis & L. A. Rosenblum. New York: Plenum Press.

Journal of the American Psychoanalytic Association (1976). Cumulative Index, Vols. 1–22/1953–1974. New York: International Universities Press.

Keller, H. (1913). The Story of My Life. New York: Doubleday.

Knight, R.P. (1946). Psychotherapy of an adolescent catatonic schizophrenia with mutism: A study in empathy and establishing contact. *Psychiatry*, 9: 323–339.

Kohut, H. (1959). Introspection, empathy and psychoanalysis. *J. Amer. Psychoanal. Assn.*, 7: 459–483.

———— (1977). The Restoration of the Self. New York: International Universities Press.

Loewald, H. (1979). The waning of the Oedipus complex. *J. Amer. Psychoanal. Assn.*, 27: 751–776.

Modell, A. (1979). Empathy and the failure of empathy. Bull. Assn. Psychoanal. Med., 18: 70–74.

Nunberg, H. (1926). The will to recovery In Practice and Theory of Psychoanalysis, Vol. 1. New York: International Universities Press, 1948, pp. 75–88.

Olden, C. (1953). On adult empathy with children. *Psychoanal. St. Child*, 7: 111–126. New York: International Universities Press.

———— (1958). Notes on the development of empathy. *Psychoanal. St. Child*, 8: 505–518. New York: International Universities Press.

Ornstein, P.H. (1979). Remarks on the central position of empathy, *Bull. Assn. Psychoanal. Med.*, 18: 95–108.

Psychoanalytic Quarterly (1969). Cumulative Index, Vols. 1–35/1932–1966. New York: Psychoanalytic Quarterly.

———— (1977). Cumulative Index, Vols. 36–45. New York: Psychoanalytic Quarterly

Rabkin, R. (1977). Strategic Psychotherapy: Brief and Symptomatic Treatment. New York: Basic Books.

Reik, T. (1951). Listening with the Third Ear. New York: Farrar, Strauss & Young.

Schafer, R. (1959). Generative empathy in the treatment situation. *Psychoanal Q.*, 28: 342–373.

Shapiro, T. (1974). The development and distortions of empathy, *Psychoanal Q.*, 43: 4–25.

——— (1981). On the quest for the origins of conflict. *Psychoanal Q.*, 50: 1–21.

——— & Stern, D. (1980), Psychoanalytic contributions to the study of infancy. In: *Infancy and Early Childhood*, Vol. 1, ed. S. Greenspan & G. H. Pollock. Washington, D.C.: U.S. Govt. Printing Office.

Sullivan, H.S. (1953). The Interpersonal Theory of Psychiatry. New York: W. W. Norton.

Whitehead, A.N. (1925). Science and the Modern World. New York: Macmillan.

Wilson, E. (1978). Abstracts. *Psychoanal Q.*, 47: 151–155.

Winnicott, D.W. (1953). Transitional objects and transitional phenomena. *Int. J. Psycho-Anal.*, 34: 89–97.

——— (1965). The Maturational Processes and the Facilitating Environment. New York: International Universities Press.

The Unconscious Still Occupies Us

(1983). *Psychoanalytic Study of the Child* 38:547–567.

Recent developments in psychoanalysis beginning with the surge of interest in ego psychology have led us into a number of areas which now account for some of the excitement of our discipline. Studies of narcissism, object relations, borderline conditions, and altered ego states are but a few of the sectors of interest that have encouraged psychoanalysts to extend their scope of inquiry and also have produced significant reformations of theory. Several of these changes have extended our models, so that some consider including interpersonalist schools, self-psychology, and other variants which the psychoanalytic method itself is said to permit. On the other hand, during the first phase of ego psychology, Anna Freud (1936) noted that prior to that time, one considered oneself an analyst only insofar as one was a depth psychologist. The question raised then also is relevant now. Is depth psychology essential to psychoanalysis? Or stated more boldly: has the proliferation of other "psychologies" led us afield from the initial aims of rendering the unconscious conscious so that the latter is less done than thought of? Has it become an aim that belongs to an antiquarian past?

Some thinkers believe that psychoanalysis became too mechanized following the introduction of the structural theory. Then Hartmann's views (1939) on adaptation became central to what is now generally considered to be the *American school*, and the lively discourse around experience-distant theorizing led some to view ego psychology as dangerous to depth psychology. Indeed, certain European analysts balked strongly; Glover (1961) even suggested that there was need for an International Association for the Protection of the Id Concept. Extreme forms of this position were taken by many Kleinians too, who are more prone to direct symbolic interpretative approaches than considerations of level of ego integration in casting their remarks to patients. The recent upsurge of Lacanian psychoanalysis, an approach that uses *The Interpretation of Dreams* as the text to be analyzed, also prescribes greater attention to the unconscious as a deeply structured, contentful organization, renaming it the Discourse of the Other.

While these positions may represent a kind of counterreformation, espousing a radical or radically conservative view of psychoanalysis, there are many who believe that ego psychology and some of its variations can very well be melded with the aim of depth analysis and restated in terms of the central requirements of symbolic transformation. It would be pitiable for the less flamboyant among us if the central spokesmen for depth analysis were cast solely in the images of Klein and Lacan. I think Marianne Kris would have concurred. There is sufficient solidity in our approach to depth understanding so that we need not discard all because parts of theory are less tenable now than earlier. Libido theory may be the stumbling block for many "moderns." It may, however, be viewed as a theory of stage- and phase-related fantasies which are anchored in the development of personality, psychopathology, and even symptom choice. We need not, at this stage, discard it as obsolete because it is closely tied to energic concepts, which unfortunately blind our way to clarity because of their tenuous theoretical status. Having supervised with Marianne Kris, I recognized in her supervisory approach a firm devotion to depth and defense analysis derived from free association and play. Many *moderns* seem to forsake free association as the means by which interpretation of dreams and symptoms and traits is achieved (see, however, Anton Kris, 1982), and have substituted instead anagogic and analogic paraphrases of observed behavior (see Stein, 1981); (Shapiro, 1982).

The technique that would permit the unfolding of the unconscious was important to Marianne Kris, as it ought to be to those of us working even in the 1980s. This aim also can be accomplished without the fanciful constructions of the Kleinians; interpretation can be brought into close relation to the conscious life of the child and, as experience grows, to include many events. Malcove's (1933) early paper that relates childhood theories of dismemberment to the cutting and mashing of food represents to me the kind of evidential base that is experience-close for human beings. Fantasies derived from such experiences are incorporated into phase-related themes that ought to be reconsidered by analysts and interpreted. How fantasies become guiding forces for life, and the source of childhood theories that lead to misinformation, also ought to concern us more than the pat reinterpretation of experiences as stale derivatives that are the hallmark of wild analysis. On the more conservative side, we dare not ignore unconscious fantasies and substitute warm, caring corrective experiences as *the* therapeutic tool.

T. S. Eliot once wrote that there are three basic experiences in life: birth, copulation, and death. Ernest Jones (1916) added four other basic universal fantasies to these three. But even if these are the base deep structures according to which we order our data, the phenomenology of play sequences, unique life events, and individual family constellations add considerable variability to the way in which these universal fantasies are organized, emerge, and dictate life's course. In this paper, I shall recount an experience that is designed to confront the issues mentioned and which reaffirms the central focus of psychoanalysis as a science of symbolic transformation and the discovery of unconscious fantasy by the use of a specific method. In applying it to children, we attempt to discover how children respond idiosyncratically and personally to universal themes that are part of growing up as a human because of the need to master life events with both symptoms and character traits. The event that will be recounted is a single meeting with a youngster. Some might view the incident to be told from the standpoint of newer theories and ask if the analyst could not have acted differently in order to help this child. I cannot redo the consultation. However, I believe that I would not have done anything differently today and that may be why I write about it. This most remarkable, poignant meeting confirmed my central conviction about what the central aim of psychoanalysis ought to be.

Although Winnicott's (1971) Squiggle game was used as a technical innovation, the essential focus of the meeting was depth-psychoanalytic and provided an important clue to understanding a cognitive confusion. Although I claim a depth focus to guide my understanding, the interpretation or, more precisely, the clarification, was presented to the child in words directed to the ego. In that sense, commonplace childhood problems and symptoms may be said to yield to an essentially linguistic intrusion. I would argue tha this procedure is not dissimilar to Freud's interpretative approach as presented in both *The Interpretation of Dreams* (1900) and in the early paper on defense neuropsychosis (1894)—namely, we use words to reveal and render accessible that which until then had been cast in nonlinguistic derivatives of action or symbolic representation. The method holds up but has been neglected in recent writing.

The strength of conviction that I believe accompanies these data derives from what I consider to be the self-evident nature of this child's productions as well as the immediate therapeutic effects of the interpretation. Moreover, the interpenetration of phase-related themes with life events should be noted. I had the opportunity to present the material to Marianne Kris briefly following the excitement of the consultation. The characteristic delight in discovery and the enthusiasm that she demonstrated were lively parts of her teaching style that was so important to the many people she instructed during her long, productive career.

The event to be described concerned a 5-year-old who developed a phase-related sleep disturbance which became more severe in a setting where she was confronted with learning the meaning of death. Her cognitive appreciation of this difficult concept was incorporated into phase-related fantasies that came into full contact with unconscious fantasies and, as Freud suggested, resonated with them just as the day residue grabs hold of a deeper organization. The sleep disturbance was most distressing to her and her parents, but the meaning of the sleep disturbance and the reason for its presence constitute the essential aspects of what had to be analyzed.

THE CASE OF EMILY

BACKGROUND

Recently, at the end of January, Emily's parents consulted me about their 5-year-old daughter. They complained about her sleep disturbance which kept her in a hypervigilant state that made it difficult for her to go to sleep and caused her to wake up frightened in the middle of the night. Once she was awake it was most difficult to help her to relax so that she could again drop off. The family feared that the sleep disturbance had been caused by Emily's learning of the recent death of two cousins, a child of 6 and his mother, in a fire at their country home.

Emily and her family had been away on a Christmas vacation. During the vacation Emily already showed some signs of restlessness and sleeplessness, but not so severe as to warrant concern. They returned to their suburban home just prior to New Year's and were told about the death of Emily's cousins. The disturbance became accentuated after Emily learned of the tragedy.

When Emily awakened she was anxious and trembling, complaining about dinosaurs who would eat her up; she also had fears and worries that the rest of the family would die while she was asleep, and she expressed concern about the possibility that her parents would make a new baby. Emily already had a younger brother, aged 3, who slept in a separate room. The parents were in their late 30s, the father a surgeon. The mother was the firmer of the two parents—more insistent that the child go back to sleep and stay in her room. The father, on the other hand, was somewhat more touched by the child's complaint, more easily cajoled into caring for her and sitting with her until she slept again. Both parents were sincerely disturbed about what had transpired and convinced of the traumatic effect that the cousins' deathbed on Emily. They could conceive of no other reason why Emily would have a sleep disturbance—despite the fact that the sleep disturbance had begun during the vacation.

The remainder of Emily's developmental and behavioral history was well within normal limits. The family could not bring Emily for consultation until mid-February, on Valentine's day. In the interim, the father wished to give the child mild doses of Benadryl at bedtime in order to see if he could not interrupt some of the desperation of the evening pattern. Just prior to my consultation with the child, he wrote me the following letter:

> Since we spoke with you, Emily's initial hysteria at bedtime has subsided. She has talked some and told me that she is not really afraid of dinosaurs, etc. Emily is afraid of dying; of the family dying. She says whenever she sees her grandmother she is reminded that her grandfather is dead. Emily has always spoken of wanting a baby sister for herself and a baby brother for Ronald. She now says she wants no more babies in the family: she doesn't want daddy's penis in mother's vagina. She spoke about death—I just listened sympathetically; she knows the answer, but does not want to hear that everyone does die. When she spoke about babies, I told her that we were very happy to have her and Ronald and at this time we do not plan to have any more children. She seemed satisfied and reassured with this answer, which is truthful.
>
> Emily now has to sleep with all the lights on and someone to stay with her (since having his own bedroom, Ronald has

slept with his room fully lit and last year requested nightly that someone stay with him; once in a while someone did, but usually he was told to wait in bed until we had finished in the kitchen, and he would fall off to sleep by himself—she had never had more than a tiny night light and went right to bed).

I believe her fear and anxiety regarding death and reproduction are genuine. However, although she seems more in control of herself, I do not think it is because she has accepted anything, rather she has chosen not to think about it. Bedtime is a long, drawn-out affair. Emily falls asleep about 9:30 to 10:00 P.M. regularly with one of us in her room, and awakens almost every night at 3:00 A.M. for 15 to 30 minutes.

It was clear that the symptom was under some control even before I saw the child, but that the anxiety persisted and that its meaning was still unknown except in the most general terms.

I had scheduled an early morning appointment for Emily. She and her father were waiting outside in the lobby as I arrived to open the front door. My first view of Emily revealed that she was a pretty, slight child, slender, with big dark-brown eyes and long dark-brown hair carefully plaited into a long braid that hung almost to her waist. She was neatly dressed in plaid skirt and tights. She hid behind her father as they entered the waiting room. Although I did not approach her as she undid her coat, she snuggled behind her father pulling at his trousers. She then smiled coyly as I attempted to greet her. She was eating a small sugared breakfast bun which was held neatly in a partially opened napkin. Dots of confectioners' sugar showed around her mouth. It was clear to me that at that moment separation from her father would be a terrible tussle and I was not about to venture a consultation with a child assaulted on first meeting by acute separation anxiety. I therefore invited both father and daughter into the office and further invited Emily to help me release a wall-held table and set up the room for our meeting. She immediately disengaged herself her from father and helped quietly. She then made her first spontaneous advance toward me as she turned her face away and held out the bun to offer me a bite. I demurred and began to puzzle about how to approach Emily. I had just been entranced at reading Winnicott's *Therapeutic Consultations with Children* (1971) and thought of the possibilities of the Squiggle game for children who will not or cannot talk. I thought that this technique might be a welcome entry in this circumstance.

As I pulled out a pack of paper and sat down on the floor with her giving Emily her own pencil, I said simply that I would make a scribble. I indicated that she could complete it and make a picture of any sort that she liked. She brightened, took the pencil in hand, looked at her father momentarily, and began. She engaged in the game directly and persistently and was not diverted throughout the entire hour of our meeting. When she finally spoke, she was fluent with speech that was marred by a slightly sibilant "s" slur. She was permitted to elaborate her answers and comments as she pleased, and I did not probe. The increase in fluency and animation was evident in her facial expressions, the music and tonal quality of her voice. In general she was a child who was quite articulate, animated, and affectively spontaneous. Within two minutes of the onset of the consultation simultaneous with the drawing of the second squiggle I casually asked her father whether he would not rather sit in the waiting room. He assented and left as Emily paid almost no attention to his departure.

THE SQUIGGLE GAME

1. I constructed an S-like structure on its side. Emily: A worm—which is all upside down. (Fig. 1.)

2. I then made horizontal and vertical lines as though beginning a square. She completed it. Emily: Pants. (Fig. 2.)

3. I then made another S-like structure. Emily: An 8 for the squiggle. (Fig. 3.)

4. I constructed another S-like figure, she crossed it, placed two zeros and an X on it. Emily: X's for tic-tac-toe board. (Fig. 4.)

5. I made a circle. Emily: A circle—a girl. [What's her name?] Arlene. [Tell me about her?] Her birthday was yesterday, she was 2 years old, she had a Snoopy party and she had a beautiful triangle cake with a standup Snoopy on it. (Fig. 5.)

6. I drew a horizontal line. Emily: A dress. [What about it?] Arlene was wearing a pretty blue dress. (Fig. 6)

7. I constructed an inverted U. Emily: It's a cup—and there were standup cups at the party. (Fig. 7.)

8. I suggested that she do the next one by herself. Emily: It's a boot. There is a zipper on it. [Who has such boots?] Mommy, but Ronald and I have little ones which you can't tell apart, which have fur inside. [Mommy has a big one and you and Ronald have little ones which are just the same!] (Fig. 8.)

9. I drew an inverted V. Emily: It's a clown's hat with a pompom. [Have you ever seen one like it?] We went to the circus and we also saw ballerinas on a horse who went in a circle and stood on top of the horse and danced. [Do you dance?] Yes, I go to dancing school, but I am going to be a *nurse* and work with my daddy in a hospital. Do you know that he takes care of little children? And does surgery on them, and puts children to sleep

with sleepy air? [Why does he put them to sleep?] So that he can take out their hernias and appendixes! [What are those?] Those are little bumps that people have. (Fig. 9.)

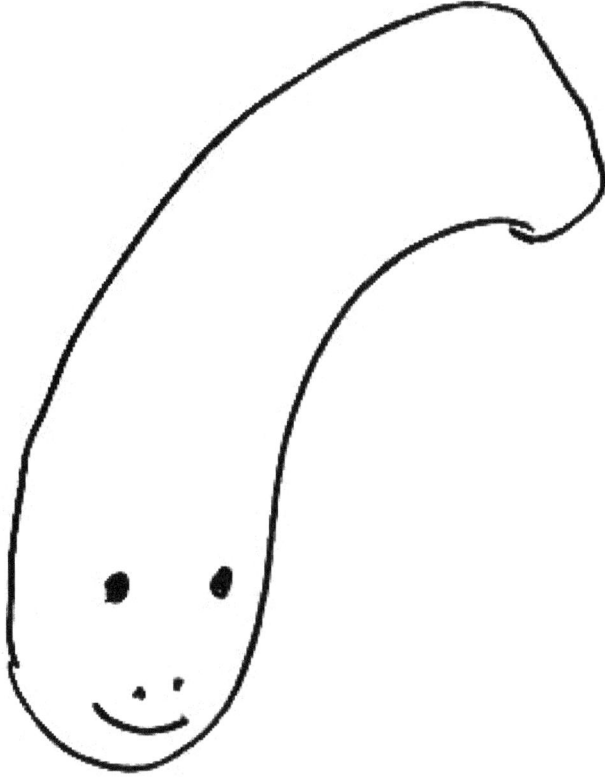

Figure 1

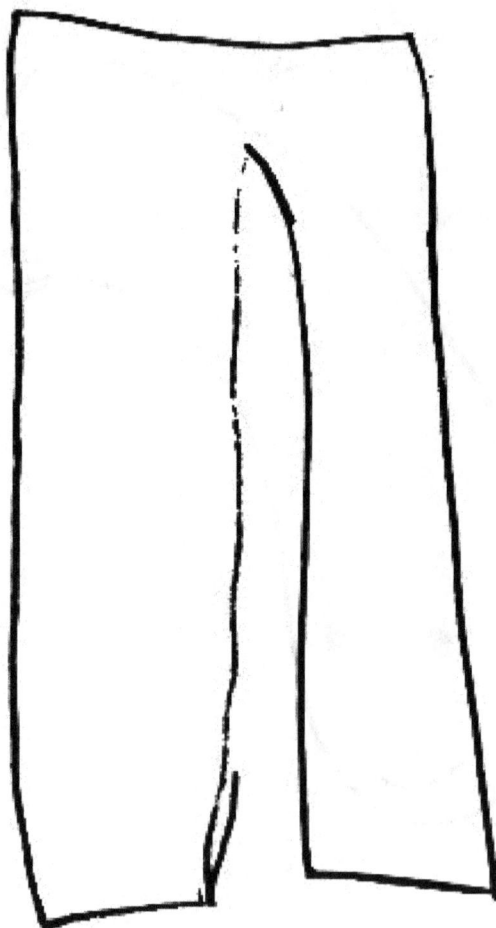

Figure 2

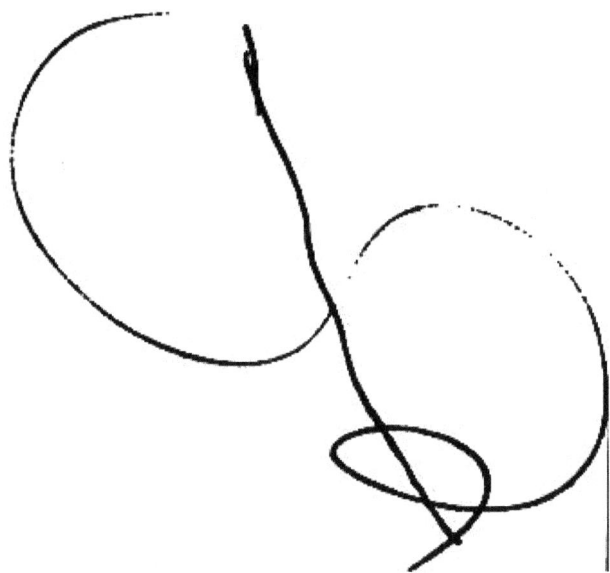

Figure 3

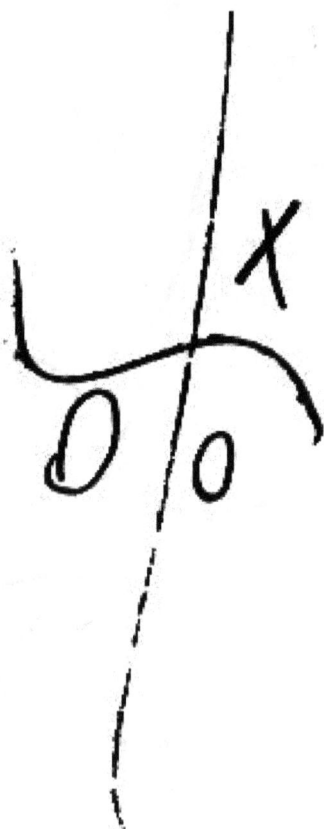

Figure 4

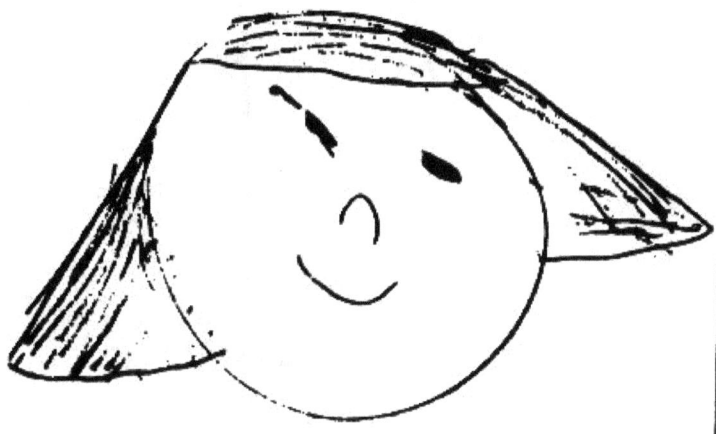

Figure 5

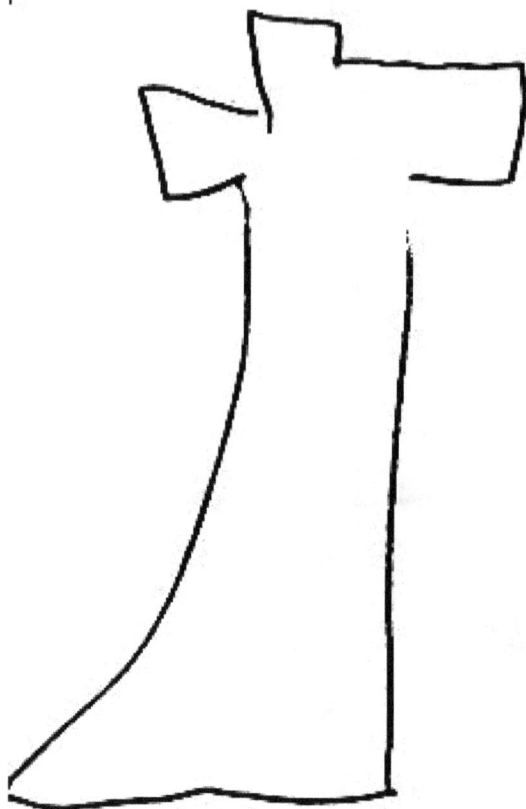

Figure 6

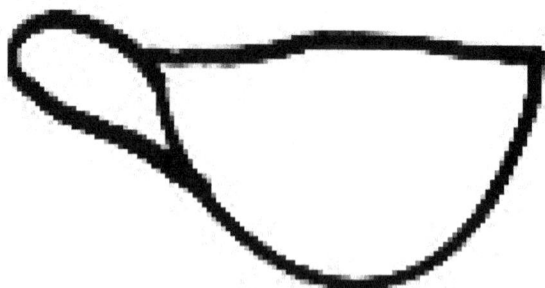

Figure 7

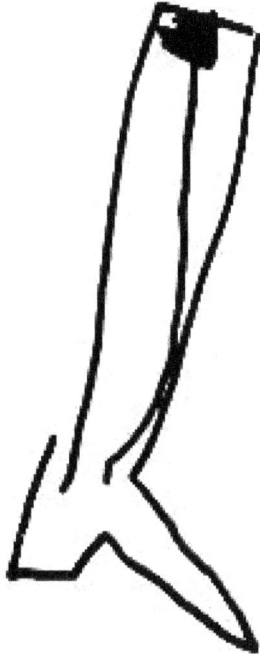

Figure 8

10. I made another S figure. Emily: A tree. [Tell me about it.] It is
going to develop apples! [Oh?] We have an uncle who lives on
a farm in Massachusetts, and an aunt, and there are two cousins
in the house. I forgot the older one's name. Do you know they
have a dog who let me pour raisins on his back when I was 2
years old [giggles]. [Such good things happen to 2-year-old!]
I'll be able to do it again. (Fig. 10.)

11. She now drew a house on her own. Emily: That's a house—Aunt
L. and Uncle B. have a house that looks like that, and it's
made of bricks, I mean wood. [Is that good or bad?] Well,
it has bricks on the outside and wood on the inside. [And
that's what makes it good?] Because bricks and wood are

good for houses. Wood is not as good as brick, because it can chip, splinter,... and rust. [And what else can it do?] It can break. (Fig. 11.)

12. I made another deeper S-like structure. Emily: A cat [Fig. 12]— my friend has a guinea pig and a cat, and I am going to get one for my birthday. [When is it?] In the spring. Ronald had a Snoopy party in November when he was 3, and a Fireman party when he was 4. [I know you like a Snoopy party, but how do you like a Fireman party?] It's okay... firemen are good for putting out fires [noticeable sadness in her voice]. [I heard that there was a sad fire recently in your family.] Yes, I felt sad that they died; you know a sister did get out... I look at my daddy's surgery book and see pictures of them doing dog surgery. My mother and Amy had their appendixes out. [Your mother and Amy?] Well, they only have it out if it is infected, and you cut a hole in a blanket when they are asleep—I saw my mother's scar. [Maybe you would like to draw it.] What if it comes out like a child? [Do it as you like to. She draws and says,] The oval part of the scar is what I'm going to show, and she has a ponytail. [You have one too! Disdainfully she says,] I have a braid. My hair is as long, no longer than my mother's. (Fig. 13.)

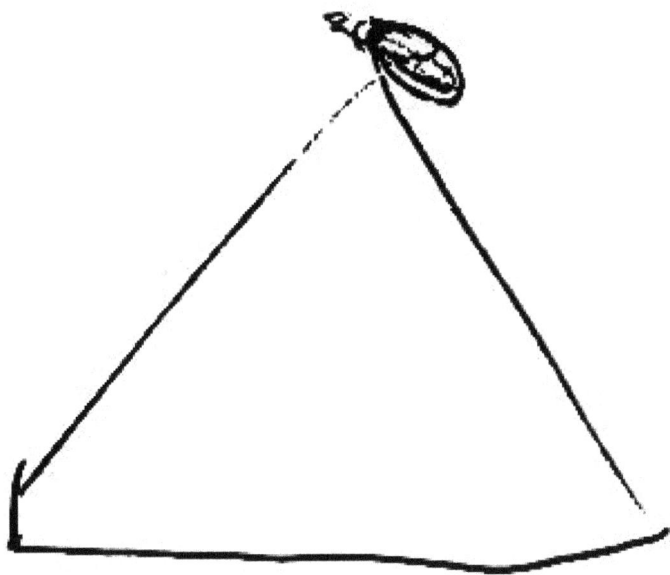

Figure 9

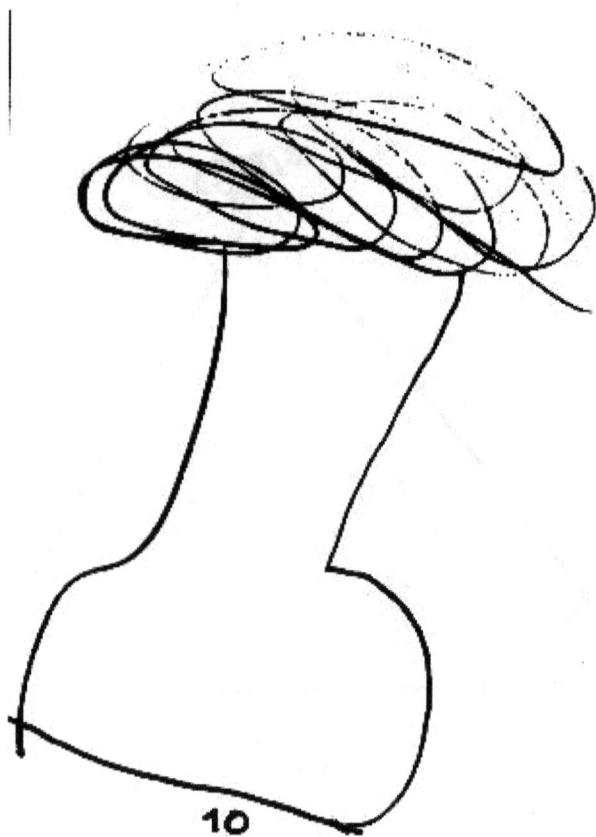

Figure 10

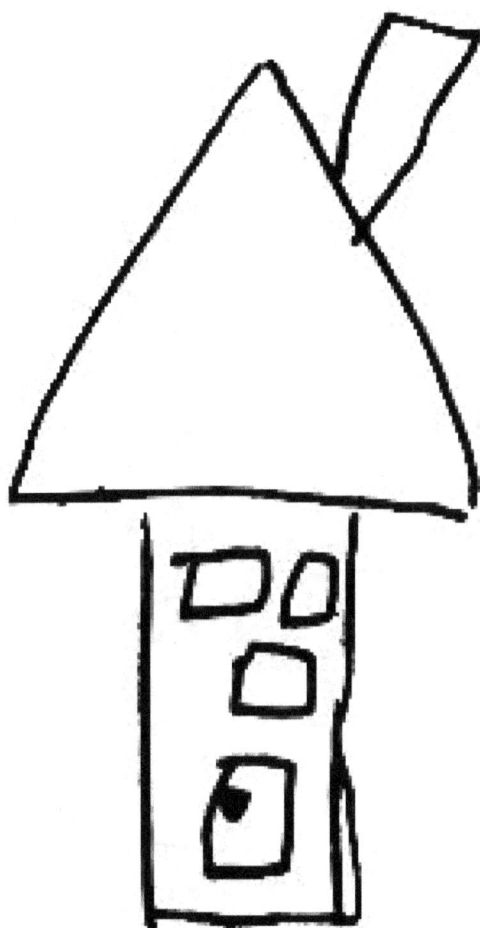

Figure 11

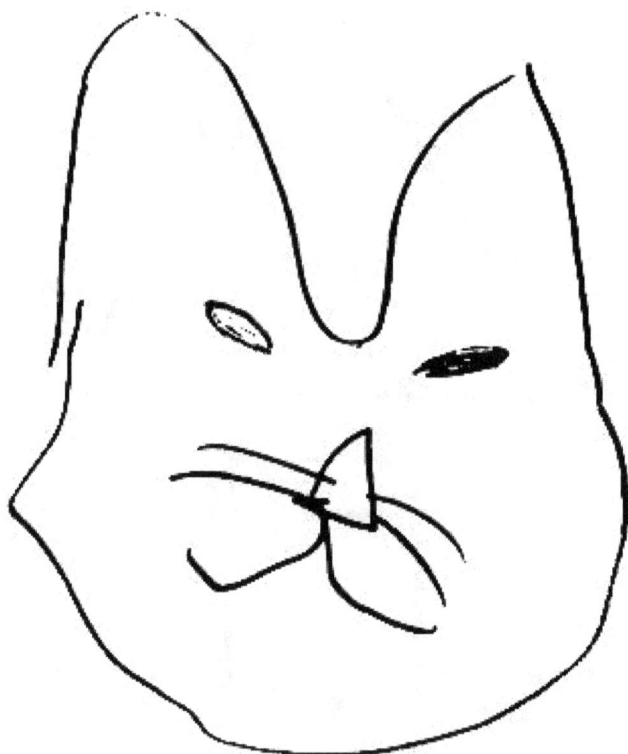

Figure 12

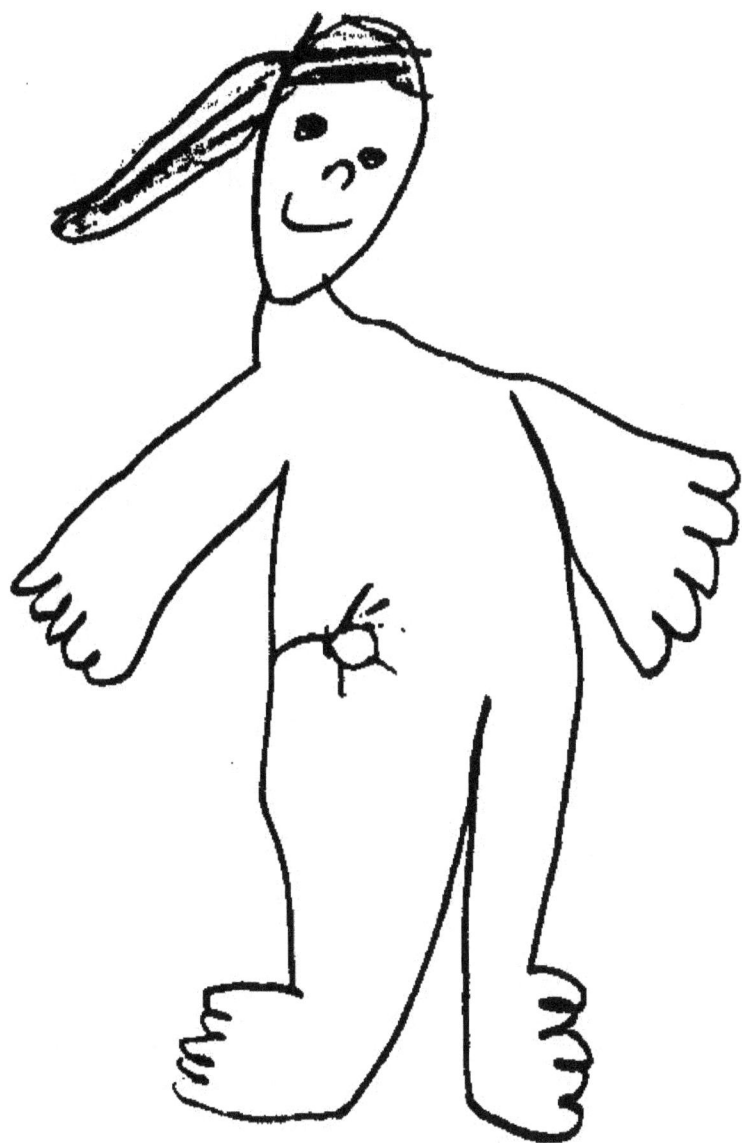

MOTHER

Figure 13

At this moment, our time was drawing to a close, and the aims of the Squiggle game had been achieved. Winnicott believes that as preconscious ideas become available to verbalization and reveal the willingness of the child to explore some of the feelings associated, enough work has been done and one need not press the child further. Moreover, the ego defenses should also be reconstituted to help master the traumatic constellations. I considered that I would have the opportunity to see her again. But I also had witnessed the emergence of defensive structures that seemed to me to be adequate to effect the linkages between death and surgery as well as the regressive pull toward the Oedipal attachment to her father. I therefore shifted ground and asked if she would like to draw a person. She responded, "Clothes on or off?" When I said, "Whichever way you like," she drew a female first, and then made a male (see fig. 14).

She spontaneously began to describe the drawings as if there was pressure to reveal more and said, "The girl is 8 years old. It's supposed to be pink and yellow in her dress, but I couldn't draw it. She is going to a party with her dress on and she is very happy." (Why?) "Because she is going to dance and she likes to do that." She then turned to the boy and said that the boy was going fishing. First he is going to go inside and get his fishing pole, and then go down to the creek and fish. And then he's got to find some worms. She made a sour face. (Oh, you don't like worms?) "They are squiggly and icky and yucky." She became animated and suggested that her brother and she once found a toad and made it jump on her mother, which made her jump, and then they made a special place behind their house, out of chicken wire to keep the toad. They supplied the toad with ample moss on the bottom, and they made a *toad bed* out of moss and *put it to sleep* one night. In the morning they found that it was so sleepy that it couldn't get up. Her father was asked to examine it, only to declare: "*The toad is dead!*"

I suggested to her that it was a hard thing for children to tell the *difference between sleeping and dying,* and that makes going to sleep very worrisome. I then added that even though children sometimes get confused, grownups know the difference very well. She exited from the meeting, smiling, attached herself to her father, and coyly reengaged him as she left.

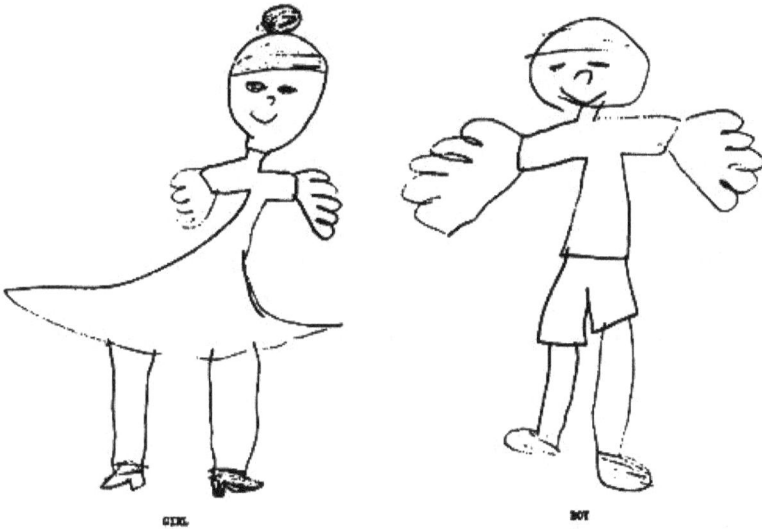

Figure 14

The second session, one week later, saw a happy, bright, and interested child. In the interim, she had sent an affectionately decorated Valentine's card. This time she was very interested in my toy closet and the materials in it; she focused most acutely on folders of other children, wishing to make her own and thereby to establish a place with me.

The subsequent meeting with the parents designed to round out the consultation revealed that Emily was sleeping well, that she was no longer as anxious, and that there was a major diminution of disturbing behavior. Since the meeting had been initiated around a single symptom, I did not feel justified in suggesting treatment, and indicated to the family that they were welcome to call as they needed. They were not eager to continue either.

DISCUSSION

I have presented this case verbally to many psychoanalysts, and have been asked: Why did you not insist on carrying the analysis further? Why did you not approach the child's narcissistic injury at having an unempathic mother? Why did you not interpret the clearly defined Oedipal constellation and castration anxiety? Why did you not approach the preOedipal ambivalence toward the mother? Why did you not do parent counseling?

These queries are legitimate and relate well to the central issue of how one practices; that is, how can our grasp of depth psychology lead to better understanding and then help us to make our interventions at the appropriate level without stirring up more sediment than is necessary, and also permit development to proceed? Moreover, when should we stop even when we understand more? The answers are determined by our theory of change and how that theory interacts with our ideas about normative development and the growth of meaning. Technique should follow directly from how we understand theory and how we use our knowledge of unconscious functioning. This case is an apt example of how a common symptom of sleep disturbance (Hertzig and Beltramini, 1983) can become a violent assault on a family and a most distressing and uncomfortable symptom to a child. The confusion of meaning between death and sleep is quite natural, given the child's wish for death to be reversible, and sleep's signifying loss of conscious control of the known world. Indeed, even our cultural tendency to refer to death in terms of sleep must add to childhood confusion and anxiety. The often-repeated bedtime prayer that admits to "if I die before I wake" is probably so ritualized that most children hardly appreciate the significance of the words; otherwise Emily's symptom might be more widespread.

The appreciation of death as irreversible and an end to which we all must come has provoked a vast literature on the stages in the appreciation of death and the capacity for mourning. While these themes are not central to my presentation, this case and other clinical experiences suggest that the understanding of death may be a discrete event in time rather than a gradual acquisition. Appreciation of its significance may occur as early as 3 and as late as the senium. The degree of cultural and personal defense that accrues is not so much existential *but*, as Freud (1926) suggested, a recasting of developmental anxieties ranging from separation to castration. Emily's case presents elements of both.

Emily wished to be in control. Her light must be on, her eyes open. She wanted a parent in her room. Her father gratified her wishes. Separation themes surely abound. Yet, her loving protector also was a "castrator" of women and children who lie helpless when they sleep. He cut holes in blankets and surgically removed bumps— her mother and Amy were living examples with their appendectomy scars. However, and fortunately, their long ponytails or big boots with fur remained testimony to the wished-for equality between brothers and sisters and mothers and daughters. Indeed, what better altruistic surrender and defense against anxiety than to become father's helper, a nurse, and participate actively in symbolic castrations while awake rather than risk sleep, passivity, and mutilation? The fire, in turn, was a trigger that caused the bitter realization that death is indeed possible for the young as well as the old, and that it is not reversible. Thus, sleep also leads to mortal danger.

It is almost a pity to belabor the obvious in this case. Emily's words are far more poetically rich as her story unfolded than a dry rehash. However, the multiple layers of this *translation* will, I think, better help us to find the appropriate level of interpretation if we spell out the trends.

If nurse Emily is to succeed, then father surgeon dare not join mother to make babies, however that is done. The regressive suggestion of oral ingestion by a dinosaur or an assault while asleep is frightening enough to wish for times when the world was happy as a warm puppy (a Snoopy party with raisins and standup everything)—a regressive paradise when knowledge of death need not even be considered.

All the foregoing is not very fanciful even to a behaviorist, given the data of our Squiggle game, but it is familiar because we have had 90 years of psychoanalysis—the derivatives and dynamics leap out at us. What might have been more remarkable in 1910 or 1930 was: why did Emily not have more than a sleep disturbance? The answer comes from within our science; psychodynamics is not psychopathology! Marianne Kris (1957) wrote in her paper on prediction in a longitudinal study, "in general we have been more accurate in predicting areas of conflict, difficulty and pathology than we have been in predicting conflict-free functioning and the use of normal defenses. This may be due to a general tendency in many of us to look for the 'defect'" (p. 186); or, as Anna Freud (1965) would put it, regressions in developmental lines. These views are useful for a modern consideration of Emily's problem. Except for her sleep problem, she was made of good stuff. Her ego functions were well in place, and she had an encapsulated anxiety that made sense psychologically.

The central theme of this presentation rests on the idea that it made sense psychologically because we could visualize the depth features of the symptom, as the child permitted us to see the layered fantasies that supported the surface manifestation. The logic of the symptom was made understandable by finding the depth fantasy. This is the age-old claim of psychoanalysis. It is also the hallmark of any structuralist model since linguistics was born. The technique of listening without excess intrusion permitted the fantasies to emerge, and the pressure of the peremptoriness of the fantasies suggests their close relation to significant drives. Were the latter not so, we would not so easily have been permitted to construct a story that makes sense. With another story, another method, another theory, our ideas might emerge differently—but I think not as self-evidently. The recent hermeneutic approach to psychoanalysis suggests that any story told to a patient might be equally therapeutic. I doubt this, because only the fit to the facts of the child's life permits conviction. Indeed, I believe that the patient's conviction does not emerge from fluff or "any story"; rather, his or her own story is a derivative of a universal grammar of stories that constitute the store of base human fantasies; these result from our ontogenesis and our prewired central nervous system that has weathered Darwinian survival.

I return to Emily and the question why I did not belabor her Oedipus complex and its regressive components once I had uncovered them. The answer lies in the description of the process and in Winnicott's claim (1971) for the Squiggle game: "The child may of course feel to have been more understood than in fact he or she was understood, but the effect will have been to have given the child some hope of being understood and perhaps even helped" (p. 5).

The description of the play reveals that the child's fantasies were emergent and preconscious. According to Ernst Kris (1956), their interpretation is then timely. Winnicott's claim is that the feeling of being understood participates in the strength of the interpretative force. I chose to limit my comments to the cognitive confusion because of both factors stated.

I had not contracted with family or child to engage in further work. I did not wish to risk the effect of a grander intervention by its too rapid association with a more far-fetched notion. The risk of defensive denial, and the question of love for and ambivalence to parents with whom the child still resides and on whom she depends, are significant here. Besides, the rules of symbolic transformation (Werner and Kaplan, 1963) would suggest that Emily's dim awareness of the source of her anxiety was sufficient for this time in her young development.

1. The fantasies were universal in form and phase-adequate, although idiosyncratic to her unique life.
2. The emergent representation in a symptom was time- and ego-bound. No other functions were encroached on.
3. Her relationships suffered only around the anxious focus.
4. Her development was proceeding.

These factors seem sufficient to have dictated the narrowness of what I told her in words.

However, some will see in this a direct counter to the purpose of this presentation, i.e., my claim that the unconscious still does and still should occupy us. I do not think so, for it seems evident that my circumscribed treatment of Emily's dilemma was dictated by the very notion that the unconscious fantasies were most relevant, and that my restraint in telling all was part of our general psychoanalytic knowledge that telling all is wild analysis and that ego factors must be considered to determine the limits of what we may convey in words.

The richness of psychoanalytic theory would suggest that every surface derivative could lead to an associative path to complete self-knowledge. Yet we cannot formularize that except in a few base forms or universal fantasies. The latter, however, are indeed empty without significant sensitivity to experiential and ego anchors. This is even more so during the current Freudian era where the excitement of the unconscious has become banal. This banalization of the unconscious is a result of common usage and popularization. For this reason special attention must be paid to interpreting derivatives within the patient's *personal* idiom. On the other hand, there is no reason for us to give up approaches centering on the interpretation of unconscious content for new theories or to suggest new models of analysis that completely overturn Freud's basic discovery.

We have come full circle to discover that the unconscious does occupy us, *but* what may be different now is the care with which we interpret it—rather than discard it. I submit that my language suggests a new reification of the unconscious. I refer to an "it." I do not intend to do so. I am using "it" as a convenient, though regressive metaphor for latent fantasies that comprise the base grammar of conscious behavior and thought. This "it" or "id" should not be neglected if we are to provide patients who are children (the ambiguity is deliberate) with a feeling that they are understood— or, to paraphrase Winnicott, that there is "some hope of being understood and perhaps even helped."

REFERENCES

FREUD, A. (1936). The ego and the mechanisms of defense W. 2.

———— (1965). Normality and pathology in childhood W. 6.

FREUD, S. (1894). The neuro-psychoses of defence *Standard Edition* 3 45–61

———— (1900). The interpretation of dreams *Standard Edition* 4 & 5.

———— (1926). Inhibitions, symptoms and anxiety *Standard Edition* 20 77–175.

———— (1937). Constructions in analysis *Standard Edition* 23 257–269.

GLOVER, E. (1961). Some recent trends in psychoanalytic theory *Psychoanal. Q.* 30:86–107.

HARTMANN, H. (1939). *Ego Psychology and the Problem of Adaptation* New York: Int. Univ. Press.

HERTZIG, M. & BELTRAMINI, A. (1983). Individual differences in the longitudinal course of sleep and bedtime behavior in preschool children *J. Amer. Acad. Child Psychiat.*

JONES, E. (1916). The theory of symbolism In *Papers on Psycho-Analysis.* London: Baillière, Tindall & Cox, 1948 pp. 87–144.

KRIS, A.O. (1982). *Free Association.* New Haven & London: Yale Univ. Press.

KRIS, E. (1956). The recovery of childhood memories in psychoanalysis. *Psychoanal. Study Child* 11:54–88.

KRIS, M. (1957). The use of prediction in a longitudinal study. *Psychoanal. Study Child* 12:175–189.

KUBIE, L.S. (1953). The distortion of the symbolic process in neurosis and psychosis. *J. Am. Psychoanal. Assoc.* 1:59–85.

MALCOVE, L. (1933). Bodily mutilation and learning to eat. *Psychoanal. Q.* 2:557–561.

SHAPIRO, T. (1982). Empathy. *Psychoanal. Inquiry* 1 423–448.

STEIN, M. H. (1981). The unobjectionable part of the transference. *J. Am. Psychoanal. Assoc.* 29:869–892.

WERNER, H. & KAPLAN, B. (1963). Symbol Formation. New York: Wiley.

WINNICOTT, D.W. (1971). *Therapeutic Consultations in Child Psychiatry*. New York: Basic Books.

Sign, Symbol, and Structural Theory

(1986). In *Psychoanalysis: The Science of Mental Conflict* (eds. A. Richards & M. S. Willick). Analytic Press: Hillsdale, NJ.

There is a remarkable conservatism of mind as well as of social form. Once a language, or a way of thinking—or more frequently a code of values—has been learned, it is difficult for individuals within a community or in a discipline to shift easily to new models or to make new interpretations of perceived nature into new categories. The Freudian (1923) shift from topographic to structural theory that became more well established with the publication of "Inhibitions, Symptoms and Anxiety" (Freud, 1926) may seem like ancient history to us in the 1980s; nonetheless, the practicing psychoanalyst during the early 1900s had become habituated to the topographic model. During my own analytic training, I remember Berta Bornstein remarking on the excitement of some analysts when topographic theory was replaced, because dynamic structural theory seemed so much easier to apply to clinical data. I also recall that during the 60s and early 70s Charles Brenner and his colleague (Arlow & Brenner, 1964) struggled to convince members of our analytic society that certain formulations of topographic theory were no longer necessary and could be dispensed with, now that we had the structural theory and ego psychology as a theoretical base. Moreover, it would be a significant accomplishment to make our theory more parsimonious by full exploitation and exploration of the range and limits of the explanatory value of structural theory.

It seems like only yesterday that rhetoric and careful exposition were necessary to convince us of such formulations. Now we find ourselves in a time when Brenner's interpretation of Freud's psychoanalytic stance that the human being should be viewed as conflicted and one's mind as structurally organized has come under new scrutiny. Even structural theory is now questioned by some who attempt to change the pace and direction of the march of history of ideas in our science. There is a long line of thinkers from Klein (1976) to Kohut (1984) to Schafer (1976) to Slap and Saykin (1983), who would have us rethink the role of structural theory and deny its clinical, heuristic value to practice. They argue that it is person-distant, remote from experience, and too mechanistic. Despite those claims, Brenner (1974, 1976, 1978, 1982) and many of his colleagues have tenaciously sought to reveal that psychoanalysis, at its best, is embedded in structural theory and that the irreducible minimum that enables us to understand patients and their minds comes from an analysis of conflict revealed in the phenomena of compromise, such as dreams, symptoms and actions. These behaviors take on meaning insofar as they are translated by analysis into the varying elements that make up psychic structure.

In this essay, I will address only one area of Brenner's work, that pertaining to sign and symbol in structural theory. It is a natural area for me to write about, since a large part of my intellectual activity within analysis has been in the study of the interplay of language and psychoanalysis (Shapiro, 1970, 1979, 1983; Shapiro & Perry, 1976). Brenner indicates in his seminal work, *Psychoanalytic Technique and Psychic Conflict* (1976), that after the introduction of the structural theory and the reappraisal of the role of anxiety in psychological conflict, the interpretation of symptoms and dream analysis were enlarged, so that even dreams not amenable to approaches described in the Dream Book (Freud, 1900) could be brought under the same umbrella of understanding common to all other psychological phenomena and symptoms. That is, symptom, dream, and behavior all represented some form of psychic compromise to be analyzed into the contributing elements of the agencies of mind and the developmental calamities that gave rise to the attendant affects. Arlow and Brenner wrote in 1964 that the essence of dreams or any other psychological manifestation is that they are compromise formations. They also showed how what had been called dream work could be understood in terms of regression to childhood mentation. Brenner went on (1976): "...a dream is from the very start, a compromise among the three systems of the mind like any waking thought, fantasy or action." Moreover any dream that is unintelligible, is a consequence of defense. From here on Brenner's argument becomes more relevant to my central theme: "What is usually referred to as the text of the dream or its manifest content is never the dream itself. It is only what the *dreamer*—in our context, the patient—tells us. In fact, one can never know the manifest content of another person's dream. After all, what is important in analysis is not a dream, it is *what the dream means*" (pp. 137–138; italics added).

In order to direct our attention to the telling of the dream and away from the dream as an event during sleep and then imperfectly remembered, we must embark on a tour into the language of the

227

patient and his idiosyncratic capacity to refer to aspects of his psychic life as yet untapped, except as a future event of the analysis. Indeed, even while a dream or symptom expresses, it also seeks to hide and lead us astray, because of the conflict about exposing or even knowing. The inability easily to understand the dream on presentation is a sign of censorship or defense. Moreover, there is a further gap between the pictorial representation and the verbal narration, which of necessity involves secondary elaboration. As Weber (1982) stated, "The distance that separates narration from narrated, like that which separates spectator from spectacle is not an empty interval" (p. 20). Writing about the naming function of interpretation from the standpoint of the analyst, I (1970, 1979) indicated that the analyst expresses in words what the patient represents in other forms. Thus, to this point my ideas are consonant with Brenner's.

To contrast this viewpoint with others currently popular in psychoanalysis, let me digress for a moment. It could be said that some current theories that postulate developmental fault, whether in the separation-individuation process or in the failure of parental empathy, sometimes provide analysts with easy descriptions of patients' symptoms that are paraphrases of experience. Such paraphrases are closely related to anagogic explanations of dreams (see Stein, 1984). They can become pseudo-explanations that further serve defense and are nonanalytic—not because they are not relevant to what was described, but because they do not break the manifest verbalizations and descriptions into simpler elements that point to the reorganization and signifying function of the symptom or dream as a surface experience or phenomenon that refers to something more remote and less apparent to consciousness. Indeed, Arlow (1981) argues that our theories of pathogenesis are themselves referential to, and signifiers of, our current theories. For example, he notes that if a pathogenetic agent is equated with a poisonous fecal substance, then the treatment mode, of course, rests on the concept of catharsis; or that if neurosis reflects the consequences of traumatic event or relationship early in life, then a corrective emotional experience might be appropriate, and so forth.

However, nowhere within these modificaions of psychoanalysis is the need for analysis of the symptom into basic structural elements more elemental than in the structural theory as interpreted in the work of Brenner (1982). He insists that the structural theory is the only one that requires us to view the contribution of id, ego and superego to symptom and dream alike and does not permit us to escape the necessity of looking at these varying phenomena as synthetic representations composed of contributions from these postulated part-structures of mind. However, Brenner (1976) notes Lewin's (1952) view that the structural theory is most useful for understanding neurotic symptoms and character traits, whereas topographic theory is probably more useful for dealing with dreams. Lewin thus seems to indicate that theories be applied to data in a complementary way.[1] In this paper, I extend this view, which Brenner discounts, in order to bring structural theory into relation with modern language theory. I will first present some evidence of the merit of reconsidering Freud's own views, expressed at the very beginnings of psychoanalysis.

Freud's earliest models were embedded in a topographic vision because of the focus on repression and sequestered memory as the pathoplastic elements in neuroses. I believe that the psychoanalytic

---

1   Actually Lewin (1952) wrote: "Nowadays most writers use both terminologies, the older when discussing dreams, the newer when writing about the neuroses. This cleavage is not deep-seated. It is due in the main to convenience and tradition" (pp. 295-296).

view of man in conflict emphasized by structural theory would suffer no harm if it also included some room for linguistic analysis in our clinical thinking; much of what goes on in structural theory must have something to do with the analysis of language and the varied signs used to represent something that is less apparent and more experience- distant, known, as unconscious wishes in psychoanalysis and deep structures in linguistics. This point was taken up by Rosen (1966), who emphasized that what distinguishes Freud's work from others is that he considered and studied the apparently meaningless experiences of life and discovered that they are meaningful when reviewed under the light of psychoanalytic scrutiny. Freud wrote to Fliess on December 6, 1896: "As you know, I am working on the assumption that our psychical mechanism has come about by a process of stratification: the material present in the shape of memory traces from time to time is subjected to a rearrangement in accordance with fresh circumstances—to a retranscription. Thus, what is essentially new in my theory is the thesis that memory is present *not once but several times over, that it is registered in various species of signs*" (E. Kris, 1954, p. 1 73, italics added). We thus have from the originator of psychoanalysis himself an early indication of his interest in signs, symbols, signifiers, and representation.

Later, in the *Dream Book*, he wrote: "If we attempted to read these characters according to their pictorial value instead of according to their symbolic relation we should dearly be led into error... A dream is a picture puzzle! (Freud, 1900, p. 277).

This point of view, reiterated throughout Freud's text, contains all the elements necessary to satisfy the definition of a structuralist model. I refer to structuralist now, not in the sense of structural theory, but from the standpoint of the philosophical concept of structure introduced by the linguist de Sausure (1911). For an elaboration of this idea, I refer the reader to Piaget's (1970) notion that structural theory must contain three elements: (a) wholeness, (b) the capacity for transformation, and c) generative activity and self-regulation. Freud's structural theory contains these three elements, insofar as it permits variation in wholeness without preformism; that is, we are not simply what we were as children or *homunculi* in sperm, but elements of the past hold on as we become unique individuals later in life. The self-psychology school may be addressing the apparent wholeness of human experience while ignoring the structural elements out of which this wholeness develops, (for example, see concepts of cohesive self, self defect, self object) Things are not merely as they appear to be on the surface but are made up of other more elementary structures. The second element of structural theory concerns the capacity for transformation that permits changes to occur, not only over time, but synchronically in concrete representations reported in a person's psychological life. They occur even within manifest experiences, so that any representation, such as a behavior or a dream, may stand for a whole group of ideas, a syncytium, or network of wishes and prohibitions. This is not only multiple function (Waelder, 1930), or the participation of conflict in each representation that Brenner (1982) describes, but the representation at different times in life of varying forms by species of defense[2] acting upon wishful elements that constitutes conflict.

Finally, the factor of generativity and self-regulation implies the homeostatic elements of any internalized symbolic structure

---

2   Species of defense refers to defense mechanisms. If I understand Brenner correctly, he would not mind the notion of an abstractly inferred series of mechanisms that permits the ego to enlist many sorts of thought and behavior in service of defense. But he thinks it misleading to segregate a single area of ego functioning as exclusively defensive. More to the point, any ego function can be in service of both drive expression and defense.

functions, in a manner that permits organismic or psychological adaptation. Adaptation takes place so that persons fit into a social environment while they are internally regulating their psychic life with regard to the meanings that dictate their behaviors and permit adaptation to their environment. Thus, a structuralist vantage point is one that not only coincides with a structural theory, but is compatible with aspects of linguistic theory. Moreover, there are elements in the topographic theory pertaining to dreams specifically that have relevance for clinical work. These could be updated in linguistic terms and made consonant with Brenner's proposition that when we deal with patients analytically, we deal with their talking about their symptoms and their talking about their dreams. I am in agreement, then, that the inner experience of the dream as it is represented may be less relevant than formerly thought. More important is the idea that what is said not only should be taken at face value (surface structure) but should be considered to signify deeper meaning, perhaps of universal fantasies and a compromise of wish and defense. There are examples in the idiom of our culture that are instructive: Patients say about themselves that they feel empty or suffer from anomie. Such expressions must be analyzed and should not be accepted as final; they are paraphrases of experience.

In 1917, Freud wrote "A Metapsychological Supplement to the Theory of Dreams" and commented on the various forms of regression that are possible in dreams. He included topographical, temporal, and formal alterations to describe the idea that there are immature methods of expression that take the place of the usual methods of presentation and can help us to understand patients' productions. Indeed they may be indispensable in alerting us to where we should carry our analysis. For example, if a past time is indicated by a setting in a dream, then the current situation may be layered on that former experience. Formal aspects of the dream that are inconsistent with current mental abilities may be referential to some disintegration of usual alert mental structures; they may lead us to other states of mind or altered ego states associated with experiences registered in such states. If the representation is pictorial or imagistic, then topographic considerations must be applied to analysis based on rebus-thinking or plastic imagery—so that the inciting thought can eventually be uncovered.

Any theory that helps us to understand our clinical work and to grasp the rules of transformation of language is complementary to structural theory and permits the inclusiveness that Hartmann (1939) espoused in his wish that psychoanalysis be a general psychology. Several language theorists have written extensively about symbol formation and are relevant to our quest for understanding. They are Jakobson and Halle, Rosen, and Werner and Kaplan.

Jakobson and Halle (1956) alerted us to the role of metaphor and metonomy in language use. Rosen (1966) used metaphor and metonomy to discuss aspects of clinical practice to show how patients with varying diagnoses reference their world. Metaphor uses the sign function of similarity as a referential shorthand. (The Homeric reference to "rosy-fingered dawn" is metaphoric insofar as we can understand the similarity in shape between the rising sun and a pointing finger; the smiling face represents yes, or permission to pass to the left of a car where such markers are used). Metonomy uses the contiguity of images or events as a means of reference. For example "the Crown" refers to the Queen; the "White House" refers to the President. Such continuities also play a major role in the formation of screen memories and in fetishism. For us to understand the relationship between signifiers and what is signified, signs must undergo a series of psychological transformations. When we break

233

the whole, (i.e. the symptom) into its elements of wish, defense, and adaptation to reality, we analyze it into the components of conflict. However, all these systems suggest the centrality of language as well as conflict and compromise.

I suggest that we tacitly use early Freudian concepts such as dream work, primary and secondary process, and thing-and word-presentation to do our work and that we can now replace those with extra analytic concepts derived from language theory.

Werner and Kaplan (1963) explored symbol formation from an academic standpoint. Every symbol derives from at least a dual building process. The classical psychoanalytic concept of word and thing presentation and the transformations of dream work are Freud's version of a similar idea. "One arm of the building process is directed towards the establishment of a referent, the other directed toward articulation of a symbolic vehicle (sound pattern)" (Werner & Kaplan, 1963) p. 123. They make a distinction between the vehicle and the referent (i.e. that which is signified), the vehicle being the acoustic, visual, or other means of expressing a concept (l shall return to this when I discuss clinical material). The relationships between vehicle and referent are at least twofold; a vehicle may have multiple meanings, that is, it may be plurisignificant. For example, a single vocable may be used to refer to several referents (ideas or things). This involves homonymy. The second mode involves multiformity of referential expression, in which several words may be used to designate but one referent. This is the common notion of synonymy. The development of these double modes of expression within a diachronic framework is relevant to psychoanalytic developmental theory; it is also relevant to how patients act in regressed states on the couch. In such states they invariably use the inferred linguistic tools of transformation that correspond to Freud's concepts of condensation, displacement, symbolization, turning into the opposite—all associated with dream work and topographic theory. These concepts, derived from both linguistic analysis and psychoanalysis, do not permit us simply to paraphrase a patient's behavior in anagogic form, but do require that we use the central tenet of free association (see A. Kris, 1982) to uncover what Freud thought was the basic referential system to which all behaviors ultimately could be reduced if we knew the coding devices used to represent the compromises made necessary by conflict.

Thus, the core of this proposal is that the structural theory that has become psychoanalysis could benefit from some complementary model that is clinically useful to alert both patients and analysts to the methods by which man symbolizes. These methods, the "symbol work," can be borrowed from linguistic sciences. Such an interpretation of theory would give us some idea of how minds organize experiences and how persons live in accord with these meaning organizations. Perhaps this exploration would also provide some understanding of why hermeneutic and Lacanian approaches to analysis have become so popular. They fill a perceived gap in structural theory, but they also ignore what remains essential to a psychodynamic point of view in the structural hypothesis and sometimes yield to ambiguity and opacity rather than greater clarity and rationality.

Brenner (1976) provides a clinical example to show the process of psychoanalytic understanding. In brief: A woman has an anxiety attack while flying on an airplane. The nub of her problem concerns competition with her youngest sibling, a boy. The idea is offered that the configuration of the joystick (i.e. the controls of the airplane) is a sign of control, which then could be referentially related to the penis as a signifier of her earlier conflict concerning her wish for equal status, represented in the current anxiety. Further on in the discussion, Brenner asked the patient what it was that had precipitated her relapse. The associations to her memories became relevant as they led to the unique line of thinking concerning her symptom, that is, how the anxiety was experienced. She described it as an empty feeling in her stomach. Moreover, "she could not remember the last time she had been sick to her stomach"; then she admitted reluctantly that the last time she had felt that way followed an episode of fellatio. The flow of her thoughts again led to the plane where she had not eaten, but she had had a large lunch earlier. She had dined on boiled sausages, which she had loved as a child. This complex flow of ideas and similarities may strike the reader as having significant categorical overlap because of our training as psychoanalysts, or because for human beings the double-entry bookkeeping in the symbolic system permits metaphor, ambiguity, double meanings, and varying symbolic transformations to register in consciousness in rapid succession. However, our surmises take on further certainty when we hear of the context of the trip and its significance to her. She had been promoted and had been chosen by her boss, an older man, above her colleagues, many of whom were men. The easy reference to that sequence in relation to her earlier childhood conflict with her brother closes the circle of our anticipated conclusion.

In Brenner's example, we are made privy to the symbolic transformations and to the multiple means of representing ideas that force us to satisfactory closure. They do not come to us with difficulty because the narrative is written in a way that makes it evident (see Spence, 1983). They are also apparent to us because as human beings we share language and a symbolic system that permits categorical overlap and use of the vehicle of language to refer to many things, some of them logical and necessary, others less logical and more peripheral or personally experiential. Multiple function, polysemy and structural elements are all working mechanisms that add up to the whole as a representation of something other than its simple designative referent. The syntax of the story is compelling. A boiled sausage may be only a boiled sausage under certain circumstances, but it certainly shares a configurational relationship to the penis, and a joystick as well. The word itself—joystick—gives the concept increased metaphoric thrust. It is the redundancy of form in this model that alerts one to the elements of conflict which make up the symptom. Those elements lead us to the current advancement in job position, the past hopes for equal treatment and the regeneration of anxiety as if the past were anachronistically active in the present. We could not have followed that route of reasoning had we not understood that things do not simply stand for themselves; they stand for referents out of sight, out of mind. To elaborate the need for not only assuming symbolic thinking, but also displaying the variant forms of symbolic transformations that go into structural analysis, I shall present a number of clinical vignettes from my own practice and experience. They demonstrate how such knowledge (which some claim as passive) is structured and indispensible as a tool for understanding how patients represent conflicts and how analysts reconstitute what is represented.

Let me begin with an example of a *homophonic* transformation that occurred in my own life. Early in my career I had a dream while in analysis. It was a pleasant enough dream in which I was led to a dock on Martha's Vineyard that I had visited the summer before. I was told that the boat at the mooring was mine. It was a large motorcraft—l was impressed, but surprised, that it was mine and protested with some ambivalence that I did not like motor boats, that

I really had been fond of sail boats. How was I to accept this boat as mine, impressive as it was? Even in the dream it was not a part of my understood wishes. I had not longed for a yacht.

It would be all too easy to carry out an anagogic interpretation of this dream, making reference to a multiplicity of simplistic yacht to body part transformations and infer that we understand its meaning. However, its significance became known to me only through an understanding of its current derivative function in the context of my life at that time regarding career opportunities and career choice. Sailing had indeed been a new excitement, and I had generated some enthusiasm for the newly learned sport during the previous summer. I also had just began a new job and my practice, both of which occupied a great deal of time; I also was going to classes at the Psychoanalytic Institute, and had a young child. Then, I was offered a highly prized position that involved close association with Marianne Kris, among others, on a psychoanalytic research project. I was sorely tempted to add yet another job to my already full work load. However, it was clear to me that it would be most difficult in terms of time and distribution of psychic energy were I to take this job. And yet, how could I turn down a position where I would be an intimate in such distinguished company? I did not understand the relationship of this dream to my life, however.

As I began to try to put the dream images into words, I described the distinctions between a motorboat and sailboat, and I described the joy I had from my new skill at sailing. I seemed to feel some pressure to help the analyst understand what kind of boat it was that I had been offered and could not be satisfied that I had conveyed the image, although the distinction between motor and sail was simple. It was only when I uttered the name of a commercial motor boat, Chris Craft, that I realized that the fulfillment of owning a boat of this sort was related to the prestige and importance that it would give me rather than what I had passionately enjoyed doing that summer. I will not belabor the homophonic relation to Kris, but it should be apparent that the elegant and prestigious new acquisition I had created in my dream stood for the ambivalent wish to take the position that would have compromised my coping in reality. The element of superego contribution to this difficulty is important in regard to how forbidden the prize might have been. To take a position (or for that matter a possession) so coveted by others so early in my career must be opposed from within. However, the referential notion of the two unlike boats' referring to the same homophone (Kris; Chris) was represented in the tension of my attempt to feel satisfied as I tried to relate the dream text. The discomfort in not being able to link the experience in life with the experience of the dream was expressed in a sense of verbal discontent in the communicative setting of the analysis itself—a kind of tip of the tongue phenomenon.

My own tension that I had not adequately represented my inner experience was paralleled by the feeling that whatever was unconscious in my ambitious strivings in my past was also forbidden. Such feelings were also signifiers of more elemental constellations in the arena of the transference. What would my analyst have thought had I appeared too arrogant so early? This had been a theme of early complaints about supervision and the relationship to the analyst himself. However, the rules of homophonic transformation somehow became the vehicle around which the symbol had been formed. Had I not been familiar with the commercial names of powerboats, I perhaps would not have been able to employ such a verbal image to represent the current derivative of an existing conflict. However, other vehicles would have been available as they always are.

In his book *Free Associations*, A. Kris (1983) indicates his conflict about becoming an analyst by recalling his intellectualized musing one day about how words could effect change in patients. Later that day he found himself daydreaming some lines from a romantic poem by Wordsworth. He vainly searched for the significance in the content of the poem until he spoke Wordsworth as words' worth— and decided to become a psychoanalyst.

The next image comes from a similar linguistic arrangement in which a patient reported a dream image of somebody with a mustache. It was a visual referent, and he described it simply. He seemed also to experience some tension in expression and began to use a more careful set of descriptors. However, one would have to know the context of his life to understand his conflict. This man was beset by anxiety concerning bodily ills, and he had focused on a minor congenital defect that marred his sense of perfect wholeness. These anxieties were used in various ways to justify passive withdrawal from sexual and other human experiences for which he said he had longed. He returned to the dream repeatedly, describing the mustache until he had made assorted circumlocutious, paraphrases of the image indicating the mustache involved hair on a lip—on the upper lip—not a beard. It was only when he uttered the word "harelip" that he remembered that he had met a friend who had a harelip, which he had thought unsightly. It marred the friend's physical beauty, and he marveled at this man's accomplishments despite his visible defect. Again, the referential system that links cleft palate to harelip to mustache brought the imagery together in homophonic unity. What was to be signified referred to his central conflict about achievement and damage. However, the reference was not clear until the words were uttered, just as verbalizing had aided my understanding of the dream from my own experience. The analytic observer who takes the view that man is in conflict within himself may be comforted that the conflictual underpinnings gain access to consciousness through a referential system that has to be deciphered, and there is a code. Indeed, the analyst and patient must find the elements of the conflict by referencing the words in unaccustomed ways. The referencing system by which words point in the direction of understanding the conflict are firmly embedded in the concept of signifiers and the rules of transformation shared by other representational systems. Knowledge of such systerns is useful in clinical practice and incompletely described in structural theory.

A more difficult reference system was used by another patient, who described a dream in which she found herself in company wearing layers of skirts. The outer skirt had a slit on the side, the under skirt had a slit in front. She felt quite comfortable in company, but also repeatedly attended to her skirt as though she were afraid that too much would be revealed. She remarked, "It should not be a problem, since the slit skirt under the outer layer of skirt was positioned differently. The top skirt, though slit also, covered the underlying slit very well." The verbal description led to a new discovery in the analytic situation not evident in prior meetings and less convincingly represented up to that time about the body ego concerns that were incorporated in both character and symptom. The referential use of the slit skirt that both reveals and covers the underlying slit permitted her to recognize the conflict about revealing and hiding her genitals. The slang expression "slit" became a paraphrase for her anxieties about what would be or would not be revealed in her current usage as well as in her conflicts about her sexual nature.

The examples used stem from dream imagery, but there are symptoms that are also importantly represented in other formal configurations and then verbally analyzed. A patient in his mid-thirties was very ingratiating and obsequious toward the analyst. This character trait was in apparent conflict with his overall sense of competence in his work. Yet he always seemed to be yielding and deferential, and more than aptly respectful. One sometimes felt that it was almost too good to be true, that behind some of these characterological and symptomatic manners lay an unsaid conviction that he was perhaps better than others. Although the feeling of superiority was not easily apparent in the analysis, it did become problematic in his life work. Given his obsequiousness, it was not easy to decipher that in his relation to the analyst, he had taken a collegial view of himself, as if both of us were observing the patient in him, but he wasn't the patient.

He told me one day that he had a fantasy that I had an impending trip that would break his usual sequence of hours. I was to visit a medical convention, and he was asked to go too in order to present his views alongside me. He left the fantasy rather quickly only to return to it later, this time to tell of a memory from the past, although he did not realize the linkage until the thought was verbalized. He had been a sickly child, frequently in the hospital and sometimes taken to rounds in front of physicians. He also had used the intellectual defense of learning a great deal about his illness as a way of coping with his anxiety about whether he would survive. He then remembered being on a pediatric ward where a little girl repeatedly asked him to look at her burns, but exposed her genitals in so doing. One conflict in his current life concerned problems in performing intercourse. He had anxieties about impotence that were related to castration anxiety represented in bodily ills. The threat of my going on vacation became another context in which his anxiety about being left behind was heightened—his dependency and his

242

illness and his sense of body infirmity might take hold during these times of abandonment. To undo his plight and deny his problem, he invited himself to the convention. He was with me as he had been as a child among the doctors who took care of him. Moreover, his deferential attitude toward the analyst was an important trait by which he covered both his anger at my leaving and his longing for our continued relationship at all costs.

In that vignette, it was clear that the fantasy had referential value. Its connection to his character trait was not easy to see, unless we can accept that there was a form of regression to a representation in fantasy of a wish that held the elements of his conflict and also a concrete reference to his personal past. The image, not immediately obvious, was related by *synonomy* to my contextual understanding of the references in the past and the symptom that appeared as a character trait. I had first to assume that these elements were part of the whole, but I dared not view them as simply standing only for themselves. We had to dissect the image into levels of organization, which permitted a transformation of a wish and a conflict into thought, which could then be analyzed. The image was related to a thought, which had a referent from the past of a scene that stood for an idea, which derived from his interpretation of damage in the visualized concatination of burn, personal infirmity, and penislessness. Both topographic transformation and temporal transformation were operative and symbolically stated. There was a time, when he was with his doctor, that he was the center of attention. If he felt threatened by his infirmity, he could deny it within the context of the pairing. The analyst became a paradigmatic phobic companion. In order to make the leaps necessary to do the analysis, the analyst had to have some knowledge of the representability of ideas—the change in medium and vehicle of representation had to be apprehended. The focus of this idea is that memories are recorded and then represented in a variety of forms. The capacity for condensation in a single fantasy that signifies broader representation is likely at the heart of why free-association is a useful technique for understanding. Although these ideas are crucial to analytic thinking and the structural theory allows for such possibilities, they offer little that is explicit to explicate the mechanisms of transformation.

Another patient struggled to discuss her sense of distress when she cheated on her husband. At those times she became even more dependent on him and increasingly solicitous. She wanted to indicate that she used being held, snuggling, as an important mode of covering up her aggressive unfaithfulness. She used the word "smuggle" to describe what she did but was uneasy because it did not sound right. Parapraxes, of course, are commonplace to the analyst. However, to alert oneself to their use as a means of representation, one should also understand the representational parameters that are involved in the formation of a new word. The word that was joined to snuggle to form "smuggle" could be inferred only if one knew that this patient also viewed her husband as somewhat overwhelming in his attentions to her. There were times when she wanted to be more distant. She struggled to find the other word that merged with snuggle and came upon it only by discussing her relationship to her mother, who intruded as she comforted. The patient experienced fear of being smothered even as she was warmed and held. Such condensations in the formation of parapractic neologisms are available only to the analyst who understands the mechanisms of symbol formation. (Of course, it could be said that the patient did manage to "smuggle" her love from one forbidden territory to another.)

Bodily sensations also have representational value for an idea as well as for a feeling state. A young woman who had been on a self-destructive binge, taking various drugs, was beginning to emerge from her difficulties by exercising greater control over her life. Sh dreamed that she had a stomach ache and went into the bathroom for an antacid. She confused the bottle on the shelf with an antiarthritic liniment named "Heat," and after she took some, her mouth became numb. She had an immediate thought within the dream that she had done something "self-destructive."

The day before she had been with her sister, whom she felt received more affection from her father than she. In a fit of rage that she did not anticipate, she began to hit her sister violently and immediately after she felt that she was bad, that she didn't fit well into the family. Nursing her psychic wounds that evening, she returned to drugs, sniffing a line of cocaine. When the drug effect wore off, she felt guilty and went to sleep. Associating to the dream and bodily sensation, she noted similarities of the word heat to "taking the heat," leading the analyst on a merry chase of seeming references that led to no satisfying understanding at all. Finally, the patient realized that the sensation of numbness in her mouth that she had associated with something self-destructive was the same sensation she felt when she took cocaine. She began to understand that the dream and the bodily sensation within the dream were overlapping references to her symptom of self-medicating to alleviate the pain of her experience. The pain invariably began with a stomach-sickening anxiety either when she realized how angry and conflicted she was about taking from her parents or when she was in a setting where she felt "bad." The self-destructive behavior itself was represented by the bodily sensation, which was the metonymic reference for a variety of guilty representations and masochistic behaviors that revolved around her disappointment at not being fully accepted by her parents.

I have introduced in the last example the problem of the merry chase of the symbol. There can be many blind alleys that seem to be plausible. They only emphasize the need for the analyst to pay close attention to the affective excitement and sincerity with which the patient receives the new information provided by symbolic analysis. Werner and Kaplan's (1963) work shows that polysemanticity and synonymy of words are equally likely ways of manipulating a vehicle as is homophony. The previous example, and the next, can be understood using that concept. Another patient referred to a recurrent image of a water pistol that he had seen a child use. As he focused and lingered over-long on the water pistol, the context of his associations permitted the analyst to raise the possibility that multiformity of referential expression was to be considered. A water pistol could be broken down (analyzed) not only as a holder of water, but also, from its configurational formal characteristics, as a reference that obeyed the *pars pro toto* rule of logic in primary process. Moreover, the equivalent genital referred to was also most frequently manipulated and played with in a place where water flow was prevalent, a bathroom. The patient's conflict concerning masturbatory activity was understood only by dissecting the obsessional imagery into its component conflictual parts.

Yet another patient in analysis, a slender black woman, was struggling in order to achieve a more prominent role in life. She presented a dream in which she exhibited herself dancing most comfortably and with pleasure. She visualized herself as plump and light skinned; and, as if this were not enough, there was the representational overkill of possessing a prominent penis. Some symbols bludgeon the observer with their clarity! But, here again, the significance of the image could be grasped only if one knew her idiosyncratic history. She provided a layered vision simultaneously and synchronically of what was valued at each stage of development. She came from poverty in an area where hunger was pervasive; being plump was important when she was three to five. Her dark skin had been a handicap when she was at college and became an asset only when the "black is beautiful" movement began. The addendum of a penis was explicable as an unconscious derivative of early wishes only in light of her competitive experiences with her brothers.

In the transference, it was clear that she presumed I would love her best if she could show me that penis envy was alive and well, just as she wished that her parents had loved her as they did her brothers. Thus, the elements of popular translation may also creep into the analytic situation and structural theory has to be applied with full knowledge of the current value of symbols within the community. A symbol that may be universal to human experience is not always part of the idiosyncratic referential system of a particular person. Moreover, the most common universal meaning may not be the most temporally salutary when other meanings are preconscious. Freud warned against the interpretation of dreams by using a universal imagery key. Instead he referred us to the idiosyncratic aspects of more immediate and personally related associations. We may yield at times to universal symbolism, such as waters standing for birth. However, these are to be used only when we find ourselves in difficult situations. On the other hand, for a presidential candidate of the 1840s to have asked, "Where's the beef?" would have made no sense at all, but it did make sense in 1983.

We can carry out our work as psychoanalysts by using structural theory as a theoretical outline to understand how the ideas that patients present are related to inner struggles and to how they use experiences defensively and as moral restraints. To do the job well, we must also be alert to the mechanisms that patients use to represent their conflicts. Sometimes the ways in which they present their problems are habitual modes of expression characteristic of personal thought patterns, or are common locutions used in a personal way. Some people are given to frequent use of metaphors. Others have more convoluted methods of dreaming. Many of us have noted that although one can catch on to styles of representation (Rosen, 1961), sometimes style gives way under the analysis, as though the patient's habitual defensive mode has been uncovered. We can wonder, for example, why, in the broader psychiatric arena, hysteria and catatonia have become in recent years less frequent as modes of representation. They seem to have fallen into disrepute, or maybe we found the key to such representations with the advent of Freudian analysis. Psychoanalysis may not permit patients to use representational forms that no longer seem to hold the attention which permitted secondary gains and adequate disguised expression of conflicted wishes, as in former years.

The mechanisms of representation are not self-evident. I think perhaps topographic theory did provide us with some of the means to help us along, especially in regard to dream representation. Although analysts may no longer use topographic theory as it was written, they remember the rules of transformation Freud described in dream work and defense analyses. We ought at least give due respect to the significance of Freud's intention that the productions of patients should be viewed as symbolic transformations in various species of signs. This is an easy complement to the structural vantage point, and one I believe most analysts use anyway. This discussion merely makes conscious a dimension of work that is part of practice, but is not talked about as much these days. It also introduces a terminology from language theory that may be useful in analyzing the symbols and signs that patients invariably bring to the consulting room.

As my argument suggests, I believe that psychoanalysts cannot escape their education in topography. However, topographic models are problematic because of their linkage to reified psychic levels full of contents and controversial energic concepts. This presentation is a reminder to analysts that modern linguistic models cannot explain psychic compromises as structural theory does, but they do have relevance to fill in the gap made by abandoning topography. Moreover, all recent theorists seem to agree that verbal texts of patients are the *stuff* of the analysis. Verbal texts are linguistic and not random. We twist and turn and alter initial language forms in various symbolic ways that obey laws of recoding and also have referential specificity. It is time we learned to absorb some of the rich knowledge derived from linguistics and bring psychoanalysis into closer relationship with its origins. After all, Freud used his knowledge of philology and aphasia to inaugurate his own early theories.

REFERENCES

Arlow, J.A. (1979). Metaphor and the psychoanalytic situation. *Psychoanal. Quart.* 48:363-385.

———— (1981). Theories of pathogenesis. *Psychoanal. Quart.* 50:488–513.

———— (1964). *Psychoanalytic Concepts and the Structural Theory.* New York: International Universities Press.

Brenner, C. (1974). Depression, anxiety and affect theory. *Internat. J. PsychoAnal.* 55:25–32.

———— (1976). Psychoanalytic Technique and Psychic Conflict. New York: International Universities Press.

——— (1979). Depressive affect, anxiety, and psychic conflict in the phallicOedipal phase. *Psychoanal. Quart.* 48:177–197.

——— (1982). *The Mind in Conflict.* New York: International Universities Press.

Freud, S. (1900). Interpretation of dreams. *Standard Edition* 4 & 5.

——— (1917). A metapsychological supplement to the theory of dreams. *Standard Edition.*

——— (1923). The ego and the id. Standard Edition 19:1–59. London: Hogarth Press, 1962.

——— (1926). Inhibitions, symptoms and anxiety. *Standard Edition* 20:75–172. Hartmann, H. (1939). *Ego Psychology and the Problem of Adaptation.* New York: International Universities Press, 1964.

Jakobson, R., & Halle, M. (1956). *Fundamentals of language.* The Hague: Mouton.

Klein, G. (1976). *Psychoanalytic Theory: An Exploration of Essentials.* New York: International Universities Press.

Kohut, H. (1984). *How Does Analysis Cure?* ed. A. Goldberg & P. Stepansky. Chicago: University of Chicago Press.

Kris, A. (1 982). *Free Association.* New Haven: Yale University Press. Kris, E., ed. (1954). *Origins of Psychoanalysis. Freud's Letters to Wilhelm Fliess.* London: Imago.

Lewin, B.D. (1952). Phobic symptoms and dream interpretation. *Psychoanal. Quart.* 21:295–322.

Piaget, J. (1970). *Structuralism.* New York: Harper & Row.

Rosen, V.H. (1961). Relevance of "style" to certain aspects of defense and the synthetic function of the ego. *Internat. J. Psycho-Anal.* 42:447–457.

———— (1966). Disturbances of representation and reference in ego deviations: In: *Psychoanalysis: A General Psychology: Essays in Honor of Heinz Hartmann,* ed., R M. Loewenstein, L.M. Newman, M. Schur & A.J. Solnit. New York: International Universities Press, pp. 634–654.

———— (1977). Style, Character and Language. New York: Aronson.

Sausure, de, F. (1911). *A Course in General Linguistics.* New York: Philosophical Library, 1959.

Schafer, R. (1976). *A New Language for Psychoanalysis.* New Haven: Yale University Press.

Shapiro, T. (1970).Interpretation and naming. *J. Amer. Psychoanal. Assn.*18:399–421.

———— (1979).Clinical Psycholinguistics. New York: Plenum.

———— (1983).The unconscious still occupies us. *The Psychoanalytic Study of the Child* 38:547–567.

———— & Perry, R. (1976).Latency revisited: The significance of age 7 ± 1. *The Psychoanalytic Study of the Child* 31:79–105.

Slap, J.W., & Saykin, A.J. (1983).The schema: Basic concept in a non-metapsychological model of the mind. *Psychoanal. Contemp. Thought* 6:305–325.

Spence, D. (1983). *Narrative Truth and Historical Truth: Meaning and Interpretation in Psychoanalysis.* New York: W.W. Norton.

Stein, M. (1984).Rational versus anagogic interpretation: Xenophon's dream and others. *J. Amer. Psychoanal. Assn.* 32:529–556.

Waelder, R. (1930).The principle of multiple function. Observations and overdetermination. In: *Psychoanalysis: Observation, Theory, Application,* ed. S.A. Guttman. New York: International Universities Press, pp. 68–83.

Weber, S. (1982). *The Legend of Freud.* Minneapolis: University of Minnesota press.

Werner, H., & Kaplan, B. (1963). *Symbol Formation.* New York: Wiley.

Words and Feelings in the Psychoanalytic Dialogue

(1991). *Journal of the American Psychoanalytic Association* 39(Supplement):321–348.

P sychoanalytic therapy requires that we render our feelings in words. Insofar as nominalization of feelings is required, we can apply a linguistic analysis to that process illuminating the range of effects that language has on these complex affective states. Syntactically, we notice the subject-object vectors of feelings. Semantically, we note the representational valence of affects as part of word definition. Pragmatically, the psychoanalytic situation provides a unique dialogic relationship not seen elsewhere. These parameters are elaborated for their significance to the process of psychoanalysis.

A character in a T. S. Eliot play fragment protests,

"But I got to use words when I talk to you" (1930, p. 152).

The painter Francis Bacon (1989) is quoted as saying,

"If you can talk about it, why paint it?"

These are just a few of many pronouncements concerning the radical argument that affective experiences are nonverbal and therefore inexpressible in words. I refer to these positions initially to provide a counterpoint to the central assertion of this essay: We live in a largely nominalist world, and Freud and his progeny in psychoanalysis continue to demand turning feelings and experiences as they occur in various states of psychopathology and everyday life into words, so that they may be dealt with rationally as propositions. This is so because we have a special interest in the affective emotional life of our patients and not despite it.

I will propose that psychoanalysts, especially Freud, were early interested in a cohesive theory of symbol formation that linked affects with the derivatives of drive discharge represented as thought. Representational modes were highly elaborated in the topographic theory, especially in the dream book (1900) where Freud labored to determine the relationship between thing- and word- presentation and representation. However, when Freud (1923) switched to the structural theory and to the concept of signal anxiety (1926) he turned his focal interest to defense and compromise formation, neglecting the nuances of the mechanisms of symbol formation, only referring back to his earlier work.

The recent advances in linguistics provide an easy map of symbol formation that can be used with profit by psychoanalysts as we integrate a modern theory with our clinical postulates and observations. Indeed, psychoanalysis as a method, I will propose, can be viewed as a linguistic interchange emphasizing man's symbolizing role as he encodes simultaneously words and narratives as a means of both emotional expression and self-protection. As such, the rich opportunities provided by linguistic analysis apply. I will proceed to use a linguistic frame to explore:

1. The contrived dialogic arrangement that is necessary to doanalysis;
2. The role of the dynamic unconscious in symbol formation and language usage in analysis;
3. Free association and transference from the vantage of a linguistic analysis.

In this pursuit the affective component of linguistic structures should emerge as a major means of comprehending the affect-laden elements of symbolic life as expressed in the analysis, and offer a mutually enriching proposal in which psychoanalysis gains and linguistics is broadened to consider a new, pragmatic sequence in the analytic method and process.

Having stated these preliminary notions, I will introduce some of the language of linguistics to see if some of the constructs of that somewhat arcane field can be melded with the language of psychoanalysis and determine if such a blend enriches our psychoanalytic understanding of how we deal with affects (Shapiro, 1979). Before I embark on purely linguistic matters, one thing is certain: In usual discourse, we generally employ other channels than speech (the phonetic shape of language) *per se* to lend emotional tone in the two-person world and to communicate feelings. Some of these accompaniments may be excluded in telephone conversations (*gestural-mimetic features*) or computer-written material (*prosody or the musical contour of speech, and tonal variation*). On the other hand, what is lost in the latter two vehicles is exaggerated in theater where communication channels include gesture and mimesis, and prosody as well as the usual broadcast transmission in words. We also employ these more fully in the cadences of poetry. Siomopolous (1977)and others have commented on the aptness of the rhythms of poetry in conveying affects to supplement the verbal rendering of feelings in metaphors which stimulate images that refer to feelings as well as to things.

There are those (as noted above) who claim that music and the visual arts are not amenable to such reductions to language, but we also try to take nondiscursive forms and render them discursively. The students of music and art certainly use a language which makes us wonder whether there are not *synesthetic* significances among the different vehicles of expression. Designations such as a *pastoral symphony* elicit pastoral images as well as pastoral voices. The Blues induce another feeling-state that goes beyond the low notes and cadences of that musical form. The words match the tones. In psychoanalysis, verbal communication is asked for from the very beginning: "Say what comes to mind!" the analyst requests. However, such a request does not keep the analyst from watching as well as listening. Indeed, we also ask for images and bodily feelings as well as thoughts and words, and they enrich the experience of the content to be explored. The analyst and the patient may experience the composite in an immediate empathic apprehension, but I proffer that the translation into a verbal form is necessary to understanding.

Although we study affects in the analytic field, empathically and in transference-countertransference modules, we dare not be misled by the false notion that words are mere labels or adornments that are arbitrarily appended to ideas and feelings. Instead, *words in use* are our most parsimonious means of rendering inner personal, subjective experience in a sound repeatable communicational system. This does not deny that there are other kinds of human communication, both proximal and far, that are important and are sensed as an "experience of community" with others, but not verbalized.

The *communion* of the religious group or the political rally, or the quiet sighing, grunting or scream of coitus, the nodding approval of the conversationalist, the commiseration and sense of unity with the bereft, all bring people together. Nonetheless, words and sentences derived from human codes and language also are a major vehicle of being together, emotionally as well as cognitively. The latter distinction between cognition and emotion is quite artificial and fraught with confusion. Indeed, we may argue that the distinction is artifactual—the result of scholars' need to make distinctions. Researchers too have exploited some of these splits in order to keep their fields simpler and clear of contamination from "nonessential data." Nonetheless, in life, feelings and thoughts are experienced together as wholes or units.

Mahoney (1987) notes that there are three forms of translation: *interlinguistic, intralinguistic,* and *semiotic.* The latter includes the translation of symbolic entities such as dream images into words; feelings into words. Thus the third of these modes is the most central to psychoanalysis and the one which analysts deal with most commonly. Indeed, Freud's (1900) treatment of dreams is apt in this argument, because he noted that we never see the dream of the dreamer, but we hear the dream report. And the dream report in words is what we deal with analytically. Trying to reimage, rethink, and reunderstand the rebus-like nature of the relationship of the images and to translate them into common thought is a major task, as we assume the surface has a deeper significance (Levy and Inderbitzin, 1990). A similar thing happens with feelings, since we never can be certain that the feeling tone expressed facially reflects the same feeling that is experienced. Necessarily, we use facial expression as well as descriptions of inner feeling-states as important data in the analysis. Because the analyst-patient arrangement does not permit so careful a view of facial expression, the analyst may have to pay particular attention to the lilt of the voice, the prosodic variation, and the gestural accompaniments to "read" the emotion. But defenses against expression in any of the communicative channels may be selectively employed, even in average discourse. If the patient wishes to hide, he/she does so, unless the involuntary expression is imminent or triggered by the analyst's tact or clumsiness. The notion of a "poker face" is too familiar and becomes a metaphor for dissimulation, *but* the "social smile" too is a dissimulation that hides, *but* less completely, because we can often decipher how it differs from the full smile of enjoyment (Ekman et al., 1983).

This distinction between *expressed feelings* and *read feelings,* as opposed to inferred feelings, is crucial in clinical psychoanalysis and one of the areas in which its practice is unique, because we can explore the experiential nuance and history of feelings as well as discrepancies between the read feelings from facial expression and experienced feelings. Indeed, this distinction can be seen as a developmental achievement in the second and third year as well. At the point when the child can dissimulate and pretend feelings we recognize that emotions as expressed may be dissociated from felt emotion—the pretend pout or smile to get one's way becomes social manipulation, just as the breakthrough of rage or laughter is unplanned and may signal a failure of mastery of feelings. The human possibility to hide or erupt perforce includes recognition that conscious and unconscious mechanisms may be at play. At the conscious level manipulative guile or even consideration of others may be at work, while affect may be isolated or displaced unconsciously from one content to another. Thus, as in the case of repressed or suppressed ideas, we are at times called upon not to permit expression to reveal inner states that may be affectively charged. The split-off affective tone of an ideational-affective complex may be expressed in a different setting by virtue of displacement (kicking the cat instead of the boss) or attached to another person by projection or, as Arlow (1953) notes, be expressed in pleasurable contentless masturbation, while unaware of the arousing ideas that are represented in disguised form in a dream.

Linguistics has its own formal traditions. It divides language into syntax, semantics, pragmatics, and its most applied anthropological branch, sociolinguistics. By and large, syntax does not interest psychoanalysts as much as the issues of reference as studied in semantics, as well as the circumstances and models recently studied in pragmatics that describe how dialogues take place and how they are interpreted (Shapiro, 1986), (1988). The latter should be of special interest because of the somewhat "unnatural" arrangements of the psychoanalytic dialogue. Sociolinguistics deals with the differences in cultural expression and how members of each culture name the elements of their affective experiences and permit expression of feelings. For example, it is said that the poverty-stricken and poorly educated may use, or rely more heavily upon, vehicles for the expression of their feelings that differ from those of the middle classes. It is an uncertain general observation that they tend more to action to express their feelings. Some developmentally disabled children, too, have difficulty putting their feelings into words and mentally designating them for discourse that requires a delay between thought and action. The impulse-ridden, organically damaged child tends more often to short-circuit the mediating effect of cognition on emotion. We also might look at the concept of alexithymia as an example of not encoding emotion in language, but rather channeling affects into bodily ills, as another variant on the inability to tolerate affects consciously. If we look at each of these areas of language study separately, we may be able to bring some order into how psychoanalytic thinking can be influenced and enriched by the data derived from linguistics and, conversely, where psychoanalysis might provide new directions for linguistic study.

Syntax and Psychoanalysis

Psychoanalysts could attend to this area well because, among other things, it provides the rules by which we verbally establish agency and object directedness, establishing the "I" as feeler. Indeed, the translation of Freud's *Ich* into ego may, according to some, be a Latin tragedy that has permitted English-speaking Freudians to forget agency and responsibility for actions by using the less personal Latin form. Schafer's (1976) notion of action language makes clear the need to "own one's feelings"—to be the "I" of the experience rather than be the passive victim of one's feelings. Fenichel (1941), too, in his book on technique, similarly alludes to the notion that patients come to therapy feeling as though they are victimized by their feelings.

Even in our more common forms of expression we create confusion about how we syntactically relate to emotion. There are common verbal forms such as "I *have* feelings too," "I have had (or seen) happiness," or there is the confusion of identity with one's feeling in "I am depressed," which seems to signify the identity of the feeling with the person. Then there is the ambiguity portrayed in being a victim of feelings or a receptacle of feelings in phrases such as "I was accosted by anger," "I am full of rage," or "He makes me angry."

All of these avoid the "I" as feeler and create semantically ambiguous references, where the patient requires redirection to understand how these common forms represent defensive disavowals of responsibility as an agent. The analytic clinician should take into account these varying syntactic forms as traps from patients and clues to understanding their sense of plight. Syntax reveals the stance of the feeler as she casts herself as first, second, or third person. Is she the feeler, are you making her feel this way, or is she a third person observing her feelings? The obvious relation of these variables to object relations is central, but the clue is in the syntax and knowledge of a person's place, if the proposition can direct the analytic interpretation.

Dahl (1978) uses a specific schema designed by de Rivera to pose a series of poles which derive from Freud's (1915) three polarities of subject-object, pleasure-unpleasure, active-passive dimensions. He uses terms such as "it, me; to and from" as important distinctions that delineate a person's discourse, creating the final common pathway of a number of decisions that emerge as "how to act toward someone." This scheme attempts to remove feelings from the romance of subjective depth and probes their relationship to inner objects and real people in a syntactic form. Each of the binary decisions that determines the end—i.e., how we act toward another—might be probed in the analytic process to determine abiding attitudes toward others or potentially in the transference. The following analytic confrontation can be considered for its integration of affect and interpersonal import: "You act injured and hurt each time I tell you that you feel victimized by your brother, and then you become quiet as if I am hurting you." Such a transference confrontation puts the affect in a syntactic field. The statement strikes parallels between current feelings in the therapeutic relationship and historical interpersonal feelings as well. It is a syntactic formula for recognizing future events and experiences. Dahl (1978) also has shown that analysts reveal their hidden wishes and countertransferential attitudes in specifically awkward grammatical constructs. I have observed the tendency of analysts to use hypothetical conditional constructions such as "You act as if..." in conveying reconstructions to patients. In this way, the analysts cover uncertainty and anxiety about their patients' acceptance of the ideas proposed.

Another vantage point derives from the development of agency in social relationships by social referencing (Klinnert et al., 1983); (Sorce et al., 1985). The establishment of social referencing by reading affects begins in the second half of the first year. When a child is placed in a dilemma involving an ambiguous choice, she looks to her mother or her surrogate for information that is read from facial emotional expression as to how to proceed. We not only socially regulate our behavior in relation to the feelings and signals of mothers, but we utilize feelings as an organizer of behavior as expressed in the words of others. Indeed, the developmental movement from responding to affective tone to being able to understand "no" as a prohibition to action is very well marked in the developmental sequences and has been studied as a hard-won achievement of the mediational power of words over motor impulse. The Soviet scientist Luria (1961) and his coworkers used a simple experiment requesting that children of 3 to 5 press a rubber bulb attached to a string gauge to record the pressure when they saw a certain color light. The younger they were, the more the children had trouble suppressing the squeeze until the light went on, and only the older children could obey linguistic interdictions of "no" to reregulate the actions. Moreover, only the oldest children could obey a change of rules in midexperiment on linguistic command, e.g., "Now *don't* press when the light is red as before, but only when it is green."

Freud's concept of acting out is clearly derived from his central proposal that thought is trial action, utilizing small amounts of energy. Mature human organisms use thought and language profitably, and do not waste action until further cognition and planning are completed. These require syntactic schemes that describe future direction. Again, the analytic situation especially calls for a translation of action potentials into words. The words are syntactically arranged in order to convey a sequenced scheme of potential action that can be avowed as deriving from the self or projected onto others, "He made me do it!" or "She made me feel guilty," or "You don't want me to have pleasure." The voice and trajectory of each proposal define the potential action sequence as it is being formed, before it is done, so that analyst and patient can experience the direction of the aim together in a shared linguistic reference. In that way, both can weigh the consequences of wishes or inhibitions on adaptation and survival. Without syntax we have no verbal vectors, but vectors need designated starting points and ends, and thus we need a means of reference. I have suggested (Shapiro, 1988) that the notion of a drive's having a source aim and object even posits a linguistic unconscious.

Semantics and Psychoanalysis

Semantically, words signify that they have meanings. They refer to feelings, things, areas in the world, and in fact, they also serve as action potentials that guide individual behavior. The distinction between and among signal, sign, and symbol has been utilized in psychoanalysis by Rosen (1961) and by Lacan (1956). *Signals* are based on contiguity between referent and reference and are the simplest of our symbolic systems. For example, a signal is represented in our psychoanalytic practice in the contiguity of the fetish to the female genital, signaling recognition of an absent, hoped-for, male genital, or the incidental remembrance in the screen memory which is an event *near to* the more frighteningly significant event that it signifies. Freud (1899) suggested it is the *sham* near the gold.

Signs are based on an iconic relationship to the signified, as the arrow shows direction or the purse stands for the female genitals, insofar as each may be seen as a receptacle. *Symbols* in linguistic terms are based on arbitrary relationships; i.e., there is no intrinsic or structural reason why "R" stands for the sound it represents, except convention. The psychoanalytic symbol is closer to the sign; e.g., sometimes a cigar is a penis; sometimes a snake is a penis. The error of *pars pro toto* is a logical one, not one that precludes an associative psychological path based on iconic likeness (Shapiro, 1979).

This tripartite analysis of symbolic form should permit analysts to consider the degree of disguise in symbolic presentation and offer an opportunity to reconsider Freud's original mechanisms described in the dreamwork, turning into opposites, displacement, etc. In fact, there is some evidence that certain character styles habitually use metaphoric (*pars pro toto* symbols) or metanymic (displaced) associative mechanisms, the former using a sign relationship and the latter signal. We may refer to our enemies as snakes, which represents a metaphoric transformation based on sign function of partial similarity, e.g., a trait of sliminess or deceptiveness. We may also refer to the President as the White House or the Queen as the Crown, which referents are based on contiguity or metonyms. A concept such as overdetermination is well rendered as polysemy (many referents or meanings attached to one sign). Reference and meaning, in general, may be grasped as a single process employing a number of mechanisms, bringing together translation and semiotics, and even such diverse figures as Webster and Lacan. Webster, the classical lexicographer, offers denotative referents for words and in addition shows the context of use within our corpus of written examples of language. He is a traditional writer of dictionaries; Lacan reaches for the connotative and even more for the idiosyncratic referents that make the patient's ramblings meaningful. The common usage is less interesting in his translations.

Since patients start their communications in words we attend— i.e., common denotative references—we also have a more complex referential receiving system that is alerted to words as embedded in meanings that have affective valence. We hover about the verbal productions waiting for cues that signal affects. Indeed, our "pay dirt" in the clinical process involves "hearing better" than others the lodestone of affectively charged unconscious constellations and resistances to their exposure.

Affects may be generated in an analysis as a signal in contiguity with a word. For example, the patient may tell the analyst any number of disparaging or unpleasant facts about a spouse. Then if the analyst suggests that he or she sounds close to divorce, a flood of tears emerges. The word "divorce" may be seen as a signal to the affectively loaded idea of divorce as a signifier of danger to the patient.

The dream may be told and described as vivid, *but* the affect associated with the referent behind the image will emerge only as the patient using the free associative process uncovers the sign function of the image. The image accompanied by the affect now is linked to an unconscious residue, up to now unknown.

The symbolically arbitrary relationship of the word to the thing does not mean that there are not significant affective components in the apparently simple definition of words. Linguists use a feature analysis as a way of defining symbols, potentially giving us a way of considering affect as a feature to be included in dictionary meaning (Shapiro, 1979). Words have dynamisms that should be included in such a feature analysis. Words are not just labels, for they may have strongly affective features which are mobilized when the hearer audits the word. There are, after all, words of opprobrium which jar our sensibilities—nigger, kike, wop, mickey! All are emotion-arousers as compared to calling someone Black, Jewish, Italian, or Irish. The latter group does not call up emergency emotions as do the former. Words and names are not merely interchangeable in the affective content. Feces is different from shit. Masturbation is different from "jerking off." Indeed, some of our comedians utilize the jarring, outrageous effect of specific words in order to titillate our emotions and stimulate these associated arousals. These examples reveal that the usual process of definition is achieved by providing roughly equivalent words to clarify meaning of the index word (what Mahoney calls intralinguistic translation). Analysts have had the experience of a bilingual patient using a word in his second language without effect on the emotions, while expression in his first language brings tears or laughter. This example provides simple evidence that emotions are linguistically as well as cognitively bound to sentences and complex thoughts. Anyone familiar with the film, *Citizen Kane*, will appreciate the evocative force of the word, "Rosebud." In analysis, we discover our patients' idiolect and in each of those personal languages their Rosebuds.

Freud (1905b) was correct when he suggested that comedy consists of loosening repression and permitting a rapid emergence of unconscious fantasy. Just as a bull rages at seeing red, we can stimulate rage in almost anybody if we knew their symbolic catalogue well enough to say the right things to trigger idiosyncratically significant emotion-thought complexes. Indeed, a common clinical situation was alluded to in the Dora case (Freud, 1905a) in which she went on interminably about how awful her father's deeds were. Instead of Freud criticizing her father along with her, he turned her complaint about and commented on how much she must love him for her to be so preoccupied with him. He thereby turned attention to another affective valence, which he recognized in the symbolic significance of her overzealous negative preoccupation. In this instance, a whole sequence of negative narratives pointed to a positive, but disappointed affective constellation: love. Indeed, the analyst's interpretation is often an exercise in naming an unnamed enemy, i.e., a warded-off emotion associated with an unconscious complex (Shapiro, 1970).

Let us turn now to the matter of how we name and categorize emotions, i.e., how we turn emotion into a shorthand verbal reference. There are a number of curious confusions in how we designate feelings. Moreover, cross-cultural distinctions and problems exist with regard to how we interpret expressed feelings, or how we attach feelings and affects to our notions of disorder, or even how we name affective disorders.

The word depression is used to designate everyday sadness and also major depressive disorders. Curiously, we also use the word *melancholia* to designate similar disorders. The latter calls up connotations of Galenic medicine, with etiologic inferences about the role of black bile in the generation of dark moods. On the other hand, depression is associated with feeling low, heavy, leaden, etc. The clinical depression of the Western world has been found to correspond to the neurasthenia of China (Kleinman, 1980). Very similar components that define major depression in DSM III are interpreted by the Chinese in a way by a term that is out of use in the West. Similarly, the alexithymia that is postulated in the individual who cannot put his feelings into words, but sidetracks them into the soma, represents a cultural variation of how people are tagged as "different" because they use different mechanisms to deal with feelings. Indeed, my very word "sidetrack" reveals a Western cultural stereotype that seems to require that we experience our affects in the usual way, i.e., in a manner to which we in the West have become accustomed.

It was brought to my attention at a WHO meeting a number of years ago that Westerners frequently talked about *somatization* of feelings, but we were brought up short when our colleagues from India suggested that we may *psychologize* too much (see section on Sociolinguistics). These polarities bring to attention the fact that concepts of affect are frequently intermingled with cognitive organizations as well as a world perspective, and that, although feelings have physiological and other components, they also are psychological, nominal entities. As we name them in the course of our experience, we also bring them into a domain where they can demand our attention and be considered, but not before categorical, nominal boundaries are drawn. The frequency range of colors is known as an empirical fact, but color-naming varies from language to language. The functional use of such language is culture-bound. Similar nuances of emotional tone may be more or less differentiated in different cultures. Freud's notion of a pleasure-unpleasure dimension might be sufficient for some purposes, but more shades of affective tone are required for a psychoanalytic exploration, because we anticipate that psychological-cognitive accompaniments of these variants will direct us to a better understanding of the person's emotion-eliciting circumstances.

Psychoanalytic and dynamic psychotherapeutic enterprises for some individuals are an attempt to bring into consonance feeling states and tones with specific cognitive elements, i.e., memories and experiences. The anticipatory anxiety that certain phobic individuals experience is indeed at times a cognitive misreading of events on the basis of unsaid and unknown, unconscious and irrational identifications between referents on the basis of their sign or signal function. The phobic object is avoided; i.e., the patient avoids circumstances and places which usually do not elicit fear. We see this referential confusion as a displacement of the feeling tone belonging to one constellation onto a different symbol in the service of defense, to shield the patient from realizing the warded-off thoughts. Thus, an affect-laden mental complex can lead to a designative error using a sign or signal as a representation that stands for the danger. This is a nonshared new vocabulary that is noncommunal and idiosyncratic.

The obsession also can be seen as a linguistic event, which represents another form of displacement that includes the compromise formation of unconscious organizations as thoughts intrude on consciousness in a barely disguised way, but the affect is isolated. These are all within our symbolic system and are linguistically relevant. That is why we listen so carefully to *how* people tell us about their lives and experiences, and why we are so tolerant of the *redundancy of the form* in the analytic situation. But we are not only listening to hear *what* is hidden, but also what emotions would be elicited if the unconscious fantasy were made conscious, thereby rendering a more complete "definition" that enhances understanding of the meaning of behavior.

I will mention, but briefly, other communicational channels for the expression of emotion and include music and other auditory experiences as well. Even within language we have a bevy of onomatopoetic expressions for feelings that carry the weight and impact of the feelings to which they refer. In fact, many expressions of strong emotion do not employ formal words, but the vocal accompaniments of emotional expressions. The *ach!* the *oy!* the *ahhhhh!* and the *aghh!* used in comic strips are related to actual nonword vocalizations that co-occur with certain feelings such as pain, fright, despair, or ecstasy. They are not words, and yet we can communicate with them. I have already mentioned the poetic in this vein and its imagistic language forms used to evoke feelings. On the gestural and mimetic side, we make commands and demands by raising or wagging our fingers. We point to things, and we accuse with our fingers as well. These have as much iconic significance as words do, and they may be expressed with words or alone. Indeed, the designation through gesture in emotional states as seen in analysis is probably more frequent than in our traditional discursive forms of discourse. One can immediately bring to mind the gesturing of the logician as he organizes, layers, counts, and cuts through the air, signifying the sequencing and margins of arguments as well.

The prosodic or paralinguistic features of language in speech remind us that, in traditional discourse and couch monologues, these elements carry the emotional tone to the auditor analyst. These matters are very difficult to represent in the written language that records the semantic-syntactic production, but are certainly available clinically on the couch or on videotape. Indeed, the flow of associations may sometimes move from words to gesture (Needles, 1959) or may include gesturing in one way, while the person is talking about something else (Grand, 1977); (Freedman, 1977). Observing a patient's foot wagging, or the replacement of the hands from one part of the torso to another, or the lack of animation in the hands, while the voice is animated, all give kinesthetic clues to what is going on in the patient's thoughts. The frequent play of a smile across the lips of the patient telling a horror story suggests that sadism might be a part of the unconscious structure to be dealt with. Thus, we watch and listen for dissonance, consonance, and sequential shifts in the vehicles of expression, for clues to understanding how emotions hide in communicational sequences, just as the child analyst watches the change in play items, while the theme does not shift.

We move now from words and gestures and their meaning to the notion of a dynamic unconscious which influences surface activity. We move into an area of questioning how complex mental structures are organized and how we deal with *potential affects*. Freud (1915) struggled mightily in the initial phases of his work with the question of whether affects could be unconscious. He initially opted for the notion that only ideas were unconscious, and then finally admitted to the limited possibility of the unconscious wish for self-punishment. This notion has been adopted by some to mean unconscious guilt, but others even espouse the notion of a whole array of unconscious affects (Pulver, 1974). On the other hand, I would offer that there are structural mental organizations that are clearly cognitive. If brought to the surface, they would yield the expression of a full range of affects when their personal significance is integrated with the context and time of life of their emergence. Traditionally, guilt as an experience, or even anxiety and glee, are feature components of organized mental complexes when they are elicited or when derivative forms emerge. Thus, just as humans in the environment and internal objects regulate emotion, cognitive organizations determine which affect is to be expressed once basic affects are mentally arranged.

Arlow (1977) noted about moods that they are

structured affective states evoked and perpetuated by the continuing influence of unconscious fantasy (p. 164).

For example, moral masochism indicates that there is an unconscious dynamism in the form of a mental constellation that dictates self-destructive external surface behavior in the service of guilt. While these are not exactly coded into words, some feelings are acted on and interacting with mental organizations that have significance and emotional valence. Returning to the area of reference in semantics again, we have many superficial displays which refer to deeper emotional signifiers. Indeed, what a patient says on the surface only partially reveals what is meant. The choice of words hides too, thereby revealing the action of wish and defense, or compromise formation, but also displaying the interplay between superficial and deeper mental organization which perforce requires an assumption of a potential emotion. The proposal that meaning is coded along with affects utilizes a linguistic frame that is explicated in the analysis. The analyst names the unconscious referent or fantasy in a syntactic for designating conflict; and elicits the experience of affect that is tied to the words we call an interpretation.

This brings us to the interposition of the defenses of repression, denial, displacement, and isolation, and how they may suggest varying feelings that are being avoided. In 1926, Freud posited that defense is instituted at the behest of the signal of anxiety. This notion has been expanded by Brenner (1982): it is not only anxiety, but depression that calls for defensive action.

Pragmatics in Clinical Psychoanalysis

The next large area of linguistic consideration to be addressed concerns emotion in psychoanalysis as *pragmatics* or the practical interactions between people in dialogue or polylogue. Within philosophy and then linguistics, the concepts of performatives and speech acts (Austin, 1962); (Searle, 1969) were introduced, providing the opportunity to consider *intention* and *motive* in the language sciences (see Shapiro, 1979). One can appreciate that grammar is most easily isolated for study from human context and interaction because, like mathematics, it is analytic and has a formal structure. Semantics adds the complication of referencing a world of things or ideas, but pragmatics, as defined by the new language theorists, requires human interaction or *language in use* as its study base. With every word expressed in an interaction we witness, or better still, infer, what is called illocutionary force. This rhetorical force is empowered either by social convention or by habitual practice—politeness, guile, cultural rules, etc. When use becomes too idiosyncratic, its force is only recognized by the few who know the individual speaker well. Loewenstein (1951) used the model of a developmental psychologist, Karl Buehler, as a parallel to psychoanalytic couch behavior. We not only *express* and *appeal* on the couch, but we also *propose*. When we arrive at the propositional aspects of language, we are free of the demand structure of the appeal and its associated needs to influence others in a ministration, but now only are we able to express those thoughts which are developmentally free of need for sharing of ideas and exchange. In analysis, the pragmatic arrangement of patient and therapist is unusual. It is not a dialogue of mutual sharing as in a conversation—the patient is expected to free-associate, and the analyst remains a receptive listener and is only sometimes a verbal contributor (Shapiro, 1988). Couch behavior in relation to permission for affect expression is similarly unique, insofar as analysts are asked to interpret the meaning of the phrases in terms of their illocutionary force, which includes affective valence as inferred, as well as their face value or semanticity. Consider the patient who says, "I don't usually use such language" and then interposes street language or frank smut or sexually provocative words. Others say, "I mean to say..." or we hear the frequent locution, "You know..." What is the patient trying to get across by these various locutions? What is the read-out for those expressions in terms of the status of the transference, or the status of unconscious constellations that are being expressed?

Pragmatics has taught us that the patron who looks at a seat in a theater and asks the person sitting next to the empty seat, "Is that seat empty?" is not only asking whether it is occupied, but is also saying, "I want to sit in it. May I sit in it?" A somewhat less circumlocutious way an individual might approach the seat is to say, "May I sit down?" to ask for permission, when a more direct request might be, "I want that seat!" Similarly, the father who states casually as his son walks into a room, "It's warm in here," is requesting that his son open the window. If the same utterance were to be delivered by the son as father entered the room, he might interpret the remark as insolent or arrogant and possibly become angry.

Let us return now to "I don't usually use such language." Is this some variety of appeal to the analyst suggesting that "I don't want you to think ill of me" or "I'm embarrassed to say what I think using the language of my thoughts?" The "I mean to say" probably and frequently refers to "I hope you don't take me wrong. This is not the meaning I wish to convey. I don't want you to infer that I am hostile, angry, lascivious, wanton, lewd, unsophisticated, prudish, or the like." Freud's (1925) essay on negation provides examples of how the associational path is intruded upon rather than repression's being effective, and the patient provides a negation in order to disavow the thought as his own. For that matter, the patient is isolating the emotions that accompany the thought because of the awareness of the hearer as a judge—a transference figure.

Speech acts add richness to semantics by including interactive fields in which psychoanalysts reveal transference possibilities as well as stereotypic affective exchanges. We read how the patient feels about us at that point of the analysis by how she addresses us in the dyad. A sudden lapse into baby talk, lisping shyness, the aggressive tone, silence and obsequiousness, all have meaning in the transference. This ought to be looked at from the standpoint of *what do these behaviors stand for?* and what do they add to our knowledge of the significance of her utterance in a traditional semantic way? We ask: what is being said that cannot be read from the grammar or the semantics of the words themselves, but must be a composite derived from context, tone, and illocutionary force as well? In the area of emotional expression, the force of the feeling may be found in the context rather than in the sentence form, and indirection or, for that matter, excessive directiveness. Each may tell more about emotional status than the clean statement "I am sad."

A clinical experience of recent vintage may highlight the discussion. There is a current trend, especially among adolescents, that evaluative statements and emotions are expressed by irony. They say "bad" and mean "good"; they say "groovy" and mean "banal." In addition, a traditional or usual form of address may be associated with an appeal function without being stated in that form. *Sir* implies obsequiousness, *man* too much companionableness, *buddy* fawning friendship. It helps to know these things, because sometimes what appears to be an unprovoked emotional storm may be instead a response to an unrequited appeal for attention or love.

I referred earlier to a woman in her 40s who was emotionally contained as she related endless details about her husband and home life, all of which had a negative, angry ring. The details also conveyed the sense of desperation about her dependent bond and lack of initiative, as well as fear of, and rage at, this man. The analyst's summary comment or clarification, "You sound angry and desperate as if you would think of divorce, but can't do it," brought a flood of tears. Analytic statements of this sort, naming the idea expressed in another way, are frequent and attest to the binding of affects to designative shorthand, naming of a set of ideas. Moreover, such simple generalizations in words have the further interpersonal impact of feeling understood, which provides a further sense of community(Shapiro, 1970),

making the psychoanalytic process a linguistic event that can be analyzed by pragmatic tools. The fit of the words to the events described are clear in the misadventures known as incomplete or premature interpretations (Glover, 1955) in which the patient evades the unconscious and acquires a new obsessional defense, rather than being fully relieved by understanding. The patient becomes part of the interpretive field as he or she feels relief. Sometimes the relief is similar to a tip-of-the-tongue phenomenon—it only occurs on recall of the missing word or phrase.

The notion of a dynamic unconscious rather than a simple cognitive unconscious may receive some warrant from recent studies and discussions from cognitive sciences on memory (Erdelyi, 1990); (Clyman, 1990). Although these investigators are not linguistics students, their distinction between implicit procedural and declarative symbolic knowledge is apposite to psychoanalytic and pragmatic inquiry. Implicit procedural knowledge concerns knowing how to do something like drive a car, or behave at a social gathering; these are like dialogic rules. Many of these procedures have never been reencoded in language in a declarative form; i.e., we usually do not iterate the procedure to ourselves or others, yet we know how to do it. Indeed, declarative knowledge seems to be a later developmental landmark, and as such it is lost in expressive aphasias. The proposition offered earlier in a more linguistic frame, that affective constellations are to be considered part of feature analysis of meaning, can be understood pragmatically for psychoanalytic analysis. It is a procedural nonexpressed feature of memory that has not been declared, but can be recognized once the dynamic barrier is lifted in the two-person field by trust and transference.

The patient's tears on hearing the word *divorce* permits a dreaded idea into awareness for consideration between two people and now is available for reworking as an ego property—the tension of suppression/ repression or isolation of affect is relieved.

Linguists could certainly take a lead from psychoanalysts by including affective determinants in their semantic and pragmatic definitions and illocutionary devices. On the other hand, analysts could certainly use such an analysis as a way of considering "potential affects" as linked to cognitively conscious, linguistic events.

Sociolinguistics

Sociolinguistic analysis is but a small step from pragmatics, because it too takes its data from language in use—this time in communities. Because the frame is larger, it may seem somewhat remote from the dyadic analytic field. Nonetheless, there are cautions and mechanisms to be learned. Common language groups share and even define ethnic separateness. However, discrete language groups also show a tendency to shift the meaning of words over time and from generation to generation. The word "fag" in the early nineteenth century was used to describe an under-classman with menial duties serving upperclassmen in English boarding schools. By the mid-1940s, it referred to gays, but remember it also is used to refer to a cigarette and is used to describe fatigue, as in "fagged out." Even within cultures, groups like adolescents develop their own idiolects, confounding their adult auditors. Many of the words are used as affective referents (Shapiro, 1985).

It is not by chance that some anthropologists have used the words *etic* and *emic*, borrowed from phon*etic* and phon*emic*, to reference sequentially the universals and the particulars of cultural habits and practices. These structural notions derive from the linguistic notion that we all make sounds for speech (phonetic), but that there is a specific corpus of sounds (phonemes) that make up the specific acoustic shape of words in specific languages in order to signal meanings.

A recent series of studies (Badad et al., 1983) show that American school children return the social smile of strangers, while Israelis do not. The implications within each culture regarding shows of friendliness and sincerity are legion. I introduce this fact because we analyze individuals who use our common tongue in ways that mark them regionally, but also in ways that mark them culturally. This is especially so when we consider how they encode their affectivity. Are exuberance and expressiveness only the mark of the southern European or Latin American? Is restraint of emotion the mark of the Anglo-Saxon, the Swede, or the Down Easterner? These stereotypes bear some notice, but we are also attuned to the specifics of an individual's style.

The analysis of an Afro-American who grew up in the South brought home the emic-etic problem entirely. She had an OedipalOedipal complex, no doubt, but her specific shame centered more fully on poverty, rather than on the universals discovered or the specifics of being black in a white world. Such specificity suggested the need for careful attunement and empathy to her verbalizations and behavior, rather than to preconceived ideas.

Doi's (1973) concept of Amai brings home the notion that rearing practices may lead to powerful changes in the constellations of early relationships that count later in life. His emphasis on mother-son ties preOedipally has significant impact, he claims, upon emotional life later. This should remind us of Kohut's (1977) almost casual comment that the closer we are to a person's cultural experience, the more empathic we can feel.

In a contrary vein, Hartmann et al. (1951) noted the completeness of Freudian metapsychology as a general plan of the vicissitudes of drives that must be adapted to cultural variation. In that sense, the etic is there in the paradigm, and the analyst is moved to reduce data from the surface. Technically, this requires a good working knowledge, not only of how resistances are organized in transferential enactments, but also of how much an individual exploits cultural variation for idiolectic reason.

The formal northern European is a stereotype, as is the hot-tempered southern European. However, within each culture there is variation. We have had enough experience in the United States with émigrés from middle Europe and elsewhere to understand that adaptation to a new language is but one feature of adaptation to

279

cultural expressiveness. Linguistically, this can take many forms with respect to emotional expression.

The analyst must become accustomed to the exuberance that covers depression or the formal serenity that covers rage. If we yield to the notion that affects may, at times, not be encoded in words, we have also to agree that simple affective displays require understanding and even curtailing as a feature of civilized action in some communities.

Within the culture of the analysis itself, we create a refuge in which safety of expression is the claim, and yet we see patients fall into habitual patterns—no, we expect and welcome such regression, for without it we could not analyze. Thus, we expect that the vehicle of expression of emotion in adults will have been acted upon by experience that is culturocentric and idiosyncratic at the same time. We learn the codes of each. If we are familiar with the former specifically, it makes some of our tasks lighter, but the latter must be learned firsthand: in the analysis.

Summary

I have proposed that the clinical process of psychoanalysis can be viewed with some advantage as a subset of linguistic experience, using a specific method. As such, the general rules of linguistic analysis and understanding apply. Nonetheless, psychoanalysis may be viewed as a subcultural experience that requires special linguistic consideration in order to account for data derived from (1) the contrived communicative pattern of the analytic situation; (2) the theoretical underpinnings of the method that includes dynamic unconscious mental functioning; (3) free association and transference as special cases of discourse. In each of these three areas, we must account for the unique role of affective experience. The contrived clinical arrangement is designed to help the patient focus within and offers possibilities to experience affects that might otherwise be overlooked. The dynamic unconscious is held in abeyance by mechanisms that are responsive to affective signals. The transferences permit the unusual possibility of experiencing affects in new contexts which seem appropriate, but which soon can become ego-alien under the scrutiny of the observing ego.

Each domain is embedded with linguistic significance that can be illuminating for understanding of how language facilitates and permits affective expression and comprehension in the special circumstance of the analysis. The events discovered can then be studied in relation to the usual circumstances or dialogue in life. Contrariwise, psychoanalysis can also contribute to linguistic analysis by adding the dimension of a dynamic unconscious understanding of symbolic function as it occurs in life. More specifically, analysis forces linguistics to include affective valence in its definitional parameters.

There is no way that we can consider affective experience only from the vantage point of the physiology of affect or the varying physiognomies that make up facial expressions accompanying feelings. We need a depth understanding of affects that includes how they are linked to conflictual constellations of ideas and the words we use. We also should be curious as to how affects deter cognitive and other expressions, and how affects determine or modify object relations—because they become the organizing feature that has the valence and countervalence that makes for significance and meaning. The language of affect and the study of the linguistic forms in analysis should be useful to systematically help psychoanalysts better grasp what they do and how they understand affective expression, using a modern interdisciplinary model.

REFERENCES

Arlow, J.A. (1953). Masturbation and symptom formation. *J. Am. Psychoanal. Assoc.* 1:45–58.

——— (1977). Affects and the psychoanalytic situation. *Int. J. Psychoanal.* 58:157–170.

Austin, J.L. (1962) *How to Do Things with Words.* New York: Oxford Univ. Press

Bacon, F.K. (1989) Quoted in New York *Times Magazine, August 20 "Unnerving Art."* by M. Kimmelman, pp. 41–76.

Badad, YE., Alexander, E.E., & Babad, E.Y. (1983). Returning the smile of the stranger: Developmental patterns and socialization factors. *Monographs of the Society for Research in Child Development*, No. 203, Vol. 48No. 5:

Brenner, C. (1982) *The Mind in Conflict.* New York: Int. Univ. Press Clyman, R.B. (1990) *The Procedural Organization of Emotions.* New York: Int. Univ. Press.

Dahl, H. (1978). A classification of emotion words. *Psychoanal. Q.* 1:269–270.

——— Teller, V., Moss, D., & Trujillo, M. (1978). Counter-transference examples of the syntactic expression of warded off contents. *Psychoanal. Q.* 47:339–363.

Doi, T. (1973) *The Anatomy of Dependence.* San Francisco: Kodansha International Publishers

Ekman, P., Levenson, R.W., & Frieson, Wv. (1983). Autonomic nervous system activity distinguishes between emotions. *Science,* 221:1208–1210.

Eliot, T.S. (1930) Sweeny agonistes. In *The Complete Poems of T. S. Eliot.* New York: Harcourt Brace

Emde, R.N. (1983). The prerepresentational self and its affective core. *Psychoanal. Study Child* 38:165–192.

Erdelyi, M.H. (1990) Repression, reconstruction, and defense. In *Repression: Personality Style and Mechanism of Defense* ed. J. Singer. Chicago: Univ. Chicago Press

Fenichel, O. (1941). Problems of Psychoanalytic Technique. New York: *Psychoanal. Q.*

Freedman, N. (1977). *Hands, Words and Mind: Communicative Structures and Psychic Structures* ed. N. Freedman & S. Grand. New York: Plenum Press

Freud, S. (1899). Screen memories. *Standard Edition* 3.

——— (1900). The interpretation of dreams. *Standard Edition* 4 & 5.

——— (1905a). Fragment of an analysis of a case of hysteria. *Standard Edition* 7.

——— (1905b). Jokes and their relation to the unconscious. *Standard Edition* 8.

——— (1915). The unconscious. *Standard Edition* 14.

——— (1923). The ego and the id. *Standard Edition* 19.

——— (1925). Negation. *Standard Edition* 19.

——— (1926). Inhibitions, symptoms and anxiety *Standard Edition* 20.

——— (1940). An outline of psychoanalysis. *Standard Edition* 23.

Glover, E. (1955) *The Technique of Psychoanalysis.* New York: Int. Univ. Press

Grand, S. (1977). On hand movements during speech. In *Communicative Structures and Psychic Structures* ed. N. Freedman & S. Grand. New York: Plenum Press

Hartmann, H., Kris, E., & Loewenstein, R.M. (1951). Some psychoanalytic comments on "culture and personality." In *Psychoanalysis and Culture* ed. G. B. Wilbur & W. Muensterberger. New York: Int. Univ. Press.

Kleinman, A. (1980) *Patients and Healers in the Context of Culture.* Berkeley: Univ. California Press.

Klinnert, M.D., Campos, J.J., Sorce, J.F., Emde, R.N., & Svejda, M. (1983). Emotions as behavior regulators. In *Emotion: Theory, Research and Experience* ed. R. Plutchik & H. Kellerman. New York: Academic Press.

Kohut, H. (1977) *The Restoration of the Self.* New York: Int. Univ. Press.

Lacan, J. (1956) *The Language of the Self.* Baltimore: Johns Hopkins University Press

Levy, S. & Inderbitzin, L. (1990). The analytic surface. *J. Am. Psychoanal. Assoc.* 38:329–349.

Loewenstein, R.M. (1951). The problem of interpretation. *Psychoanal. Q.* 20:1–14.

Luria, A. (1961) *The Role of Speech in the Regulation of Normal and Abnormal Behavior.* New York: Liveright.

Mahoney, P. (1987) *Psychoanalysis and Discourse.* London: Tavistock.
Needles, W. (1959). Gesticulation and speech. *Int. J. Psychoanal.,* 40:291–294.

Pulver, S. (1974). Unconscious versus potential affect. *Psychoanal. Q.* 43:77–84.

Rosen, V.H. (1961). Relevance of "style" to certain aspects of defense and the synthetic function of the ego. *Int. J. Psychoanal.* 42:447–457.

Schafer, R. (1976) *A New Language for Psychoanalysis.* New Haven: Yale Univ. Press

Searle, J.R. (1969) *Speech Acts: An Essay in the Philosophy of Language.* New York: Cambridge Univ. Press

Shapiro, T. (1970). Interpretation and naming. *J. Am. Psychoanal. Assoc.* 18:399–421.

——— (1979) *Clinical Psycholinguistics.* New York: Plenum Press

——— (1985) Adolescent language. In *Adolescent Psychiatry* ed. M. Sugar. Chicago: Univ. Chicago Press, 12:297–311.

——— (1986) Sign, symbol, and structural theory. In *Psychoanalysis: The Science of Mental Conflict.* Hillsdale, N.J.: Analytic Press

———(1988) *Language Structure and Psychoanalysis.* Madison, Ct.: Int. Univ. Press

Siomopolous, G. (1977) Poetry as affective communication. *Catro* 46:499–513.

Sorce, J.F., Emde, R.N., Campos, J.J. & Klinnert, M.D. (1985). Maternal emotional signaling. *Devel. Psychol.* 21(1):195–200.

On Psychoanalytic Listening:
Language and Unconscious Communication

Coauthor: George Makari

(1993). *Journal of the American Psychoanalytic Association* 41:991–1020.

ABSTRACT:

The authors review past and recent perspectives on psychoanalytic listening, then present a synthetic model founded on psycholinguistics and semiotics. They argue that the analytic listening process can be broken down into nonlinguistic communications and—most important—linguistic categories pertaining to narrativity, symbolic reference, form, and interactive conventions. In each of these areas of signification, the authors present the ways in which the technique of psychoanalytic listening attends to unconscious meanings, thereby differing from ordinary listening which "hears," at best, only denotative and connotative meanings.

> "Wherever we are, what we hear is mostly noise. When we ignore it, it disturbs us. When we listen to it, we find it fascinating."

John Cage—*Silence*

Listening is the most basic of our skills, and yet our theories of *psychoanalytic listening* are narrow and poorly articulated. For the beginner, surprisingly little is taught about how one listens psychoanalytically. How do we listen to another's unconscious? How is the not-listening of Freud's "evenly suspended attention" listening?

In the past, little attention was paid to this technical issue, because many believed the kind of listening that was required of psychoanalysts could not be taught. Recently, however, the ways one listens to another's unconscious have emerged as an area of greater concern. In this paper, we shall review past perspectives on analytic listening, and then present a tentative synthesis based on semiotics and psycholinguistic theories as they apply. No doubt our model will only approximate the nuanced experience of analytic listening. However, the fullest articulation of the ways psychoanalysts listen to conscious and unconscious processes should lead to further modifications and tests of the propositions we employ. Furthermore, it is our belief that psychoanalytic listening can be taught, and it is the goal of this paper to put forth a theory that articulates the principles to be mastered. With this goal in mind, we shall err on the side of exploring the elements of listening that can be described in an empirical, rational context.

Historical Beginnings

Freud never wrote his textbook on technique, but he did write a series of papers in which he made technical "recommendations," and in one of these papers he articulated his notion of psychoanalytic listening. Freud called for evenly hovering attention (the German is *gleichschwebend* and could also be translated "evenly suspended" or "evenly floating"). Rather than focus intently on any one thing said, Freud advocated placing equal value on all the patient's words. In this way Freud (1912) hoped to prevent the analyst from following his expectations and making selections from the patient's story. Freud wisely cautioned that "things one hears are for the most part things whose meaning is only recognized later on" (p. 112). Here we see that listening, for Freud, was an early stage of data gathering, which preceded understanding.

Freud's straightforward advice became more complicated when he discussed the analyst's use of his own unconscious processes: "He should withhold all conscious influences from his capacity to attend, to give himself over completely to his 'unconscious memory'" (p. 112). The difficulty this advice imposed on the analyst was articulated by Ferenczi (1919): "Analytic therapy, therefore, makes claims on the doctor that seem directly self-contradictory. On the one hand, it requires of him the *free play of association and phantasy*, the full indulgence of his own unconscious... [in order to] *grasp intuitively* the expressions of the patient's unconscious that are *concealed in the manifest material* of the *manner of speech and behavior*. On the other hand, the doctor must subject the material submitted by himself and the patient to a *logical scrutiny*, and in his dealings and communications may only let himself be guided exclusively by the result of this mental effort" (p. 189; italics added. This prescient text teases apart the elements that are now seen to be essential to the task of analysis, and places the process of analytic listening in a logical, orderly communicational field.

The idea of a shifting duality between free play and focused analysis at the core of psychoanalytic listening was challenged by

Reik (1948), who proposed his romantic notion of listening with the metaphoric "third ear." Reik shifted Ferenczi's balance between reason and fantasy by suggesting a more immediate communion between minds. "The psychoanalyst," Reik claimed, "has to learn how one mind speaks to another beyond words and in silence. He must listen with the third ear" (p. 144). For Reik the analyst's attention to nuance and aside, to what is "whispered between sentences and without sentences" was not teachable (p. 145). These ideas have received more recent attention in the work of certain French analysts, e.g. Viderman (1979).

Reik's attempt to designate the subtle nonverbal communications in the analytic situation was developed in a less romantic way by Otto Isakower. In 1963, he introduced the term "analyzing instrument" to describe the evocative communications that occur between the thought processes of a regressed analysand and a regressed analyst in the treatment setting.[1] Balter et al. (1980) have attempted to operationalize this notion, and use it as a model for how one listens to unconscious communication.

Empathy and Listening

A different stream of listening theory originated with Kohut's (1959) paper, "Introspection, Empathy, and Psychoanalysis." Kohut distinguished psychoanalytic listening from other listening; psychoanalytic listening, he argued, allowed for an imaginary attunement to the mental position of the patient. While such

---

1   Minutes of Faculty Meeting, New York Psychoanalytic Institute, November 20. Unpublished.

a feat was prescribed, Kohut provided little instruction in this process, save for his call for an attunement to breaks and changes in empathy between patient and analyst. He claimed that "vicarious introspection" or "empathy" was the *sole* tool by which an analyst might know the inner state of another. He called this mode—in conjunction with the patient's own introspection—"the essential constituents of every psychological observation" (p. 461). Kohut claimed that "our thoughts, wishes, feelings, and fantasies cannot be seen, smelled, *heard* or touched" (p. 459; italics added); only by vicarious introspection can the analyst observe a "psychological fact" (p. 461).

Listening, for Kohut and his followers, is the ability to imaginatively take the position of the speaker, to listen as if one were in fact the other who is speaking. Kohut concedes that the reliability of this method declines "the more dissimilar the observed is from the observer" (p. 467). We would add that even similarity of surface does not guarantee common experience or internal structure, by the same argument.

Kohut's work has engendered much discussion on "empathetic" psychoanalytic listening (Lichtenberg, 1983); (Ornstein and Ornstein, 1985). In an unusual tangent to Kohut's work, Schwaber (1983), (1984), (1986) has refocused attention on how an analyst listens, and has thereby invigorated our careful attention to this data-gathering process. She has asserted that empathy is a "specific, scientifically trained mode of perceiving data" (1984, p. 144). However, the specificity of empathy, its scientific status, and the manner in which one is trained to be empathetic are not elucidated. She faults notions of an "objective outside observer" and seeks to put in their place an "observer from within" (1984, pp. 149–150). She shows how she attends to the patient's subjectivity via careful observation of surface behavior. However, her description of the cues in listening, we think, is incomplete. Her careful attentiveness to finding the meaning of another's subjectivity leads to a paradox; she offers a means of knowing another's subjective experience. The myth of the purely objective outside listener deserves skepticism, but it is hardly less realistic than the notion of an observer who imaginatively can shed the fetters of subjectivity and *be* inside another. We have no choice of ontological position, nor can we choose to abandon our own subjectivity for that of another. We must admit the difficult epistemological position we are in, as psychoanalysts trying to know the intricate inner workings of another. But that is no reason to assume "empathy" can rescue us from the imperfect position of being an outside, subjective presence in the curious and tenuous position of having to decide, as does any scientist, what are to be considered data.

Empathy is a Germanic reification of a rather fluid concept—literally "feeling in"—which might be better understood as a common pathway that occurs in various forms, at different times in the course of everyday life and in an analysis (Shapiro, 1981p. 430). Hence, empathy is both too broad and too narrow (in its dismissal of linguistic ordering and communication) a concept to be precisely tracked and theoretically useful as a model of listening. Like Reik's third ear, empathy can too easily be reified into an organ, and therefore become mystified. It seems more judicious to say that under the banner of empathy go countless transient identifications and shared unconscious fantasies (Beres and Arlow, 1974), as well as countless false transactions of pseudo-understanding, countertransference enactments, and projections. Shapiro (1974) suggests that such transactions should be analyzed, as are other psychic compromises. Spence (1984) terms distortion under the banner of empathy the "pathetic fallacy," in which attempts at knowing are replaced by "a sympathetic projection onto the object" (p. 54). Buie (1981) considers empathy to be the end result of a complicated process consisting of (1) perception of another's cues, (2) matching of these cues with those from one's own experience, and (3) inference. In all of these realms, as Buie points out, there is ample room for miscues, mismatching, and false inference, leading to false knowledge.

These critiques seem particularly relevant to a notion of empathy that considers itself *the* form of listening permitting unconscious data gathering. For in the word empathy we find a metaphoric composite that does not explain, but mystifies, how we distinguish *what* the data are in psychoanalysis. This concept is not sufficient to provide grounds for a rational theory of listening which must be, after all, selective and directed in the end.

To call psychoanalytic listening empathetic radically marginalizes the importance of linguistic and paralinguistic communication in the process of listening. In Schwaber's writings, empathy seems to make discussion of what one actually listens to—words and other sounds—less than important. She may argue that these are things studied better by other sciences. However, if we omit these dimensions from our purview, it will be no surprise to find, at the extremes of discourse on empathy, discussions of mental telepathy (Major and Miller, 1984). Empathy seems to provide a way past the wall of words, and in our worst hands becomes a somewhat mysterious, unmediated, intuitive route into the world of another. Moreover it should be noted that, like listening, empathy itself is to a great extent predicated on linguistic and symbolic communications. With the possible exception of the earliest mother-child relationship, we must hear the words "I feel so bad" or see the tears to empathize.

How much empathy could be generated and how much could be psychoanalytically "heard" in an analysis with a patient who speaks only a foreign tongue or one who shows no feeling or one who only lies? Indeed, one of our premises is that we lie to ourselves and obfuscate by not telling what is central in our lives, because we cannot bear to express it directly in words. We need it to be interpreted. A theory of psychoanalytic listening that ignores the very stuff we listen to does so at great risk. It is essential to examine these "surface" data, for these materials are transformed into the inferences upon which any psychoanalytic interpretation relies.

The Linguistic Turn

Around the same time Kohut was formulating his concepts of empathy, other psychoanalysts were turning toward linguistics, in the hope that this might root theoretical advancement in the material soil of language. One of the first to embrace this line of reasoning was Lacan (1968), (1977) who, in the 1950s, attempted to fuse structuralist linguistics and psychoanalysis. Lacan's theory of psychoanalysis, as well as his notions of listening, were enmeshed in his unique adaptation of Saussurian structural linguistics with *fin de siècle* Freud. In his 1953 Rome report, Lacan (1968) described the dearth of psychoanalytic work in linguistics, and proposed his model of analytic listening. We must know what we are directing our attention to and that, he asserted, is "the Word of the subject" and not any object beyond the word (p. 15). In so privileging language, Lacan concluded that the analyst must attend to the details and nuances of words themselves. Lacan would call this process the play of signifiers, for it was in this assortment of signifiers (and not necessarily the concepts they signified, much less any "real" referent) that one found unconsciously encoded messages. Lacan understood repression to be the block between a signifier and what it truly signified (pp. 43–44). For Lacan (1977) the unconscious itself was structured like language (p. 147).

Later in the U.S., a group of psychoanalysts used linguistics as an informing science to look at their discipline. In parallel with Lacan, Rosen (1961), (1974), (1977) used linguistic formats such as R. Jakobson's metaphor-metonymy bifurcation to explore various referential styles of patients. Edelheit (1969) similarly applied linguistic deep-structural elements to enable us to grasp the limited structures that could generate a bevy of surface fantasies. Shapiro (1970) argued that interpretation can be thought of as naming, then developed this focus into a survey of linguistic approaches which may pertain to psychotherapy. He also argued that psychotherapeutic transactions could be fruitfully understood along the tripartite model of syntactics, semantics, and pragmatics (Shapiro, 1979). Edelson (1972), (1975) used Noam Chomsky's theory of generative grammar to argue that the syntax of dreams is like that of language. Furthermore, Edelson argued that psychoanalytic listening is primarily linguistic and based on an internal and unconscious competence in the listener: "I have come to believe that… much of the understanding the psychoanalyst attributes to conscious and unconscious extralinguistic competence actually derives from his own internalized linguistic competence" (Edelson, 1975, p. 28).

Schafer (1983) moved the linguistic focus to a more macroscopic level by calling attention to the importance of narrative structure in the psychoanalytic process. In his opinion, psychoanalytic histories are provisional and continually undergoing modification, till at the end of analysis there is a "radically new, jointly authored work or way of working" (p. 219). Spence (1982), (1984) developed Schafer's narrative approach in what is one of the most thoughtful readings of the problems and paradoxes of psychoanalytic listening. The Freudian paradigm in which the patient free-associates and the analyst hovers in evenly suspended attention is flawed, Spence argued, in that when the patient is truly freely associating, the analyst must listen actively and try to supply narrative context to these fragmented primary-process utterances. Conversely, it is only when the patient supplies a censored, contextualized secondary-process narrative that the analyst can freely and passively float along (Spence, 1982, p. 30). This critique is congruent with the commonly held notion that free association as a goal is only imperfectly achieved and that is fortunate, for otherwise the product would be hard to distinguish from word-salad.

While accepting active listening as necessary to the analytic endeavor, Spence, like Edelson, adapted the Chomskyan notion of linguistic competence to psychoanalysis and sought to make explicit the conventions by which a competent analyst searches for meaning and hence structures his listening. For Spence (1982) these interpretative axioms are (1) the assumption of unity of thematic meaning (which leads us to look for commonalities rather than disruptions), (2) the assumption of therapeutic urgency (which assumes crucial issues are always being discussed), (3) multiple function or meaning, (4) transference, (5) empathy (pp. 109–113). These are the ways we listen, according to Spence, and they are by their very nature, active, potentially distorting forces, especially if they are not self-consciously employed, for then silent "unwitting interpretations" are made in these registers (p. 102). Spence's concern with the analyst's need to project meaning onto phenomena has led him to propose a "post-Freudian metaphor," in which a patient's associations are heard as belonging to no theoretical structure (Spence, 1987).

This brief and selective overview of recent psycholinguistic approaches forms the basis for the synthesis we propose. We agree with Edelson's (1975) assertion that psychoanalysis as a science is essentially the study of symbolic systems and therefore must avail itself to semiotics in general, and linguistics in particular (p. 19). We shall attempt to schematize psychoanalytic listening along these lines. In so doing we shall no doubt be vulnerable to the accusation of oversimplification or reductionism, but we hope this work will be read in the spirit of building a rational framework on which later modifications, expansions, and refinements can occur.

A Model of Psychoanalytic Listening

All listening begins by distinguishing sound from silence. Silence and the meanings it can hold are profoundly important in psychoanalytic work, and so the first challenge for a model of listening is to account for the converse of sound (see Panel, 1959).

Silence only has significance in relation to sound and other contexts. While nothing in itself, it means and signifies in its dynamic relation to the surround of signifying sounds. It is, for example, the background that structures or patterns sound, leading to rhythmicity of utterance or a pause that gives emphasis. Furthermore, silence may take on meaning in relation to discursive roles, or the particular utterances that accompany it. If we ask a patient for his or her father's name, and the patient responds with silence, it is a meaningful silence insofar as a normal discursive role is shunned, and insofar as the patient's silence gives meaning to our question. If a patient is

297

free-associating, then suddenly stops, the patient's silence takes on meaning relative to the preceding and subsequent free associations. Early on, we are sometimes led astray by overgeneralizing our schooling on angry silences. But in the end, silence has no specific meaning and means in relation to the network of other semiotic elements in which it is enmeshed. A silence is "pregnant" only insofar as the semiotic elements that surround it have impregnated it with meaning.

What are these other semiotic elements? When silence is broken, we hear sounds that are either *signs* or *noise*. If a low rumbling is heard as a snort, it reveals contempt, thus it signifies. If a low rumbling is nothing but a far-off sound, for the time being it is noise. Over time this noise might take on a context that gives it meaning; at that moment it is no longer noise, but has become a sign. This basic semiotic distinction should be familiar to those with medical training; according to Eco (1979p. 11), medicine's emphasis on signs and symptoms represents the oldest semiotic tradition.

This seemingly transparent distinction between an auditory sign and a noise marks a crucial distinction that separates everyday listening from psychoanalytic listening. In a "normal" conversation, we might consign our own internal associations, the errors our partner makes in a word choice, the slightly pedantic phrasing or loud, booming voice, to the realm of noise. We might not attend to these things, and consider them relatively meaningless or unnecessary observations in the face of this speaker's intended meanings. One of psychoanalysis' accomplishments has been to rescue a whole host of such meanings from aural meaninglessness, and redefine these noises as *unconscious* signs. So in a psychoanalytic theory of listening, it must be understood that our definition of noise will be fundamentally different from a general listener's and will follow our (psychoanalytic) codes of listening. This difference cannot be more extreme, for a basic tenet of psychoanalytic listening is precisely the *reversal of value* between the conventionally held relation of sign to noise, so as to privilege the unconscious meaning possibilities of "noise," and diminish the normal totalizing impression of the foregrounded "consciously intended" sign. Perhaps this is what supervisors mean when they counsel candidates to listen closely, but not only to what the patient is saying. Furthermore, the rule of psychic determinism can be seen in this light, as not so much a law of nature, but a technical device that ensures this reversal of value and keeps the analyst attuned to what the ordinary ear dismisses as noise. Psychic determinism does this by proclaiming that theoretically there is *no* noise in the system of conscious and unconscious mental processes.

Insofar as a sound signifies something, its meaning can be understood by employing three broad semiotic categories: *paralinguistics, kinesics,* and *linguistics.*

Paralinguistics is the study of those auditory signs that corroborate, embellish, or contradict linguistic communication, and it remains very much part of the art of psychoanalytic listening. Without these cues—one finds this difficulty when reading the written texts of analytic hours—much meaning can be lost. Tropes of language may be missed if we do not attend to the accompanying music of the words. We miss the cues for irony, sarcasm, contempt, tenderness, love. A crucial element of psychoanalytic data is contained in the realm of paralinguistics, for these cues frequently are the best signals of a shift in a patient's inner affective state (Horowitz, 1979).

G. Trager (cited in Eco, 1979p. 10) has attempted to systematically look at paralinguistic elements. He distinguishes the speaker's "voice set" (determined by sex, age, and infirmity), the speaker's "voice qualities" (such as pitch and range), and, finally and most important for us, "vocalizations." This last category is further divided into "vocal characterizers" (laughing, crying, whimpering) "vocal qualifiers" (intensity, pitch height) and "vocal segregates" (noises of the tongue, lips, grunts). It is artificial to simply segregate these elements of communication, since so often their meaning results from their interface with each other, kinesics, or linguistic communication. For instance, if a man laughs while telling of an attempt on his own life, he means something that emerges only by listening to the disparity between two sets of signs (semantics and vocal characterizers).

Kinesics is the study of the meaning of gestures and physical movements that accompany speech. Insofar as these cues are fundamentally linked to a linguistic communication, they also are important accompaniments to psychoanalytic listening. For example, raised eyebrows may signify an ironic intent that reverses the meaning of the words spoken. There is a substantial early literature on gesture in psychoanalysis (Reich, 1949); (Feldman, 1959); (Scheflen, 1963). For instance, Gostynski (1951) proposed that stereotypical gestural behavior constitutes a "sign language"; these movements, he argued, once lent weight to words at a particular moment, then became permanent aspects of character structure. Needles (1959) points to the gestural associations that lead to the interpretive mark as they follow and interdigitate with verbal precursors. More recently, Jacobs (1991) has shown how attending to our own gestures can direct us to interpretive understanding.

Freedman and Steingart (1975) distinguish between *representing* and *focusing* gestural behaviors. Representing behaviors accompany spoken descriptions; for instance, the hand movement that might help describe a spiral staircase. On the other hand, focusing behaviors may be self- or object-directed and are meant to weigh or color a representation in a certain manner. Freedman (1978), (1983); (Freedman and Grand, 1985) also proposes a kinesic axis for the listener. *Shielding* behaviors are self-stimulations like doodling or the tapping of fingers, which, in Freedman's opinion, are a mechanism for dealing with the stress of being in the "receptive mode" of listening. *Contrasting* behaviors are movements such as weight shifts or foot kicks which Freedman argues are related to a shift from the receiving mode of listening to the refocusing mode. Contrasting behaviors do this by creating stimuli at the edge of conscious experience that stimulate the self and hence help the self distance from the speaker (1983, p. 415). Such signs are not necessarily indicative of countertransference; in fact, they merely may be the shift from listening to formulating an interpretation and preparing to speak. However, contrasting behaviors may also signal intrapsychic distress and the need to distance oneself from the analytic situation.

The integration of both paralinguistics and kinesics with verbal communications presently remains a complicated and fascinating area in need of further study. On the other hand, the third and most important category for comprehending a sound-sign—*linguistics*—has been studied extensively. There are different frameworks for understanding the verbal communicative process, but let us start with a macroscopic focus.

Intended and Shadow Narratives

Generally speaking, we first hear a patient's words as if they were not words at all, but invisible, undistorting avenues into another's mind. As Wittgenstein (1969) wrote: "If someone says, 'I know that that's

a tree' I may answer: 'Yes, that is a sentence. An English sentence...
'" (1969, p. 46). We are surprised by Wittgenstein's veracious but
unusual retort, for the first level of listening ignores the thingness of
spoken utterance and attends to the meanings signified by words. We
do not hear signifiers, but rather stories, complaints, difficulties with
a husband or a wife. In short, we attend to the world of the referent.
And in listening to this level of meaning we become immersed in
what we shall call the patient's *intended narrative*.

The intended narrative is predominantly conscious; it is the
meaning the speaker thinks he is conveying. The lines of intended
narrative not only include the patient's presentation of his personal
history; they also include all the conscious themes of, among other
things, his past, his dream and fantasy life, and his experience in the
here-and-now of the analytic setting. The analyst listens and, like any
listener, sticks common meanings onto these signifiers and narratives.
He tries to grasp the analysand's intended themes and meanings.
In so doing, he will, like any attentive listener, note discrepancies,
repetitions, strands of narrative that do not cohere (Spence's
convention of thematic unity is not particular to psychoanalysis),
motivations that seem unconvincing or overstated, characters that
are extensively or scantily developed, themes that are not borne out.
He notes the affect and mode of the tale, whether tragic, romantic,
ironic, or comedic (Schafer, 1976). Furthermore, he free-associates
along with the patient, at times attending more to his own thoughts
than the analysand's as the intended narrative unfolds.

The psychoanalyst listens with an attentive openness and a
suspension of the need to make hasty other meaning. But as the
patient's story progresses, it eventually juts up against (1) itself
(confusions, halts in association, contradictory themes, scotomas),
(2) the transferential experience in the here-and-now (i.e.,

transference resistance), and (3) our theory. Though many would hesitate at the epistemological implications of our third claim, it seems hard to dispute. As Friedman (1988) points out, this is one of the fundamental frustrations of the analytic dialogue; the patient seeks to convince the analyst of his (conscious) meaning, whereas he knows that the analyst has a theory that decodes meaning differently. This is not at all to say that the analyst attempts to enforce the acceptance of a perceived "objective" reality, at the expense of the patient's subjective experience. It is not by comparing the patient's narrative to any "normal schema," but rather insofar as we experience and register unconscious strands of narrative that are communicated but left out of the patient's conscious story, that we attempt to listen to and make conscious untold narratives that adhere to, and are inferred from, the intended narrative.

But how does the transformation of an *intended narrative* to its unconscious or *shadow narrative* take place in the analytic listener and, it is hoped, in the patient? What are the semantics of unconscious meaning? Merleau-Ponty (1964, p. 39) argues that all linguistic signification is indirect and ultimately metaphoric. Following this philosopher, we may say that unconscious data are also indirect communications, but of a different order. Shadow narratives do not come to awareness from the analyst's intuitive grace or telepathy, but are the result of hearing many bits of frequently recurrent, indirect communication.

Listening for unconscious communication on the level of narrative is based on this assumption that repetitions in material, either at a narrative level or metanarrative, thematic level, can be inferred to have overdetermined unconscious meaning. Repetitive, indirectly meaningful, strands that adhere to intended narratives are clarified through the trials and errors of analytic interpretation.

Hearing this indirect communication comes about in part from empathy and the analyst's use of his own associations, but essentially it is rooted in language. Unconscious communication is the story that emerges again and again despite the storyteller; paradoxically, it is also the tale the storyteller validates.

An analysand made repeated references to a series of men who were solicitous of his mother during different stages of his development. The analyst became aware of the repetitious signifying function of the proper names involved; they were all variations of surnames relating to horses. This indirect communication of another element adhering to the patient's intended narrative manifested its shadow narrative later on in the analysis, when the analysand spoke warmly of an intimate vacation with his mother during his Oedipal years. He described proudly sitting up on a great horse for a photo that subsequently held a central place in his mother's album of remembrances. The shadow narrative's little horseman had entered the intended narrative, transformed into a redundant suitor.

In this manner, the analyst and analysand begin to reweave the meaning of the *intended narratives* with their unconscious *shadow narratives*. Over time, signs from the unconscious cohere to form an interpretation, a way of naming the fragmentary and indirect linguistic communications that have occurred (Shapiro, 1970). That *naming* results in the movement from unconscious to conscious is something Freud recognized when he placed word presentation in the preconscious. Along with confrontation and clarification, interpretations allow for linguistic constructions that paraphrase unconscious meaning. During the course of an analysis, these interpretations undergo repetitive modification and refinement.

Any system with explanatory value relies on a relatively small number of "deep" constructs that reduce "surface" data that otherwise seem heterologous. The signs that need such deciphering are ones that are meaningful in terms of the listener's theory. Freud's earliest linguistic codes of interpretation were for dream work. Linguists give them other names, but displacement, condensation, and turning into the opposite are good enough. They help us, while listening, to attend in a way that permits further decoding of the unintended message. Arlow and Brenner's (1964) drive, defense, compromise model articulates the condition for narrative interpretation in accord with Freud's structural theory. In the years since Freud, many other perspectives on interpretation have been put forth. Chessick (1989) discusses "channels" with which a narrative can be constructed in psychotherapy: Freud's theory of drive/conflict/defense, object relations, self-psychology, the interactional school of H. S. Sullivan, and the sociocultural approach of E. Fromm, J.-P. Sartre, and others. Recently, attention has been paid to the kinds of experience-near interpretive work that can be made at the analytic "surface." These codes of listening include Gray's (1973) "defense analysis," Gill's (1982) transference analysis, and Anton Kris' (1982) focus on free association. Spence's (1982) conventions for psychoanalytic interpretation have already been mentioned. Schafer's (1983) psychoanalytic "story lines" fall into the categories of drives, free association, resistance, and reality testing (pp. 224–226). The grammar of each of these interpretive modes may differ, but in general the semantics are similar, for each code ultimately refers to man in conflict or to the deficits of early rearing.

Of course the registration and deconstruction of signs will be, to varying degrees, dependent on the kind of psychoanalytic code one adopts. A discussion of these different interpretive codes and their relative value is beyond the scope of this paper. But we do not mean to imply that any of these codes is as good as the next.

Luborsky's (1984) core conflictual relationship theme (CCRT) and other dynamic empirical approaches suggest that the pure relativism of such an attitude is not warranted. And it should be added that the availability of numerous interpretive narratives without one unifying, generally accepted grand narrative may seem lamentable, but it is not a dilemma restricted to psychoanalytic theory. Some have argued that this is the general state of knowledge in the "human sciences" in post-modernism, a condition J. Habermas has called the "crisis of legitimation" (Lyotard, 1984).

In listening to *intended narratives* and gradually listening for and constructing with the patient his or her *shadow narratives*, we rely on sources of unconscious data other than those supplied by (1) empathy, (2) our own free associations, and (3) the analysand's intended narrative. There are frequent moments in a patient's narrative when the illusory transparency of language fails, and words turn opaque. In these moments, which are frequently heralded by a sense of surprise or confusion in the listener, a signifier becomes problematized; a sign becomes charged with noise. Thus, we have stumbled onto a mini-narrative, the affectively charged story, desire, or memory buried under the apparent obviousness of a signifier.

If a patient continually refers to his mother as a "bird," he may mean a devouring eagle or a showy peacock, or a sexy woman, or many other personally ascribed features. There is a history to that patient's metaphoric equation of the words "mother" and "bird." Words are learned as a way to name the world, and so in a person's language we hold the clues to how that person once sought, and still seeks, to describe and divide now-forgotten individual realities.

As De Saussure (1959) first pointed out, signifiers are only arbitrarily related to that which they signify. Therefore, the room for "slippage" between signifier and signified is potentially great.

We all live in a net of signifiers, many of which we rightly believe have general cultural currency, ignoring that they may *also* have profoundly individual histories that carry and convey unconscious messages. A signifier first has a *denotative* meaning, which is (ideally) the unique referent it signifies. In this denotative realm there is, of course, more arbitrariness than perhaps we would like, but it is via this shared system of codes that human communication generally proceeds. Second, a word has *connotative* meaning, that is to say a meaning that relates to the signifier by a more subtle, historical, and contextual relation (see Shapiro, 1970). The room for "slippage" is greater here, since differences in culture and history can lead to misunderstanding. A California surfer might refer to his nonsurfing friend Bill, as a "Fred," and in so doing adhere to a shared connotative meaning that this signifier held for his social group. Figures of speech such as similes, metaphors, and metonymies bank on such connotative meanings, but as any analyst knows, their meanings can be idiosyncratic and often unconscious.

While denotation and connotation are the staples of semantic usage and are the ways in which the psychoanalytic listener hears the intended narrative of the analysand, where does the unconscious meaning of words reside? Thass-Thienemann (1983) argues that the unconscious meaning of words can be discovered by a diachronic, etymologic analysis. Without denying the power of such historical inflections to convey concealed meaning, we (and we believe other psychoanalysts) take a broader and more perspectivist approach. Linguists distinguish a third level of meaning beyond denotation and connotation, in which the signifier refers to the user's own essentially idiosyncratic, personal store of meaning. Psychic reality is manifested in the private store of unconscious meaning that adheres at the level of the signifier, which we shall call, following Barthes (1968p. 21), "ideolectic." Indeed, in the unusual setting that constitutes the psychoanalytic dialogue, the context is designed to permit slippage into personal codes and such ideolectic meanings.

Since we are interested in understanding the analysand's psychic reality in psychoanalysis, we approach these three levels of semanticity differently than a normal listener. Insofar as possible, psychoanalysts hold a listening convention which is that signifiers that surprise or confuse us, may have personal, previously unconscious tales to tell. We proceed *as if* such signifiers must be *ideolectic*. Following Nietzsche, we believe that on some level every word is a private prejudice.

Such a theory of linguistic relativity takes one step beyond the Whorf-Sapir hypothesis. After studying Hopi and other Native-American languages, Whorf (1956) concluded that language structured space and time relations in such a powerful manner that it was reasonable to conclude that one's language structured one's worldview. Although Whorf might not have agreed with this psychoanalytic extension that relativizes not only language groups, but also language users, on an unconscious level we might say that all language has an ideolectic component. This is not an argument for solipsism; the denotative and connotative aspects of language carry communication on their backs; everything else, whether ideolectic meaning or verbal slip, is heard by the ordinary listener as noise.

Frequently, attunement to such ideolectic language is heralded by surprise or an ambiguity in meaning that shatters routine signification, sending us back to the signifiers themselves. Certainly, malapropisms and slips of the tongue based on articulatory similarity offer the listener ways into unconscious meanings and idioms. Isay (1977) discussed the most frequent linguistic ambiguities he encountered in the psychoanalytic setting. Pronominal ambiguity may take the form of depersonifying a part of the body. For example, we have observed one patient who referred to his nose and his penis as *the* nose and *the* penis, and was thereby enacting the isolation from urgency he felt, and the objectification of his body as things, because he feared confronting his dangerous sexual thoughts and feelings. Words with multiple meanings provide common modes of semantic ambiguity. As Isay notes, in these situations the linguistic data point the auditor in two or more directions.

We need not think of this focus on the word as overly intellectualized or barren of feeling. As Shapiro (1991) notes, affective tone is a feature of word meaning in use. Recent and continuing studies in multilingual analyses, under the guidance of Amati-Mehler (see Amati-Mehler et al., 1990), highlight how shifting semantic codes may involve shifting affective content. The implications for analysis here are broad, for it is not only that a particular word may hold connotations and affective meaning not easily translated into another language; more generally, analysis attends to the personal associations words carry from a specific time and place. In that sense we are all multilingual, speaking at varying times baby talk, adolescent slang, and various adult dialects. For this reason two words naming the same thing can feel different; "Mommy" does not hold the same resonance as "Mother" for most of us. And that is just the most obvious example of the power of "childrenese" to contain and indirectly convey unconscious affective meaning.

For example, an analysand recalled that as a child he referred to his mother alternatively as "poome" and "pooher." Only later in the analysis did we learn the context for these unintelligible terms; they referred to his mother's illness and his own suffering as two sides of the same coin. "Poor me" and "poor her" were his contrivances to name these persons, their plight, and their linkage. In this way, words can be like old songs whisking us back to particular feelings and moments in the past.

For all these reasons the psychoanalytic listener must hear the analysand's language as slightly foreign, a dialect no one else speaks, in which numerous histories animate the all-too-familiar words in that speaker's mind. Listening at this microlinguistic level ("the play of signifier" as Lacan called it), can take place not only in relation to a particular sign or group of signs (semantics). It can also be fruitful to examine the manner in which signs are ordered. This study of sign relations can be broken down into the *syntagmatic* and *associative* axes (De Saussure, 1959pp. 122–127).

The *syntagmatic* encodes the rules of secondary process, based on commonly held rules by which we structure our language. But syntax can also be an individually charged manner of ordering the relation of subject, object, and action, and therefore can reveal unconscious meanings. Schafer's (1976) work on "action language" was, in part, an attempt to exploit such a syntagmatic approach to unconscious communication. Dahl et al. (1978) postulated that "each speaker has available a variety of syntactic options, and the particular syntactic structure which he chooses reflects, among other things, the inventory of wishes that he is motivated both to conceal and to express" (p. 344). These investigators examined ten statements by an analyst on a taped analysis and showed how latent meaning is encoded in 12 specific syntactical strategies. For instance, accusatives may convey a sense of interrogation, or "trial by syntax," as these authors call it (p. 348). By using the agentless passive voice, one may be disavowing action or hostilely murdering the subject that was to be referred to. The analyst's syntax can serve to reinforce unconsciously communicated psychic realities; we play into our patients' sense of their own victimization by using phrases like "you are assaulted by your rage."

Syntax should break down as a patient's associations approach primary process, a situation that never occurs and is not even desirable, because it does not permit a coherent thematic statement, as noted earlier. But relatively free association can be characterized by what De Saussure called "associative relations" between signs. In *associative relations*, normal rules of syntax are suspended in favor of, among others, the rules of contiguity in time (i.e., memory), relations of signs based on likeness or contrast, interdependence, or perceived necessity. Of course this is the linguistic process with which psychoanalysts gather much data regarding unconscious fantasy organizations.

"Artist" might be followed by the conceptually similar "painter" then the similarly sounding "pain" in a chain of associatively related signifiers. In such a string, signifiers that previously were opaque in their denotative or commonly connotative usages now take on individual metaphoric meaning in relation to each other. An analysand may use the word "artist" in a manner that never varies from the most commonly held denotation. However, while free associating, he displays personal unconscious accretions of meaning. For this reason, too, we can assume that in psychic reality words have a fundamentally ideolectic meaning. Even if a word does not reveal ideolectic significance in itself, in the store of associations that this signifier holds, it can.

Insofar as the analyst can unpack the history of signs in which the analysand lives, he will be making conscious that which is unconscious, and gathering data from which a coherent and mutually validated narrative can be constructed. He listens for noises that signify in psychoanalytic terms: slips, metaphors, similes, archaic or

311

idiosyncratic usages, repeatedly used words, words used in the wrong context; he listens for odd syntax, passive voice, obsessively formed sentences; in short, he listens for the poetics that structure another's signifying repertoire. In so doing he gains data with which to name and interpret, confront and clarify, all of which helps the analysand piece together his own shadow narratives.

Pragmatics and Transference

Up to this point—having discussed narrative, semantics and syntactics—we have treated listening in analysis as if the analyst were listening to a monologue. This brings us to a final linguistic category which is crucial to the psychoanalytic process of listening—*pragmatics*.

Pragmatics relates to the indirect metalinguistic communications that occur between speaker and listener, and hence structure interlocutionary discourse. It is that aspect of linguistics that sees language as a tool for affecting the world and listener. Pragmatic communications can be thought of as second-order significations that are implicit, not in the actual signifier, but in the relationship between the speaker and the listener.

While the basic rules of dialogue (e.g., topic maintenance, turn-taking, intentionality, social rules) generally apply, pragmatic communications are based on more subtle rules that operate ate at interpersonal levels. An elderly grandfather says to his fifteen-year-old grandson, "It's hot in here." The boy opens the window, for he has read the older man's intention as a need to act, though his grandfather's statement was not in the form of a request. This indirect communication is predicated on an unspoken conception of the roles of speaker and listener. Pragmatic communications are truncated; part of what is to be communicated is verbally produced, but the rest relies on the listener's understanding of the discursive roles at hand. There is an ellipsis present—a communication not spoken, but inferred. Based on all the speaker and listener know about each other, the listener must "hear" the implied next utterance.

Pragmatic concerns in the psychoanalytic dialogue must be considered from within the very unusual constraints of the analytic encounter. The general rules of discourse become more specific and idiosyncratic within the analytic situation. For example, a patient who was given to the tendency to become aggressive, rather than report embarrassing associations, came in one day and verbally attacked the analyst with no clear provocation and without portent from the previous hour. The analyst's familiarity with the patient's defensive style in their dyad alerted him to this indirect communication, and led to a confrontation that elicited the embarrassing conscious fantasy.

The most salient structure in analytic discourse is the mandated role of the analyst (listening more than speaking, abstinence and neutrality) and analysand (speaking more than listening, the rule of free association). Insofar as this is a mandated structure, it in itself holds no individual unconscious meaning. It is a ritualized sequence, like a phatic greeting. But each patient comes to these discursive roles with a history of dialogic interaction, as well as a whole set of fantasies about what *might* occur in this relationship. Thus hopes, fears, and desires about the role of the analyst are frequently expressed in second-order signifiers which, linguistically speaking, would be called pragmatic.

Friedman (1988) refers to attempts by the analysand to affect the analytic listener as "seductions." In psychoanalysis, the conscious and unconscious assumptions about who the listener is are conveyed in these attempts to mold the analyst into a shape that would actualize certain *a priori* assumptions. Like Ulysses, the analyst will not stop up his ears, but theory has tied him to the mast and he will not enact these fantasies. Instead, he is committed to analyzing them. These indirect communications, the discursive structures by which the analysand organizes the telling of their intended narrative, and the information that this unconscious molding provides in the here-and-now, are described by the psychoanalytic concept of transference.

Transference, put in these linguistic terms, is not to be restricted to a dyadic situation; it is the other (i.e., internalized object, ego ideal, superego) whom we imagine ourselves talking to, even when we are only talking to ourselves. It is the "listener" inscribed in the analysand's language, the he, or she, the analysand speaks to when in fact speaking to the analyst. In this pragmatic realm, the analyst experiences the way language is used by the patient to define relationships and affect others. For instance, a schizoid man routinely leaves his session with the parting words that reestablish a feeling of distance more appropriate for a passerby; these discursive roles are experienced by the analyst. They provoke responses which the analyst must then subject to scrutiny. And so an unconscious scene of the shadow narrative is staged in the analyst's office.

Here we have entered into another important tenet of psychoanalytic listening. So as to be attuned to all the possible dialogic conscious and unconscious pragmatic transactions that may be occurring on the most subtle of levels, it is crucial for the analyst to attend to his own fantasies and associations, especially the manner in which he completes certain indirect utterances. However, it is not adequate to call the analyst's associations "free," for they are provoked; they are part of a dyadic system, as Isakower noted. As the analyst comes to know the unconscious discursive roles the analysand employs, his attunement to this communicative realm can become quite accurate. That having been said, in this realm of secondary signification the possibility of miscommunication remains substantial; it is based fundamentally on inference and must be held up to the light of verbal examination.

In our previous example, the grandson, on hearing his grandfather's words, is provoked to complete the communication. By understanding his relationship to his grandfather, he infers a silently communicated desire. Via a pragmatic communication based on the actual utterance in the context of a relationship, the grandson infers thoughts which he *attributes* to his grandfather. Whether in fact he is correct in his inference is questionable. So he asks: "Do you want me to open the window?" Here the pragmatic communication shifts to a purely semantic one that enacts the grandson's doubt and hence can receive confirmation or refutation. In the same way, an analyst makes an interpretation to try to name the unspoken pragmatic transferential communication that he believes is occurring in the here-and-now of his office. Object-relations theorists view some enactments as provocations set up by projective identification. In these circumstances, the analyst must become aware of his tendency to become party to the analysand's self-object constellations.

In this pragmatic realm, subtle or overt disruptions of listening can easily occur. Firstly there may be a loss or disruption of empathy, which mars the analyst's ability to understand the implications of the *intended narrative* and hence disrupts any movement beyond the conscious realm. Going back to our original example, let us imagine that the grandson had just gotten up to close the window, only to hear his grandfather exclaim: "You're lazy!" At this point his ability to empathize and "hear" his grandfather may be impaired.

There are, of course, countertransferential issues that originate not only from the discursive interaction between speaker and listener, but are in part derivatives of the conflicts of the listener alone. This is the more narrow, earlier usage of countertransference (Abend, 1989). Countertransference in the narrow sense of a disruption of listening (rather than all the responses of the analyst) would cause failed communication, due to the intrapsychic distorting noise within the analyst. A discussion of these countertransferential distortions is beyond the scope of this paper.

Conclusion

We have tried to situate psychoanalytic listening within the realm of a linguistic and semiotic analysis. We believe this model has the advantage of articulating the assumptions we employ to grasp unconscious meaning, without postulating a reified homunculus in the analyst or resorting to nebulous, mysterious explanations. The formal analysis we offer may seem lacking in the poetry of immediate experience in analysis. However, what we have attempted to do is explicate the poetics of analytic listening. We have left out much that is complementary in psychoanalytic listening that may come under the rubric of the intuitive. These domains are not so easily captured, nor are the effects of shifting states of consciousness on our listening. Along with countertransference, these are important areas of future study.

We have suggested that psychoanalytic listening is distinct from ordinary listening, insofar as it employs certain rules to hear indirect unconscious communication. Like ordinary listeners, we become immersed in the analysand's *intended narrative*, but then, based on the patient's flow of signification, we shift among gestural, paralinguistic, semantic, syntactic, and pragmatic modes so as to gather the fullest understanding of the analysand's unconsciously intended *shadow narrative*.

We have proposed that the psychoanalytic tenets of listening include: (1) open-minded, caring attention; (2) relative reversal of sign-noise value for all signs; (3) the assumption of a signifier's "ideolectic" meaning at the level of psychic reality; (4) a psychoanalytic theory of associative relations based primarily on contiguity, as well as attention to subtle psychodynamic meanings contained in syntagmatic choice; (5) the assumption of the overdetermined nature of repetitious signs or groups of signs (e.g., word, gesture, theme);

(6) employment of a chosen psychoanalytic interpretive code; (7) attunement to one's own associations as they reveal, among other things, pragmatic discursive secondary-order communications such as disruptions of empathy and transference.

Psychoanalytic competence then would be the *ability* to employ these tenets when one of them is relevant to the patient's discourse. Freud's warning of selecting particular meanings *a priori*, of course, still holds.

The model we have presented is intended to make explicit the ways an analyst can hear how language and its accompaniments convey unconscious data. By attending to these signs, the patient's symbolic world can increasingly be heard by the psychoanalyst as a coherent, mutually validated narrative that testifies to what was once forgotten and silent.

REFERENCES

Abend, S. (1989). Countertransference and psychoanalytic technique. *Psychoanal. Q.* 58:374–395.

Amati-Mehler, J., Argentiei, S. & Canestri, J. (1990). *La Babelo dell Inconscio.* Milan: Rafaello Cortina.

Arlow, J.A. & Brenner, C. (1964). *Psychoanalytic Concepts and the Structural Theory.* New York: Int. Univ. Press.

Balter, L., Lothane, Z. & Spencer, J. (1980). On the analyzing instrument. *Psychoanal. Q.* 49:474–504.

Barthes, R. (1968). *Elements of Semiology.* New York: Hill & Wang. Beres, D. & Arlow, J. (1974). Fantasy and identification in empathy. *Psychoanal. Q.* 43:26–50.

Buie, D. (1981). Empathy: its nature and limitations. *J. Am. Psychoanal. Assoc.* 29:281–307.

Cage, J. (1973). *Silence* Middletown, CT: Wesleyan Univ. Press, p. 3. Chessick, R. (1989). *The Technique and Practice of Listening in Intensive Psychotherapy.* Northvale, NJ: Aronson.

Dahl, H., et al. (1978). Countertransference examples of the syntactic expression of warded-off contents. *Psychoanal. Q.* 47:337–363.

De Saussure, F. (1959). *Course in General Linguistics.* New York: Philosophical Library.

Eco, U. (1979). *Theory of Semiotics.* Bloomington, IN: Indiana Univ. Press.

Edelheit, H. (1969). Speech and psychic structure *J. Am. Psychoanal. Assoc.* 17:381–412.

Edelson, M. (1972). Language and dreams: the interpretation of dreams revisited. *Psychoanal. Study Child* 27:203–282

——— (1975). *Language and Interpretation in Psychoanalysis.* New Haven, CT: Yale Univ. Press.

Feldman, S. (1959). *Mannerisms of Speech and Gestures in Everyday Life.* New York: Int. Univ. Press.

Ferenczi, S. (1919). On the technique of psychoanalysis In *Further Contributions to the Theory and Technique of Psycho-Analysis.* New York: Basic Books, 1952 pp. 177–189.

Freedman, N. (1978). The bodily manifestations of listening. *Psychoanal. Contemp. Thought* 1 157–194.

———— (1983). On psychoanalytic listening: the construction, paralysis, and reconstruction of meaning. *Psychoanal. Contemp. Thought* 6 405–434.

———— & GRAND, S. (1985). *Shielding: An associative organizer. In From Research to Clinical Practice,* ed. G. Stricher & R. Keisner. New York: Plenum, pp. 353–373.

———— & Steingart, I. (1975). Kinesic internalization and language construction. *Psychoanal. Contemp. Sci.* 4 355–404.

Freud, S. (1912). Recommendations to physicians practicing psychoanalysis *Standard Edition* 12.

Friedman, L. (1988). *The Anatomy of Psychotherapy* Hillside, NJ: Analytic Press.

Gill, M.M. (1982). *Analyses of Transference Vol. I. Psychol. Issues Monogr. 53.* New York: Int. Univ. Press.

Gostynski, E. (1951). A clinical contribution to the analysis of gestures *Int. J. Psychoanal.* 32:310–318.

Gray, P. (1973). Psychoanalytic techniques and the ego's capacity for viewing intrapsychic conflict. *J. Am. Psychoanal. Assoc.* 21:479–494.

Horowitz, M. (1979). *States of Mind: Analysis of Change in Psychotherapy.* New York: Plenum.

Isay, R. (1977). Ambiguity in speech. *J. Am. Psychoanal. Assoc.* 25:427–452.

Jacobs, T. (1991). *The Use of the Self* Madison. CT: Int. Univ. Press.
Kohut, H. (1959). Introspection, empathy, and psychoanalysis. *J. Am. Psychoanal. Assoc.* 7:459–483.

Kris, A. (1982). *Free Association*. New Haven, CT: Yale Univ. Press. Lacan, J. (1968). *Speech and Language in Psychoanalysis.* Baltimore,

MD: Johns Hopkins Univ. Press.

———— (1977). *The agency of the letter in the unconscious, or reason since Freud In Ecrits.* New York: Norton, pp. 146–178.

Lichtenberg, J. (1983). An application of the self-psychological viewpoint to psychoanalytic technique In Reflections on Self Psychology, ed. J. Lichtenberg & S. Kaplan. Hillsdale, NJ: Analytic Press, pp. 163–185.

Luborsky, L. (1984). *Principles of Psychoanalytic Psychotherapy.* New York: Basic Books.

Lyotard, F. (1984). *The Post-Modern Condition* .Minneapolis, MN: Univ. Minnesota Press.

Major, R. & Miller, P. (1984). Empathy, antipathy and telepathy in the analytic hour. In *Empathy II* ed. J. Lichtenberg et al. Hillsdale, NJ: Analytic Press, pp. 227–249.

Merleau-Ponty, M. (1964). *Signs.* Evanston, IL: Northwestern Univ. Press.

Needles, W.F. (1959). Gesticulation and speech *Int. J. Psychoanal.* 40:291–294.

Ornstein, P. & Ornstein, A. (1985). Clinical understanding and explaining: the empathetic vantage point In *Progress in Self Psychology* ed. A. Goldberg. New York: Guilford Press, pp. 43–61. Panel (1959). The silent patient, H.F. Waldhorn, reporter. *J. Am. Psychoanal. Assoc.* 7:548–560.

Reich, W. (1949). *Character Analysis.* New York: Noonday Press.

Reik, T. (1948). *Listening with the Third Ear* New York: Farrar, Straus.

Rosen, V.H. (1961). The relevance of "style" to certain aspects of defense and the synthetic function of the ego. *Int. J. Psychoanal.* 42:447–457.

——— (1974). The nature of verbal interventions in psychoanalysis. *Psychoanal. Contemp. Sci.* 3 189–209.

——— (1977). *Style, Character and Language,* ed. M. E. Jucovy & S. Athens. New York: Aronson.

Schafer, R. (1976). *A New Language for Psychoanalysis.* New Haven, CT: Yale Univ. Press.

——— (1983). *The Analytic Attitude.* New York: Basic Books.

Scheflen, A. (1963). Communication and regulation in psychotherapy. *Psychiat.* 26 126–138

Schwaber, E.A. (1983). Psychoanalytic listening and psychic reality. *Int. J. Psychoanal..* 10:379–392.

——— (1984). Empathy: a mode of psychoanalytic listening. In *Empathy* Vol. 2 ed. J. Lichtenberg. et al. Hillsdale, NJ: Analytic Press, pp. 143–185.

——— (1986). Reconstruction and perceptual experience: further thoughts on psychoanalytic listening. *J. Am. Psychoanal. Assoc.* 34:911–932.

Shapiro, T. (1970). Interpretation and naming. *J. Am. Psychoanal. Assoc.* 18:399–421.

——— (1974). The development and distortions of empathy. *Psychoanal. Q.* 43:4–25.

——— (1979). *Clinical Psycholinguistics.* New York: Plenum.

——— (1981). Empathy: a critical reevaluation. *Psychoanal. Inq.* 1 423–448.

———— (1991). Words and feelings in the psychoanalytic dialogue. *J. Am. Psychoanal. Assoc.* 39 (Suppl.) 321–348.

Spence, D.P. (1982). *Narrative Truth and Historical Truth.* New York: Norton.

———— (1984). Perils and pitfalls of free-floating attention. *Contemp. Psychoanal.* 20:37–76.

———— (1987). *The Freudian Metaphor.* New York: Norton.

Thass–Thienemann, T. (1983). *Understanding the Unconscious Meaning of Language* New York: Aronson.

Viderman, S. (1979). The analytic space: meaning and problems. *Psychoanal. Q.* 48:257-291

Whorf, B. (1956). *Language, Thought and Reality,* ed. J. Carroll. Cambridge, MA: M.I.T. Press.

Wittgenstein, L. (1969). *On Uncertainty,* ed. G. E. M. Anscombe & G. H. von Wright. New York: Harper & Row.

APsaA 100th Anniversary Papers

Psychoanalysis in the U.S.: Recovered Memories and New Experiences of a Former Editor

(2011). *Journal of the American Psychoanalytic Association* 59:471–482.

Psychoanalysis in the first decade of the twenty-first century seems a very different discipline than it was during my tenure as editor of *JAPA* (1984–1993). As a former editor, I will take this opportunity to examine the scene today, in contrast to what was, and thereby mark our current boundaries by comparison. I will describe what I experienced at the end of my tenure and then review the ten-year period of that tenure, referring to some of the issues that seemed important then, before moving to the present.

I wrote somewhat coyly in my final editorial, "A View from the Bridge" (Shapiro 1993), "Now there is no such thing as an analysand without an analyst" (p. 926). This paraphrase of Winnicott suggestively indicates what I then thought was the change in focus in psychoanalysis at the end of my term. I specifically did not say whether it was healthy for psychoanalysis or a regression to a less formed, even amorphous, infantile state. As an editor, I was viewing the transformations I had witnessed in a brief ten years from the earlier experiences of the first editor, John Frosch, and his successor, Harold Blum. I also noted in that final statement that self-observation had become as central as patient observation and that a two-person psychology and subjectivity seemed inevitable for future theories.

This strongly subjective point of view was challenged by a cautionary exhortation from the Committee on Scientific Affairs (cited in Shapiro 1993). They wrote that the traditional case reports and cases as exemplars of theoretical principles could not serve as data for any scientific compilation or metaanalysis that psychoanalysts might wish to use to demonstrate a proposition. The cases presented had been disguised and focused to make a point and thus were biased. Such warnings seemed irrelevant to the writing psychoanalyst of my time. In addition, hermeneutics had taken hold. Some of our star theorists, including Roy Schafer, frequently graced our pages with the new Kleinians, while others wrote closely detailed case histories and process accounts, without any suggestion as to their import for further generalization. We seemed to have succumbed to the specific and, in contrast to the past, left the grand ideas of Hartmann and other *echt* ego psychologists behind.

In that same valedictory summary statement I noted that "on the horizon we see new interest in enactments, two-person systems, and interaction, as well as the power of fantasy construed as narration" (p. 928). I added that there was also interest in autobiographical memory as a construct rather than a replay of events experienced. Prospects for empirical opportunities were not as prominent, despite the recent work of Wallerstein, Kernberg, Luborsky, Dahl, and Thomä and Kächele, as well as Emde and Stern, who were doing exciting work in the developmental arena by directly observing babies and mothers. At term's end, prospects for a more traditional scientific future seemed dim. But at the same time there was rising interest in the incipient "Decade of the Brain," and hopes for a neuropsychoanalysis were in the air, even before the journal of that name emerged. Study groups sprang up with the intent of exploring the neuroscientific aspirations of Freud's earliest work, now influenced by knowledge based on neuroimaging and molecular biology.

In my plenary address to the American Psychoanalytic Association in 2003 (Shapiro 2004), I offered that psychoanalysts had put their hopes for the future in two distinct areas, one employing the neurosciences, the other embracing the hermeneutic aim of careful interpretation of texts. The latter was devoted to studying individual treatments as part of the *Geisteswissenschaften*. The reductionist hopes of the former pole were dismissed quickly as premature and irrelevant. Parenthetically, some of our most distinguished psychoanalysts also dismissed the relevance of developmental propositions derived from direct observation, thus bypassing some of our most creative psychoanalytic thinkers, including John Bowlby and Daniel Stern. Despite the revolution in attachment theory that followed, Bowlby was alienated from his own London psychoanalytic community and found his most friendly reception in the arena of American developmental psychology.

The hope that developmental studies would offer a better understanding of the origins of pathology was then displaced in some quarters by the hermeneutic search for *reasons* rather than *causes*. Psychoanalysts of that conviction were not interested in the ontogenesis of psychopathology or in mechanisms of change, or in the possibility of using process analysis to empirically demonstrate a treatment's contribution to good outcome. Retrospective outcome studies were also shunned. In the computer age, with tools for counting and categorizing ready to hand, the intersubjectivists and those devoted to hermeneutics retired to the consulting room and the "single case," rather than considering the probative aims advanced by Grünbaum (1984) as a challenge to American psychoanalysts of the late twentieth century.

In an editorial in 1985, I had responded to the challenge of Grünbaum's volume, calling for probity and clear scientific goals. I cited Arnold Cooper's 1984 presidential address, which argued for more research and better accommodation to the realities of the age of Prozac. I also cited the plenary address of Morton Reiser (1985), whose career was devoted to promoting empirical goals and the field's integration with neuroscience; it reads like a call from the young Freud himself. Interestingly, both these APsaA presidents had found a home in academic settings during the heyday of psychoanalysis within medical schools.

The tidal wave of the Grünbaum storm included Frederic Crews' Freud-bashing polemic (1985), an article that elicited a strong psychoanalytic response. I recall a large forum assembled in New York featuring Crews, followed by Robert Michels and Jonathan Lear in defense of psychoanalysis. These issues were even more salient following a talk by the future Nobelist Erik Kandel (1999), a friend of psychoanalysis who noted that although our field had been at the intellectual center in the first part of the twentieth century, due to the competitive excitement and interest created by developments in biological science, very few were listening now.

Grünbaum's and Kandel's confrontations were heard by few, because at the time no one in the profession had yet to feel the backlash that would come from a new generation of effective psychopharmaceuticals and from the evidence-based therapy movement, or to anticipate the economic crisis they would engender. These confrontations were reminiscent of the initial phase of my tenure as editor, when I reached out to what I had hoped would be a broader constituency of authors and readers engaged in doing and reading about empirical work as well as clinical work. In my initial editorial I wrote: "In short, a journal should be diverse and familiar, but also exciting so that it stimulates new ideas and sharpens both certainty and doubt. A journal is the recorded history of the ideas of a profession during the time of its publication. We can make it an extraordinary time if we believe that ideas are not static or objects of reverence. The Editor's job is to foster the most scholarly, well-argued and well-studied presentations of phenomena, cases or interdisciplinary efforts. The Editor's job is to shepherd the intellectual vitality of psychoanalysis" (Shapiro 1984, p. 10).

The response to this invitation did yield an increase in submissions concerning a broader variety of issues, including research. During the ten years from 1983 to 1993, we saw an average of 120 submissions a year and a rate of acceptance of about 20 percent. A thematic change was evident in many, as was true of the presentations at our semiannual meetings. Ego psychology was still strongly with us, but Kohut and his followers moved quickly to center stage. I wrote of the slow but real decline of papers in the Mahlerian idiom, and I am sure a citation count would document that. As much as the word *symbiosis* had dominated earlier volumes, by the middle of my term it was not to be seen on the printed page. On the other hand, Mahler's work had been subjected to greater scrutiny using empirical observational studies that somehow ceased to flourish after her death. I searched also for uses of the word *insight* and found it had been replaced by *empathy*, the central instrument and soundbite of self-psychology. Kohut's ideas were in their heyday. "Transmuting internalization" and "empathic listening" were everywhere, as analysts, reassessing their ego-psychological precursors, found their ideas too mechanistic and formulaic for work with patients. At the same time, there also were more submissions of papers based on systematic research.

Internationally, more analysts were focusing on psychic reality, and Kleinians worldwide contributed to that trend. Psychoanalysis seemed to embrace a new pluralism. Robert Wallerstein (1988), then president of the IRA, delivered, to the thirty-fifth International Congress in Montreal, an address with the provocative title "One Psychoanalysis or Many?" In statesmanlike manner, he traced our history from the divisions during Freud's life through the theoretical battlefield encompassed in the Controversial Discussions between Melanie Klein and Anna Freud. He concluded that we were all close enough in our central aims and essentials to qualify as "one psychoanalysis." The glue that bound us was transference and the consideration of unconscious mentation.

During this period of skirmishes concerning "who we are" and "where we are going," there was evidence that systematic empirical work was still being done. Judith Kantrowitz, Mardi Horowitz, Hartvig Dahl, and others published their findings in the journal. In collaboration with my associate editor, Robert Emde, we published a *JAPA* supplement on research (Shapiro and Emde 1995). Some of the empirical papers included there did not satisfy statistical requirements for optimal protection from bias, but in their spirit and intent they were sound enough to be called observational in the mode of the early naturalists. In some cases psychoanalytic researchers carefully studied mechanisms and processes, using taped analyses and new methods of looking at the dyad by measuring and codifying interactions. Others sought new knowledge regarding outcome and searched for evidence that could be tested without bias, so that psychoanalysis might at some future time be considered evidence-based and be compared with other treatments.

In addition, APsaA's semiannual meetings were host to a unique coming together of scientifically minded analysts attending the George Klein Forum hosted by Hartvig Dahl and others. Those Thursday morning meetings were packed with some of the most competent minds in psychoanalysis, and the data were fascinating and closer to a scientific ideal than the general forum provided. Nonetheless, most analysts showed a preference for clinical presentations, evincing a tacit split between clinicians and investigators that continues today. The establishment of a distinct research forum within APsaA in 2009 may bespeak the gradual removal of our science-minded colleagues from the larger clinical body, as they seek to interact with one another to enrich their hypotheses.

The climate described thus far soon waned, as a new wave of interest came crashing on the scene. Just past the midpoint of my tenure, the meetings began to feature "single-case presentations" viewed from various perspectives. Clinicians had an opportunity to show their technical virtuosity and sensitivity as they carefully described their clinical work in front of large audiences. They were critiqued and supervised from the audience. Many of these presentations were reported in the journal. This movement, of course, continued and flourished under the editorship of my successor, Arnold Richards.

It also should be remembered that during my term "the lawsuit," which led to a change in our heretofore exclusively medical association, was a prominent distraction. Psychoanalytic organizations subsequently became professionally hybrid. In my final report to the membership in 1993, I wrote: "During my tenure, the Gaskill amendment, the lawsuit with the psychologists, the relations with institutes, changes in our semiannual meeting… have all occupied our leadership."

Since 2001, graduates of non-APSA-approved institutes have become voting members of the organization. Now psychologists, social workers, and other nonmedical members have become our new scholars, investigators, readers, and constituency. The enrichment is obvious at our meetings and in our subscriptions. One would think that our ranks would have swelled by such action, but they have remained static, or have declined. This is so not only in the U.S. but internationally. During my tenure (in 1990) our subscribers numbered 7,100, while the membership stood at 3,021. We now claim 7,504 subscribers (2009). Submissions to *JAPA* have fallen significantly, though not for want of major efforts on the part of editor Steve Levy. Both *Psychoanalytic Quarterly* and the *International Journal* have experienced a similar falloff in submissions. That leads me to the inquiry that began this essay. Who are we today? What is American psychoanalysis (apologies to the other Americans to our north and south for my parochial usage) in relation to our compadres in Latin America, in Canada, and across the Atlantic? Who are the psychoanalysts of this and the next generation, and what drives our candidates to undertake our laborious and expensive education and join the "impossible profession"?

My view is parochial, because I see the field from my perch as a former editor and also from the vantage point of a physician who has been part of a large medical school in a university setting. This confession is apt, given the new stress on countertransference. I, in fact, cannot escape the bias of my commitment and my continuing devotion to a quest for better understanding, more knowledge, and a firmer basis for conviction. I have come to distrust what I call romantic coziness and the facile arguments of bedfellows of less rigorous thinking. I dread the call of some Lacanians who boldly indicate that understanding is not the aim of treatment. I have also been a coauthor, with Barbara Milrod, of three psychodynamic treatment manuals for panic disorder in adults and anxiety disorders in children and adolescents. I am in addition a co-principal investigator on a study of anxiety in children and adolescents using a treatment manual funded by APsaA's Committee on Research. I have been continuously active in the psychoanalytic arena, both at the New York Psychoanalytic Institute and the Columbia University Center for Psychoanalytic Training and Research. I have been book editor of the *IJP*, served as program chair of the 1999 IPA Congress in Chile, and have been contributing to the psychoanalytic literature for fifty years. These commitments help to explain my frame of reference and the description of our field that follows.

My history and biases recorded, I will approach my view of the current status of psychoanalysis in America. I will first make a distinction between the professional and the therapeutic aspects of psychoanalytic practice with patients; this will be followed by a broader consideration of the impact of psychoanalytic ideas on twenty-first century thought and culture. Perforce, I will refer to how the American scene differs from others and will describe the uniquely American influences in recent years.

As I have noted, the size of our professional group has remained static, despite the broader array of practitioners who have become psychoanalysts and the various new treatments now in use. I am, of course, not including in my count practitioners on the periphery, who work outside any monitoring agency, such as a certifying committee or an established psychoanalytic educational organization.

The reasons for our failure to grow are many, including the increased number of competing treatments, changing ideas about which populations could benefit from treatment, the financial crunch, and the social factors that dictate which disorders are considered amenable to psychoanalysis. Currently, we are a last outpost for intervention for those who suffer nonspecific personal misery of long duration, or serious personality disorders not amenable to other treatments. We tend to treat those who recognize their problems in achieving intimacy and adapting to stress. Many of our patients suffer emotional dysregulation in the form of anxiety and depressive affect, sometimes without meeting the diagnostic criteria for the full disorder.

The increased number of active and more directed interventions that have been subjected to double-blind, time-limited randomized trials, yielding evidence of their efficacy, remains the gold standard of modern therapeutics. These treatments stand up in contrast to other interventions and are less confounded by therapist bias. These treatments include CBT, which began as an intervention for depression and now is used for disorders including the classical anxiety disorders and OCD. Psychopharmacological treatment has been successful for symptom relief for many disorders, including depression, anxiety, OCD, and other neurotic disorders, as well as the psychoses. (We should remember here that Freud did not intend psychoanalysis as a treatment for psychoses or severe character problems.) Those with borderline personality disorders do well with a modified form of dynamic treatment; this is an area where such treatment has stood the test of head-to-head comparison with Dialectical Behavior Therapy. It must be said that other personality disorders fit well into the prolonged treatments that many analysts conduct.

The impact of recent financial concerns has been great, particularly for psychoanalysts who prescribe sessions at a frequency of four or five times weekly, without adjusting their fees. We should not be surprised that in the current economic climate, with fewer jobs and lower incomes, many patients balk. Economic constraints have always made analysis less available for lower socioeconomic groups. Moreover, the hundred years of psychoanalysis and its solid fifty years of dominance in the U.S. have not necessarily given the current generation a stronger conviction concerning its efficacy.

There are patients who do claim much benefit, but by and large they are now a small group, and word of mouth has not increased referrals.

The fact is that there are fewer patients available today, and that candidates seeking even low-fee referrals are having a difficult time getting training cases. Some newly trained analysts, in turn, have been accepting lower-fee patients, but also are doing more dynamic psychotherapy to balance out their practice. This situation of less demand creates a strain on the professional identity of analysts and diminishes the number of those seeking psychoanalytic training. It is a long, difficult, and, yes, expensive path toward a professional role that may be hard to sustain now and in the future. In addition, the increased number of nonmedical psychoanalysts has driven the price of treatment down for the physicians among us. Consequently, the number of physicians seeking careers as psychoanalysts has seriously diminished, because of lowered expectations for a reasonable economic return on the great investment of time and money required for medical education. Charles Fisher once told me that psychoanalysis needs an "economic re-analysis." There are some, including Karl Menninger, who in the past argued that psychoanalysis, a treatment performed by a rare small group, should be reserved for those who would themselves become mental health practitioners, rather than its being a broadly available intervention.

On the intellectual and humanistic side of the coin, it seems clear that Freudian ideas have continued to influence the larger academic and intellectual community. Post-Freudian thinkers such as Lacan and his ilk have been influential in literary criticism and cultural theory. Ricoeur continues as the hermeneutic patron, supportive of the Freudian model and idiom. Both of these important thinkers ignore empirical possibilities. Despite this presence, however, there has been a decline in Freud's influence, both in the social sciences and in academic psychology. Within the literature of psychoanalysis, a new variety of theories is popular. Two-person psychology is clearly central, as are themes of intersubjectivity and the analytic third. Some continue to discover the experiential love affair with the "case," and there is some overlap between the clinical report, literary criticism, and cultural applications. In this last area, there has been some healthy enrichment across humanistic disciplines, as well as in the field of intergroup conflict.

The Zeitgeist of twenty-first-century America may support many of these trends. While we are thought to be a pragmatic and technologically sophisticated society, we are also steeped in the humanities and the arts and are thus subject to infiltration by a romantic, antimechanistic, emotion-driven individualism that valorizes introspection and venturesome attitudes. This trend is curiously vital within the large urban communities where psychoanalysts tend to work, yet this romantic remnant is small, and its members are less likely to be economically solvent. They may not be able to afford an analysis or to take time from work to attend sessions. Curiously, Freud's own history is marked by his departure from the intellectually challenging academic laboratory to the consulting room, due to economic stress, only from there to discover a new science. He wished for scientific rigor in his discovery and exploration of conflict within the mind.

Despite the waning practice of psychoanalysis, Freud biographies and histories of psychoanalysis remain popular and are widely read. Some of these are Freud-bashing, but not all. In 2008, George Makari's book about the context and historical influences on Freud's ideas and the professional development of the psychoanalytic movement received broad acclaim. Psychoanalysis will continue to be a mainstay of our cultural and intellectual pursuit, but I am not sure its practitioners will be at the center of the Freudian movement. Norman O. Brown (1959), in a chapter called "Couch and Culture" in his Utopian tome *Love against Death*, predicted the demise of the treatment but the triumph of the ideas.

On the empirical side, there are continuing attempts to redis-cover and exploit the Freudian devotion to careful observation and systematic study. Process research remains popular, and there have been some studies of efficacy and even double-blind randomized trials. Recently *JAMA* and *The American Psychologist* have published metaanalyses of outcome studies of psychodynamic treatments (Shedler 2010; Leichsenring and Rabung 2008). Some have even tried to demonstrate, in fMRI studies, brain changes coincident with behavioral changes ascribed to psychoanalytic work.

The recent climate of professional pluralism and diminished enthusiasm is not unique to the United States. My travels abroad are fewer than in the past, but from the literature and from my continuing international contacts, it seems that elsewhere the scene bears close resemblance to what we are experiencing here. However, I believe the central figures in Latin America and Europe have remained steady, their practices more homogeneous than those in the U.S. South American analysts (especially in Argentina and Brazil) seem committed to theoretical elaboration and continue to espouse the work of Bion and Klein. In Europe, especially Germany, there has been a thirst to study dynamic therapies empirically (e.g., Thomä, Kächele, Beutel). This seems related to the public financing of treatments there, and to university-based psychoanalytic professorships, especially in psychosomatics. The British Society (largely in London) appears to be less theoretical and more case-centered, as British analysts maintain a serious devotion to careful clinical work, fostering constructs such as projective identification, which according to some American theorists is overapplied. This extravagance leads to more subjectivism and further therapeutic ambiguity. There are a few bright islands for investigators in London, however, largely at University College London and the Anna Freud Centre, where Peter Fonagy and Mary Target work, but also at the Tavistock Clinic, which has a mixed psychoanalytic representation and therefore more possibility for controversy.

I am not sure the contrasts I have provided for the American scene illuminate our psychoanalytic community, which I see as variegated and in flux. But in that diversity there seems little zeal for a coming together. In the past more energy was devoted to establishing a dominant school of psychoanalysis, a "movement" that would still bear the overriding qualifier *psychoanalytic*. In the recent past we have spoken of Freudians, Jungians, Kohutians, Mahlerians. Perhaps that is just part of the natural history of any new science. Not many twenty-first-century physicists call themselves Newtonian or Einsteinian. However, our recent theoreticians *do not challenge us with evidence*, but only with new ideas. Such lack of probity and failure to demonstrate better outcomes can be destructive of our future, because it leads to sectarianism and case-centered narratives, lacking generalizability on the basis of better outcome or even heuristic use. It promotes variation in practice, with no clear means of guaranteeing selection and survival. Indeed, much of the current climate is consonant with the American dream of individualism and the recent surge of libertarian conservatism. Perhaps psychoanalysis is an inquiry so personal, so directed to the inner life of the individual, that its survival will be found in a small group of analyzed persons. That last sentence may reveal the core of my problem. While I accept the limitations I have noted, I cannot but hope for a more optimistic future for a generative, ever-changing progression. I have never given up the idea of psychoanalysis as a science of the mind with universal implications. In that sense, I may seem out of step and be looking toward a time that has not yet arrived or, as many of my fellow analysts suggest, a metatheory that may be inappropriate for so intimate and personal an interaction. I believe that the current popular idea that the aim of exploring the inner life of *a person* cannot be expanded to more generalized ideas about *all persons* is a lazy solution to the more difficult path of engaging in the hard demonstration of generalized theories yet to come.

REFERENCES

Brown, N.O. (1959). *Life against Death*. New York: Basic Books.

Bucci, W. (1985). Dual coding: A cognitive model for psychoanalytic research. *Journal of the American Psychoanalytic Association* 33:571–608.

Cooper, A. (1984). Psychoanalysis at one hundred: Beginnings of maturity. *Journal of the American Psychoanalytic Association* 32:245–267.

Crews, F.C. (1985). The future of an illusion. *New Republic*, January 21, pp. 28–33.

Grünbaum, A. (1984). *The Foundation of Psychoanalysis: A Philosophical Critique*. Berkeley: University of California Press.

Horowitz, M.J., & Becker, T. (1982). The difference between termination in psychotherapy and psychoanalysis. *Journal of the American Psychoanalytic Association*41:765–776.

Kandel, E. (1999). Biology and the future of psychoanalysis. *American Journal of Psychiatry* 56:505–524.

Leichsenring, F., & Rabung, S. (2008). Effectiveness of long-term psycho-dynamic psychotherapy: A meta-analysis. *Journal of the American Medical Association*300(13):1551–1565.

Makari, G. (2008). *Revolution in Mind: The Creation of Psychoanalysis*. New York: HarperCollins.

Reiser, M. (1985). Converging sectors of psychoanalysis and neurobiology: Mutual challenge and opportunity. *Journal of the American Psychoanalytic Association*33:11–34.

Shapiro, T. (1984). Editor's introduction. *Journal of the American Psychoanalytic Association* 32:1–2.

———— (1985). Psychoanalysis, philosophy, and the public. *Journal of the American Psychoanalytic Association* 33:5–9.

———— (1989). Editorial: Our changing science. *Journal of the American Psychoanalytic Association* 37:3–6.

———— (1993). A view from the bridge. *Journal of the American Psychoanalytic Association* 41:923–928.

———— (2004). Use your words. *Journal of the American Psychoanalytic Association* 52:331–354.

———— & Emde, R.N. (1995). *Research in Psychoanalysis: Process Development, Outcome*. Madison, CT: International Universities Press.

Shedler, J. (2010). The efficacy of psychodynamic psychotherapy. *American Psychologist* 65:98–109.

PART III.

DIALOGUES
(USING LANGUAGE IN TREATMENT)

The three presentations that encompass this section continue the theoretical and practical applications of linguistics to psychoanalytic treatment elaborated in the prior section. Each essay was written for an invited occasion. The first, "Language Structure and Psychoanalysis," was my contribution to a symposium of the American Psychoanalytic Association on *The Concept of Structure in Psychoanalysis*. It appeared in print as a special self-edited volume of *JAPA* when I was Editor-in-Chief. The next contribution, "From Monologue to Dialogue," was presented as the 1999 Brill Lecture of the NY Psychoanalytic Institute and then as a paper in *JAPA* in 2002. The third, "Use Your Words," was the Plenary of the 2003 America Psychoanalytic Association meeting and appeared in *JAPA* in 2004. While discrete in focus, they cluster in time and significance as attempts to explore the cross-fertilization of linguistics and psychoanalysis during the shifting sands of psychoanalytic theory and practice from depth psychology through ego psychology to relational themes .

The extension of the theme of structure has a didactic purpose, linking the structure of language to the structure of the Freudian mind, insofar as it addresses the idea of structure in the work of the French linguist, de Saussure (considered to be the father of linguistics) and its relation to Freud's unique tripartite structural theory of mind. The theme was already in focus, as it is also addressed in the prior section of this volume. Psychoanalytic observation of surface behavior encountered in narratives from the couch during the psychoanalytic sessions can be subdivided into the contributions of hypothetical structures (id, ego, superego) of the Freudian structural theory of mind. In Freud's first topographic theory the sub units were organized in terms of conscious and unconscious elements (Cs, Pcs, Ucs). Saussure provides a representational model of our linguistic code in terms of signifier and signified and Chomsky later adds his model, referencing surface and deep structures in syntactic analysis, that encompasses the structure of any possible syntactic narrative. Incidentally, Lacan borrows significantly from Saussure's and Freud's topographies, creating a too-complex version of both of his teachers, who attempted to honor lucidity rather than ambiguity. Each and all theories noted thus posit transformational rules in order to illustrate the various ways in which the observer may interpret and understand any number of surface communications, from dreams to sentences and signs and symbols. The overlap of postulated structural mechanisms in both theories is striking, but also augments our tools, which aids better understanding. They are complementary in use, to help us further grasp meaning.

Communicative distortions such as transference, counter-transference, and also the salience of affect and need for defense and dynamic conflict, must be disentangled to be encoded in interpretive remarks that obey the rules of cognitive coherence. Summed up briefly, deep structures and the cognitive unconscious are not guarded against in a dynamic struggle for representation, as in the psychodynamic model, but they provide a structured cognitive scaffolding that provides rational description of the sometimes irrational dreams, parapraxes and symptoms we encounter at clinic.

The second paper, "From Monologue to Dialogue," is a response to the changing world of psychoanalytic interest, initially ranging from free association with a neutral analyst (a fiction) to the increasing participation of the analyst during the current revolution of "two-person psychology," steeped in dyadic models to account for enactments and distorted communicative sets. This move became relatively urgent beginning in the eighties through the first decade of the 21st century. Concepts such as intersubjectivity, coconstruction and various field theories such as the "analytic third" permeate our literature and panels. It was not difficult to see a similar overlap of revised focus within linguistics, away from intrapsychic models featuring transformational mechanisms to solve semantic and semiotic problems and the new role of inbuilt grammar and narratives, to what linguists now call pragmatics: speech acts or language in use and in action as performatives.

Meanings had to be interpreted in context to be fully understood, rather than as abstract transformational out-of-site formulas of mental work. The grammar and the references were more complex and related to social and personal expectations, indirect referencing, and social hierarchy, to name a few. This idea that meanings change with use in a dynamic field could be applied to analytic dialogues, reintroducing diachronic models as opposed to synchronic abstract structural models, which dominated the high period of the Chomskian revolution. Communication tropes had to be understood, and indirect intention and forms of verbalization that are known as performatives had to be recognized and analyzed as such.

The third paper, "Use Your Words," is a riff on the frequent demand by nursery teachers encouraging preschoolers to express their feelings and intentions verbally rather than in action. (I owe thanks to the Italian analyst Jacqueline Amati-Mehler, who had this paper translated into Italian for publication abroad). It is an early attempt to civilize the pre-latency students to a common goal using verbal appeal. The parallel injunction within psychoanalysis was to request uncensored monologue by the patient, in hope that these utterances might yield easier access to hidden intentions and aims and story sequences that were not within conscious intent or ken. The parallel junction during analysis was "do not act out," i.e. carry out your wishes into action and miss an opportunity to analyze the unconscious meanings.

While Freud's initial intent was to unveil unconscious wishes, he was confounded by defense and transference, which resistances were to be undone within the analysis. The shift of focus from patient to analyst permitted the observational field of interest to focus on the dyad and the reciprocal nature of the interaction. The civilizing function of language during development permits a linguistic analysis to become the instrument of discovery. New ideas were introduced to analysis that were intermingled with developmental linguistics and greater understanding of the way in which memories are stored at various stages of life, and enacted and dyadically expressed during therapy. Concepts such as role-responsiveness and words as substitute actions presented as performatives could intermingle in the jargon of the therapeutic encounter. This intermingling of language and development are further themes of this presentation, as well as the new adaptations in technique that require new tools for interpretation. The following section elaborates on my work in the arena of developmental time—from early years to later stages—and the persistence of patterned signifying fantasies.

Language Structure and Psychoanalysis

(1988). In *Structure and Psychoanalysis*
(ed. T. Shapiro) New York International Universities Press.

ABSTRACT:

De Saussure (1911) inaugurated the structural analysis of language at about the same time Freud began his seminal thinking about the structure of the mind. Nonetheless, roots in a common *Zeitgeist* has not led to an overlap of the fields of linguistics and psychoanalysis. Yet each discipline has a knowledge base that should be explored with respect to opening our minds to new findings in each field, on the basis of cross-disciplinary investigation.

There is a parallel course in attempts to understand language and psychology. This parallelism, and sometimes congruence, justifies study of the history of ideas in both domains in order to determine the roots and mutual influences between psychoanalysis and linguistics during the early part of the twentieth century. Freud, de Saussure, and Lévi-Strauss are among the most influential and generative thinkers who tacitly or explicitly have made this an era of structuralism. Structuralism is defined as "The systematic attempt to uncover deep universal mental structures as these manifest themselves in kinship and larger social structures, in literature, philosophy and mathematics, and in the unconscious psychological patterns that motivate human behavior" (Kurtzweil, 1980, p. 1). This definition brings us directly to the contribution of Lévi-Strauss as he has influenced our concept of structure during the twentieth century. However, Lévi-Strauss, himself, paid obeisance to Saussurean linguistics by applying that scholar's studies of language to the social sciences. Indeed, Lévi-Strauss' broader application included a debt not only to de Saussure, but also to Freud. Kurtzweil (1980) writes, "He [Lévi-Strauss] justifies the mixing of personal experience with intellectual interpretation by claiming geology, psychoanalysis and Marxism for his 'three mistresses'" (p. 14). Most psychoanalytic readers recognize Freud's influence on Lévi-Strauss, but may not have come upon Ferdinand de Saussure, who wrote little, but whose impact on linguistics and structuralism is universally acknowledged by the claim that he is the undisputed father of modern linguistics. He published fewer than 600 pages during his lifetime, but influenced many. Not only Lévi-Strauss, but Lacan and most modern linguists trace their roots from this brilliant professor who taught both in Paris and in Geneva. *Course in General Linguistics* (de Saussure, 1911) was taught from about 1906 through 1911, and parallels a period in Freud's own development during which he elaborated the theories of infantile sexuality and the role of unconscious functioning, and the beginnings of his metapsychological musings after the enormously influential case histories. The linguist's Course parallels exactly the period of Freud's interest in the beginning sway of the reality principle over the pleasure principle, and also corresponds directly to the time of writing when he drew parallels between linguistic theory and psychoanalytic theory. Freud was concerned not only with the structure of dreams (1900, 1917), but the structure of language and how memorial traces were organized in linguistic and visual imagery in screen memories (1899) and neurotic enactments (1914). It is unlikely that these men had read each other at that early juncture. We certainly do know that de Saussure's son later became a psychoanalyst. Nonetheless, the points of affinity between Freud and de Saussure were incorporated into Lévi-Strauss' work and that of later structuralists. Such an intellectual development requires some probing into the views of each progenitor toward the problems of language and psychology, in order to determine the mutual enrichment that evolved into the broader movement of structuralism and its countermovement, deconstructionism, that has emerged during the second half of this century.

De Saussure was an academic, a philological scholar; Freud started as a basic laboratory scientist, who then became a clinician. De Saussure dealt with texts and historical linguistics, originally. Freud dealt with animal models of the nervous system and then with individuals and their life histories. Yet de Saussure (1911) states, "Everything in language is basically psychological, including its material and mechanical manifestations, such as sound changes; and since linguistics provides social psychology with such valuable data, is it not part and parcel of this discipline?" (pp. 6-7). In order to bring home the overlap of interests, let me quote Freud in his letter to Fliess of December 6, 1896: "Thus what is essentially new in my theory is the thesis that memory is present not once but several times over, that it is registered in various species of 'signs' " (Freud, 1887-1902, p. 173; italics added). In *The Interpretation of Dreams* (1900), Freud wrote, "If we attempted to read these characters according to their pictorial value instead of according to their symbolic relation,

we should clearly be led into error. . . . A dream is a picture puzzle . . ."!
(pp. 277-278; italics added).

Each of these seminal thinkers believed there was much to
recommend the interrelation of the study of language and the study
of mental organization; and that the illumination of one area of
study impenetrably demanded constructs isomorphic to the second
level. Indeed, the notion of structure creates an ambiguity as to what
its referent is. Do we mean the structure of the product or of the
substrate? Linguists ask the question, "Does my analysis of language
and language as produced have a basis in the structure of mind, or
are the analyses the most parsimonious product of a fanciful analytic
system?" At the same time, psychoanalysts have asked, "Can my
understanding of human representation be construed as a species of
language—a theory of signs—and if so, is that system all-inclusive,
or do we need additional complementary knowledge to construe a
patient's productions?" A third issue that emerges is which system is
the more complete way of looking at mental functioning—linguistic
or psychoanalytic. *Webster's New Collegiate Dictionary* (1981)
defines structure as "the arrangement or interrelation of parts as
dominated by the general character of the whole." The *Oxford English
Dictionary* (1971) expands the idea defining structure as "the mutual
relation of constituent parts or elements of a whole as determining
its peculiar nature or character." Complementarily, the *American
Heritage Dictionary* (1982) indicates that we require structures to
construe, i.e., to analyze the structure of something is to place a
central role on meaning, on data, or to interpret. Thus, if we can
discover the orderliness in human experience and mental products,
we may be able to apprehend a mental organization that subsumes
such products. Such a supraordinate organization will permit us to
grasp redundant and significant elements that then can be considered

independent of the producer and lead to more universal models and themes than simple examples of a particular moment. Heterologous events will then become part of a representative or recurrent theme, or an index of a more basic unity known as a structure. De Saussure wrote, "Language, unlike speaking, is something that we can study separately" (p. 15). And again, "Whereas our speech is heterogeneous, language as defined, is homogeneous. It is a system of signs in which the only essential thing is the union of meanings and sound-images and in which both parts of the sign are psychological. Linguistic signs, though basically psychological, are not abstractions; associations which bear the stamp of collective approval—and which added together constitute language—are realities that have their seat in the brain" (p. 15).

With these remarks, de Saussure permits us to introduce the notion that each particular sentence uttered by an individual—each word—can be looked at from the standpoint of its organizational features and can be studied as musicians study a symphonic score. The metaphor of the symphony should be used to refer to language as an abstract whole, rather than any particular performance of that symphony, which would refer to an analogous speech utterance. Freud provided us with a similar metaphor by suggesting that any particular expression of a patient at a specific moment—whether symptom, slip of the tongue, or repeated action—can be studied from the standpoint of its hidden intentionality, as a representation of an unconscious wish. Moreover, each moiety of expression partakes of the various mental elements and agencies (id, ego, superego; thing- and word- presentation) required to make such a transformation at the time of a particular event. It could be said, in short, that every psychologically determined event has an unconscious precursor which has been acted upon in accord with topographic and/or structural[1] requirements of mind, so that each event refers to deeper elements. The surface manifestations stand for something else that is to be discovered in the analysis. Thus, protean forms of expression are reduced to a few unconscious structures according to rules of mental organization that can be stated as laws.

Freud's forays into mythology and historical analysis portray a similar propensity to use the concepts of regularity of mental structure toward the goal of finding out what is, and has been, common in the varied experiences that men report diachronically, i.e., over time spans. Lévi-Strauss' (1962) anthropology borrows a similar format and set of assumptions both from de Saussure and from Freud. Indeed, from the agreement of format between Freud's and de Saussure's ideas about the study of language, we could also say that Freud would qualify as a structuralist—and yet such a categorization would deny his primacy as progenitor of the movement and the debt admitted to Lévi-Strauss. Perhaps it is a *Zeitgeist* that gives rise to a particular kind of theoretical construct or method of construing the world and mind. Perhaps the "great man theory" of history has to be tempered by an overriding readiness to nurture an "idea whose time has come," and the person who spawns that idea becomes the midwife that Socrates said the philosopher was. De Saussure and Freud clearly were following similar paths from different perspectives, devoting their efforts to what was cramming—although Freud was the more innovative in moving away from the tasks he was trained to do. Whatever the reasons for the congruence between the thought of these two figures, the commonalities recommend that we call them structuralists while begging the question of prior or mutual

---

1   *Structural* is used here to refer to Freud's second theory of mind, with its tripartite division into ego, id, and superego.

influence. In order to look at how psychoanalysis parallels language theory, we have to see how the models match each other, even though the originators of the models studied different texts.

Both systems accept that there are certain fixed properties in the way the mind works to symbolize and to create signs. Moreover these properties are universal, although different cultures may give preference to certain variants of any basic mechanism. The mechanisms can be studied by methods that address different levels of organization, which in turn reveals the underlying orderliness that defines each system. It would be less important for psychoanalysts to designate how their structural theory is in line with more general structuralist ideas than it would be to look at how the psychoanalytic situation and psychoanalytic process obey the rules of language organization and use. It may indeed be amusing, if not enlightening, to pinpoint how psychoanalysis has unwittingly created a parallel science to linguistics while not being within a particular linguistic school, but rather part of a school of its own, called psychoanalysis. Some have alluded to Piaget's idea that any structure has a general set of organizational features (see Pulver, This Volume; Shapiro, 1979). Piaget (1970) indicates that any concept of structure includes the ideas of wholeness, of transformation, and of self-regulation.

Wholeness demands that we recognize that we apprehend whole perceptions rather than grasp smaller units that make up such a whole. This notion is similar to the *Gestalt*ist idea that one cannot analyze the experience of a whole in terms of small events or particles without destroying the overriding effect of whole experience. Moreover, the smaller units, even if understood, do not permit the whole to be understood. Self-regulation involves the possibility of a feedback mechanism so that the whole as experienced can be maintained or reexperienced over time, or the individual can regulate himself in relation to perceived structures and maintain a state of adaptiveness to external events. The interplay between homeostatic mechanisms and interactive mechanisms becomes paramount in such a self-regulatory system, and has more specific salience to the repetitive nature of psychological expressions. The concept of transformation presumes a set of mechanisms available to the symbolic producer. Defensive functions or signal affects may qualify. These mechanisms of transformation permit symbolic changes, such that an individual may represent a small body of mental algorithms or paradigms in a large number and variety of actions, symptoms, or behaviors—in the same way that a small set of grammatical rules may be applied to a very large array of lexical items (words) in order to create or encode an infinite array of particular sentences, which in turn relate to a very small number of paradigms.

Linguists might say that the surface structure of any particular sentence is heterologous, but that each possible sentence can be related to a deep structural organization which is necessary to presuppose its formation by a human being. Chomsky's (1975) notion of the split between production and competence is central to this notion, as is Freud's idea that any number of enactments are related to a deeper mental organization that dictates the repeated expression of an idea. Both require a structural theory made up of wholes, transformations, and self-regulatory possibilities. What are the circumstances of a symptomatic idea or act being brought into awareness at a particular moment? What are the particular mechanisms at work and what elements at what level of organization are transformed in order to bring the experience or enactment about? How are all the agencies of mind represented in each enactment so that we regularly discern more basic themes? What are the symbolic processes that permit representation in imagery or words or actions?

These queries and their answers indicate that structure permeates our psychoanalytic thinking; else, we could not even represent our methods and models of work in a parsimonious way. If we had no structural theory, everything that happened would be heterologous and unrelated. There has to be a core conceptual relation between the content experience and the conceptual frame that functions as our model of mind.

Our familiarity with the traditionally stated models of psychoanalysis (topographic, structural, genetic, dynamic, etc.), so well outlined by Rapaport (1967), fixes us in a frame of reference that has yielded much. However, it might be refreshing to see if another frame, that of traditional linguistics, could give us a new way to look at our data. Sometimes we can learn more about ourselves by looking through the eyes of another. Indeed, there is a naturalization of experience that evolves out of too-persistent use of the same language (used as a metaphor). Jespersen (1964), the Scandinavian linguist, tells of a German woman who remarked "How come the French call them étoiles and the English call them *stars*, when everyone knows they are *Sterne*?" Perhaps we can evade the assumptive trap of "everyone knows" if we turn our attention now to the language of the linguist and see if we can gain new insights from the way he looks at data.

Linguistic scientists require a reduction of data and a series of vantage points from which to work. They deal initially with sounds and their organizations into phonemes (the minimal differences in sound that natural speakers recognize). The next level is represented as morphemes (the minimal unit of sound that has significance in signaling meaning in a particular language) such as the terminal "s" sound which signifies either possession or pluralizes. The latter are called grammatical morphemes, because they are required to make well-formed sentences. Individual lexical items (words) and sentences are the next two levels to be recognized. While the linguist studies these varying units as they are represented in the transformations he postulates in the creation of discourse, the psychoanalyst studies symptoms, events, slips, and dreams in accord with a number of Freudian systems. Initially, there was the topographic theory, then the structural model, and finally the elaboration of a polysemantic system embodied in the concept of multiple function took hold (Waelder, 1930). We talk of defense and resistance and compromise formation that are evident in how patients express conflicts in surface phenomena. Similarly, if we invoke an object-relations model, we come to see how mental objects are represented and substituted for in varying symbolic systems.

In addition to the stated operations performed on the contents of language expressions, linguists trifurcate their studies into systems that are pursued as separate domains. They study grammar, or syntax, representation or signification, and pragmatics, which refers to the study of dialogues and how intentionality is conveyed between and among speakers—it is the study of language in use. Although these linguistic studies are free of concepts such as unconscious mental functioning in a dynamic sense, they do postulate processing out of awareness, and provide a systematic *entrée* to their subject which we can, perhaps, apply to psychoanalytic data to determine if such application adds to our understanding. By use of parallel processing in linguistic and psychoanalytic terms, we may enrich our view as well as make complementary conclusions (Shapiro, 1979). Similarly, it will be of interest to suggest how dynamic considerations may enrich the more formal linguistic structures. In order to review some of the overlapping and parallel functioning and demonstrate how such a construal (explication of structure) might work, I shall consider an event that occurred in my own analysis.

Early in my career I had a dream while in analysis. It was a pleasant enough dream in which I was led to a dock on Martha's Vineyard that I had visited the summer before. I was told that the boat at the mooring was mine. It was a large motorcraft—I was impressed, but surprised, that it was mine and protested with some ambivalence that I did not like motorboats, that I really had been fond of sailboats. How was I to accept this boat as mine, impressive as it was? Even in the dream it was not a part of my understood wishes. I had not longed for a yacht.

It would be all too easy to carry out an anagogic interpretation of this dream, making reference to a multiplicity of simplistic yacht to body part transformations and inferring that we understand its meaning. However, its significance became known to me only through an understanding of its current derivative function in the context of my life at the time regarding career opportunities and career choice. Sailing had indeed been a new excitement, and I had generated some enthusiasm for the newly learned sport during the previous summer. I also had just begun a new job and my practice, both of which occupied a great deal of time; I also was going to classes at the Psychoanalytic Institute, and had a young child. Then, I was offered a highly prized position that involved close association with Marianne Kris, among others, on a psychoanalytic research project. I was sorely tempted to add yet another job to my already full workload. However, it was clear to me that it would be most difficult in terms of time and distribution of psychic energy were I to take this job. And yet, how could I turn down a position where I would be an intimate of such distinguished company? I did not understand the relation of this dream to my life, however. As I began to try to put the dream images into words, I described the distinctions between a motorboat and sailboat, and I described the joy I had from my new skill at sailing. I seemed to feel some pressure to help the analyst understand what kind of boat it was that I had been offered, and could not be satisfied that I had conveyed the image, although the distinction between motor and sail was simple. It was only when I uttered the name of a commercial motorboat, Chris-Craft, that I realized that the fulfillment of owning a boat of this sort was related to the prestige and importance that it would give me rather than what I had passionately enjoyed doing that summer. I will not belabor the homophonic relation to Kris, but it should be apparent that the elegant and prestigious new acquisition I had created in my dream stood for the ambivalent wish to take the position that would have compromised my coping in reality [Shapiro, 1986, pp. 115B116].

Reference

From the standpoint of semiology or the theory of signs and reference, we must determine how the signifier relates to the signified. The point of tension presented in the dream centered about the inability to find the link between the pictorial representation of a large motor craft which ultimately was designated as a Chris-Craft and that became

a representation of the person who offered a position that further signified fulfillment of an ambitious aim.

Were it not that I, as dreamer, had had an opportunity offered by a particular person whose name happened to be a homophone for a trade name of a boat, and had that boat not been known to me as a culturally available lexical property that was included in my general information store, I could not have created or drawn upon either the imagery in the dream or the phonetic shape of the sign in order to make reference to the larger idea that finally emerged in the interpretation. Thus, the polysemanticity of the reference system and the high specificity of the particular vehicle of representation and its vocal designation were both in consciousness in one form, but were formed unconsciously. The emergence of the idea and its particular mode of formation were dependent on a set of fixed relations between sign, meaning, and phonetic shape, as they related to significance. The affectivity that emerged is important to us as analysts and requires attention, because linguists do not traditionally attend to such noncognitive representations unless they take literature or poetry as a text. I have argued elsewhere (Shapiro, 1979) that any system of reference that does not include the possibility of considering affective valence as a feature of definition is incomplete.

Freud's (1900) early foray into the study of thing- and word- presentations in *The Interpretation of Dreams* takes on new importance in this context, providing the essential elements in our method of understanding such a referential sequence. The imagery of signification was already well established in his paper "Screen Memories" (1899), bringing us closer to the visual configurations as they relate to words. Perhaps Lacan (1956) was the closest to the mark when he suggested that we return to Freud, circa 1900, in order to find the tools to understand man's complex referential system. It was he who reminded us that the science of psychoanalysis bears a close relation to textual analysis in the reading of symbols. He, too, claimed a strong reliance on the Saussurean method, even using de Saussure's terms signifier and signified. However, Lacan's elaborate system leads to confusion, because of his tendency to aphoristic nonlinear paradox and metaphoric explanation rather than rational elaboration. As he sought the meanings of presentations, he also sought to upset traditional and fixed formulaic thinking.

Approaching the referential system from a more straightforward Saussurean view suggests that linguistics can provide psychoanalysis with an elegant understanding of definition, denotation, and connotation.[2] If we finally add personal idiolectic references, we can round out the limits of semantic analysis as a complement to the psychoanalytic view of symbols.

Linguists provide us with a system of definition or denotation in which one can break definition into a feature analysis. Words are defined by a limited number of fixed elements called features. Thus "bachelor" becomes, by feature analysis, unmarried male, but by extension to common usage and connotation, we have to make an adjectival or adverbial addition to refer to women who are similarly unmarried. A woman bachelor is sometimes called a spinster, but the latter confuses us further because the word has taken on additional meanings (connotations) that are culturally

---

2   *Denotation* refers to the strict definition of the sign. It is meaning in its narrowest sense:a pointable. *Connotation* refers to the richer associative meanings of a sign, broadening its significance in accord with usage and cultural accretions. *Idiolect* refers to linguistic forms or words that have highly personalized, even autistic, significance.

and temporally determined, making the word not equivalent to the relative neutrality implied in bachelor. Now if we add that the feature analysis may include idiosyncratic or culturally limited aspects of affective valence to define the word, then the word can be fully represented (at least within the confines of a temporocultural period). In some cultures being a bachelor is equivalent to being a bum or a homosexual or a repressed male, and socially discriminatory features have been known to be associated with the word if not the person. Thus, for a complete referential analysis, psychoanalytic concepts such as affective significance may be added to our linguistic feature analysis to give a more complete description. However, the central task of making the unconscious conscious and rendering the symbols understandable requires both psychoanalytic and linguistic parsing. Thus, the emergence of the word that described the boat was crucial to the emergence of the significance of the representation. Moreover, the relief was experienced only in the expression of the word, not the image, as though the breakthrough into consciousness was achieved at the moment of phonetic encoding. Only then could the correspondence be secured. The sequence seemed roughly as follows: The image referred to the word that was a homophone for the person who represented a tempting fulfillment. The latter was certainly idiosyncratic to me, the dreamer, i.e., an idiolectic reference that would not hold universally across persons.

Syntax

From a syntactic viewpoint, we must construe the grammar of the dream as well as the structure of the sentences used in the discourse. These elements are frequently ignored and lost, unless the analyst attends to such formal characteristics as an area of curiosity, or has been alerted to such features as carrying a message. The visitation to the dock; the information that the boat belonged to me; the attempt to envision the gift-giving as a process; the flow of my own ideas of gratitude and surprise; the pride, the rejection, and dismay, all have to be put in some organized format that could be read from the standpoint of *I*, as an agency and subject of a sentence and author of the dream. The process of being granted something must also be considered, i.e., of being an object of a sentence and a recipient of a wish. This is all grammatical formalism up to this juncture. If one were to pin it even more squarely to the language of the unconscious, how could I wish for something so prestigious and reject it at the same time, i.e., wish not to receive it? What elements of my psychological makeup would be included in this grammatical formula? In addition, what early wishes corresponded to the sequence presented? How do they parallel or resonate with current wishes? What elements of my mental apparatus participated in the grammar of conflict presented in the imagery and in my ultimate verbal summary of the manifest dream?

The grammatical format is complicated by both an acceptance of the honor implied in the gift and the clear rejection of it by my uneasy explanation that I like sailing, not cruising. Another contrast can be drawn between my life circumstance as it existed and the relative immutability of wishes that stem from childhood and their expression at the time of the dream, as if current circumstance did not count. There is no doubt that I wished for early achievement and recognition. If we search for the most parsimonious grammar of that wish in a human circumstance of growing up in a family, Oedipal wishes are as paradigmatic as the general grammatical form of subject, verb, object is to any possible sentence. In addition, if we are to trace the agencies of the mental apparatus that participated in the syntax, we must account for the rejection of the offer in the dream discourse as the injunction, "Perhaps you should not have it"! "You are too young; you do not wish to be envied; you need more work before you are given such a possibility for intimacy with so prestigious a senior colleague."

A competitive element also rose to awareness following the dream between my allegiance to my established position and the job offered. It may also represent a competitive element within my own ambition that had to be recognized. What was the moral commitment to a job accepted as opposed to a job that came later, but provided such a visible entrée to an arena that seemed to be forbidden until one was of age? All of these must enter into the formation of the dream that could represent so much in so brief a moment of dreaming. These all suggest an elaboration of what might be construed in its most basic form as an Oedipal conflict. One might even ask or consider further whether the boat itself represented a body part imaged as an external possession to be gratuitously given. With that elaboration we may even conjecture that now a possibility of reunion with the earliest representation of the source of life itself, the original mother, might be possible. The fantasy may even have been that such reunion or new union might result in the creation of the perfect baby and other creative products that might naturally ensue.

Arlow (1988) has indicated that representability as construed in the topographic theory obeys linguistic structural models more than the psychoanalytic structural theory does. I believe that he is correct, if we consider the concept of structure as a referential system rather than as a syntactic system. He notes further that we gain in the use of a structural theory of representation insofar as every mental content representing conflict should show the evidence of all three agencies.

Thus, psychoanalysis as practiced in the light of structural theory must derive its meaning from a representation of compromise itself. A syntactical analysis would permit all agencies to be represented as well, because grammar permits the representation of relationships among the nouns of a sentence. Moreover, it would not require that the modes of transformation, i.e., defenses, be anything but unconscious and function automatically, out of awareness, almost as brain cells function automatically to do the brain's work. In short, the dream as presented managed very well to present a wish, an injunction against its fulfillment, and a compromise. These are syntactic structures insofar as they represent sequential relationships.

Pragmatics

The third area of linguistic analysis, Pragmatics, is the study of intentions and language in use in communication. Conscious intentions are read from elements in a speech event. However, such a reading or interpretation requires more than a grammatical or semantic analysis. The dialogue that takes place between patient and analyst must be viewed pragmatically. Pragmatics also shares certain structural elements with the other vantage points, this time interpersonal organizations. Dialogues involve turn-taking and the expression of intentionality, and draw on the complexity of social rules of discourse and topic maintenance. To obtain a complete linguistic understanding of an event, it is insufficient to know only the grammatical and referential format of that event. For example, ironic statements grammatically and semantically say exactly the opposite of what is meant, therefore requiring knowledge of context for interpretation. Similarly, consider the casual comment of the father as his child walks into the room, "It is cold in here!" The child then closes the window. The grammatical parsing of the sentence uttered *per se* does not provide adequate information to decipher the message and the intention of the message that led to the child's action. These are embedded in social conventions which are to be understood in the context of dialogues. The rules of such dialogues within our culture are by now fairly well-described and have certain fixed determinants. The relationship of the analyst to the patient and the patient to the analyst also is structured by conventions that are fairly well known.

How patients use or misuse these conventions constitutes part of the work we do to help patients see the defensive or resistant significance of their actions.

For example, there are patients who will not ask about the analyst's personal life because they know they are not supposed to know about such matters. Such patients frequently disobey the cardinal rule of saying what comes to mind, because they consider such wishes as deviations from the rule structure of the analysis. We thus lose opportunities to analyze, because such patients omit data we need to know in the service of ostensible compliance. There may be gaps in the productions which we can notice, but we are never sure what is in mind until the patient ventures commentary on what has happened. Let us return to the dream example that we have been considering and now look at the pragmatics of the presentation. What could the dream have meant transferentially? In what role was I placing the analyst, given the context of my ideas? Initially, I felt discomfort in my inability to describe the boat adequately. I was unable to come to rest mentally with a feeling of satisfaction until I was able to utter Chris-Craft, suggesting both to myself and to my analyst that I had continued mental tension, that I was not communicating, that there was a message in the dream image that was not conveyed in the language and lexicon I had used up to the point. I had not come to mental closure in relation to my wish to convey an idea to him. Only when I was able to realize the linkage between the name of the boat and the name of the person who offered the job was the tension relieved. From the standpoint of pragmatics, why did I have to disguise this element of conflict, which was available to me at some level, since I was consciously mulling over my choice? After all, I had made the choice not to take the job, I had weighed the elements of its practicality, the potentials for advancement, the ambition, all consciously. What I had not weighed, however, was what would my analyst think—where would he stand? Did he represent the forbidding and cautionary father saying, "You have time for such ambition" and thus, be in favor of not taking the position? Would he have been partial to the more psychoanalytic of the jobs? How would I show my intention to follow a path he took and would wish for me? In so childlike a concern, would I defensively have shielded my more aggressive Oedipal ambitions? Where could I come to rest in my dialogue with him in revealing my intention without revealing my ambivalence and hostility? It seems apparent that the structure of the transference is also a linguistic structure couched in terms of dialogue. Indeed, the *who* of the transference and its reference to a personal past becomes an element in the translation of the meaning of the interaction, just as the dream image becomes the representation in a visual vehicle of a referential token from the repressed past. In that sense, the notion of intrapsychic conflict enriches the understanding of linguistic dialogues, but the dialogic format and its formal restraints should help psychoanalysts to realize formerly missed elements of interaction that can enrich psychoanalytic alertness.

CONCLUSIONS

It should be apparent from the foregoing that the levels of linguistic organization, grammatic, referential, and pragmatic, handily fit into the analysis of a psychoanalytic event. Moreover, analysis of the unconscious meanings significantly adds to our grasp of the underpinnings of the signifier. Thus, the dimensions of the event are more than linguistic, but also psychoanalytic. Can we bring the two together, as others have tried to do, by suggesting that the most complete description of that moment or process can be derived from application of the concept of structure in its many dimensions? Structure must now be seen to include unconscious features as well as conscious aspects of linguistic organization, thanks to psychoanalysis. It is not by chance that Freud's (1891) initial interests, which evolved into psychoanalysis, included a strong affinity for J. Hughlings Jackson's work on aphasia and the curiosity that led to his further interests in language (Freud, 1910, 1913, 1925). These movements around Freud permitted him to make the shift from biological curiosity to psychosocial exploration. His creative involvement in both areas led to psychoanalysis. Psychoanalysis shares with linguistics its interest in semiology and the modes by which human beings represent their ideas, their memories, and their histories. Linguistics is the mother science of structuralism, and Freud shares many affinities with structuralism. Indeed, most structuralists pay him some obeisance along with de Saussure. It seems appropriate that even as we consider structure within psychoanalysis, we also should consider what the most current theory of language structure purports. Because of its structural regularities, language can be construed and speech events interpreted. If to construe means to interpret, then psychoanalysis itself is of necessity a part of the linguistic sciences, and if language structures are psychologically mapped, the linguistic sciences are a part of psychoanalysis.

As I bring this essay to a close, I venture that the current wave of deconstructionism should be seen as antithetical to structuralism. Its very popularity stems from similar roots to any intellectual movement that negates or undoes that which came before. Although we may respect the possibilities of multiple readings of a text, we must also define the rules of discourse that permit such diversity. Structuralism provides such limits and therefore remains within a rationalist tradition. Deconstructionism threatens such limits by its potential Babel of tongues and by extension a Babel of meanings. It does not postulate a deep structure that permits a reading and therefore the core underpinning of events, and utterances cannot be discovered and uncovered. Such a mode may be well and good for literature, but not for a human science of the mind that is at least in part deterministic. Both Freud and de Saussure sought such rigor amidst their broader humanistic concerns, and each fathered a fruitful generation of students of structure.

REFERENCES

Arlow, J. (1988). in *Structure and Psychoanalysis* (ed., T. Shapiro) New York: International Universities Press, pp. 283–294.

Chomsky, N. (1975). *Reflections on Language.* New York: Pantheon Books.

De Saussure, F. (1911). *Course in General Linguistics.* New York: McGraw-Hill, 1966.

Freud, S. (1887B1902). *The Origins of Psycho-Analysis: Letters to Wilhelm Fliess,* ed. M. Bonaparte, A. Freud, & E. Kris. New York: Basic Books, 1954.

———— (1891). *On Aphasia.* New York: Int. Univ. Press, 1953.

———— (1899). Screen memories. *S.E.,* 3.

———— (1900). The Interpretation of Dreams. *S.E.,* 4 & 5.

———— (1910). The antithetical meaning of primal words. *S.E.,* 11.

———— (1913). The philological interest of psycho-analysis. *S.E.,* 13.

———— (1914). Remembering, repeating and working through. *S.E.,* 13.

———— (1917). A metapsychological supplement to the theory of dreams. *S.E.,* 14.

———— (1925). Negation. *S.E.,* 19.

Jesspersen, O. (1964). *Language, Its Nature, Development and Origin.* New York: Norton.

Kurtzweil, E. (1980). *The Age of StructuralismCLévi-Strauss to Foucault.* New York: Columbia Univ. Press.

Lagan, J. (1956). *The Language of the Self: The Function of Language in Psycho Analysis.* Baltimore: Johns Hopkins Univ. Press.

Levi-Strauss, C. (1962). *The Savage Mind.* Chicago: Chicago Univ. Press, 1966.

Piaget, J. (197()). Shucturalism. New York: Harper & Row. Rapaport, D. (1967). *Collected Papers,* ed., M.M. Gill. New York: Basic Books.

Shapiro, T. (1979). Clinical Psycholinguistics. New York: Plenum.

———— (1986). Sign, symbol and structural theory. In *Psychoanalysis: The Science of Mental Conflict—Essays in Honor of Charles Brenner,* ed., A. Richards, & M. Willick. Hillsdale, NJ: Analytic Press, pp. 107–125.

Waelder, R. (1930). The principle of multiple function: observations on overdetermination. In *Psychoanalysis: Observation, Theory, Application,* ed. S.A. Guttman. New York: Int. Univ. Press, 1976, pp. 68–83.

From Monologue to Dialogue: A Transition in Psychoanalytic Practice

(2002). *Journal of the American Psychoanalytic Association* 50:199–219.

During the latter part of the twentieth century, psycho-analysts of various stripes espoused the move from free association and neutrality to various forms of intersubjectivity and dialogue. This shift is studied from the vantage point of conversational rules in terms of the shift from monologue to dialogue, using the concepts of semantics, syntax, and pragmatics. Viewing the data of analysis in this manner offers a means of evaluating the contributions of both monologue and dialogue to our understanding of the conduct of an analysis and the kind of information that can be expected to emerge. Exclusive devotion to either stance, it is argued, renders less understanding than would emerge from a balanced use of both.

The recent shift within psychoanalysis from what has been called a one-person psychology to a two-person psychology parallels the change in emphasis from intrapsychic to intersubjective phenomena over the past century. Some believe the shift is from a focused positivistic study of mind from outside to a dynamic equilibrium of rapidly changing states and a participant observational stance. The shift seems absolute to some and simply a refocus within ego psychology to others. Some hover between the two positions (Wasserman 1999). In what follows I will present a perspective that promises to bypass the paradox of a two-person psychology.

I will examine our evolving psychoanalytic psychology by looking at these changes in terms of a linguistic analysis of monologue and dialogue. These conversational modes designate how persons communicate. Each is, however, incomplete if we are also to understand the human psyche as an emotionally charged cognitive-linguistic entity embedded in a person within a social matrix.

David Riesman (1950) noted a somewhat parallel shift of emphasis in the sociological domain, in the changed focus from inner-directedness to outer-directedness. Alvin Toffler (1970) added the idea of postmodern modular man as a late-twentieth-century addendum. I will dwell mostly, however, on the excitement and new knowledge within our discipline fostered by the study of semantics during the earlier part of the century through the Chomskian 1950s and 1960s, when syntax was paramount, to the more recent focus on the pragmatic study of language in use between persons. Each approach complements the others. Each has provided important data that inform the theory of therapeutic action. I will briefly traverse the significant events in the march within psychoanalysis as I see it, and then shift my perspective to an analysis of psychoanalytic practice from the standpoint of language theory. Finally, I will summarize the linguistic methods of inquiry available and their limitations.

Psychoanalysis

We all know that Anna O., Breuer and Freud's first psychoanalytic patient (1893–1895), described her progression out of hysteria as a "talking cure." Her talk was largely a soliloquy uttered in altered states of consciousness. Freud's subsequent theories encouraged monologues in free association. He admonished patients to rid their talk of censorship in order to reveal their inner life and psychic conflict. Under the rubric of automatic writing, a similar movement was rampant among authors in the early decades of the twentieth century.

Initially these monologues were thought to be a means of making the unconscious conscious, and of discovering symbolically transformed neurotic compromises. Anything that stood in the way of revealing unconscious fantasy was considered a defense or, later, a resistance.

For Freud every utterance revealed but also hid. The analyst was advised in a series of metaphors not to gratify the drives (Freud 1912, 1916-1917). Neutrality, evenly hovering attention, and relative silence supported the patient's monologue, expressed in safety with a non-judgmental therapist. That cure or relief did not always follow from such uncovering troubled Freud and, later, others, leading to changes in technique.

Freud's first discovery leading to a changed stance and ultimately to the intersubjective and two-person model was transference, followed later by countertransference. Freud's first designation of transference was that of transference resistance, i.e., an intrusion in the process of uncovering, and therefore antitherapeutic. The impact on psychoanalytic technique of the discovery that the transference enactment could represent an unconscious fantasy was itself revolutionary. This now historic moment of shift became the basis of Strachey's extravagant proposal (1934) that only transference interpretations are mutative.

If we are to study transference we must focus also on the analyst's countertransferences. The loop is closed; the positivist stance of observing the patient now includes observing the analyst as well. This additional focus on the analyst has generated a variety of technical recommendations that together have become the "new psychoanalysis."

Dialogical interpersonal trends, represented by Sandor Ferenczi, Clara Thompson, and Harry Stack Sullivan, were in the air even during the middle years of the last century. Until very recently, Sullivan's interpersonal theory had been separated from traditional psychoanalysis. By contrast, the Lacanian and other French schools, more than others, maintain a one-person monologue with an almost silent analyst. Changing patient populations have also had their effect on technique. Stone's widening scope (1981) formally introduced the more talkative analyst into dealings with borderline patients. In addition, ideas such as the therapeutic alliance and the holding environment have supplemented transference interpretation as potentially mutative forces.

As two-person psychoanalysis took hold, the modern Kleinians' focus on projective identification (see Schafer 1997) and Sandler's reframing of this phenomenon into "role-responsiveness" and the phenomena referred to as "enactments" (1976) certainly attracted attention. Every enactment requires a collusion that reinforces the belief of each participant about the other. The analyst must bring this matter to attention for analysis. This technical maneuver brings the analyst's vulnerabilities into sight but nonetheless offers a contribution from both parties and an opportunity to ask, "Can we learn from what just happened?" A cooperative inquiry!

The analyst, now vigilant of self as well as other in the new Kleinian mode, may too readily assume that the patient has caused him or her to think or act in a certain way responsive to that patient's habitual patterns. It is important to remember, however, that the analyst's ideas derive also from personal sources (Boesky 2000).

There are many recent examples of how the new psychoanalysis focuses on both analyst and patient; some new theories view their interactions in terms of a "field theory" focusing on the dyad. Theodore Jacobs (1986) has given us exquisite replays of his own subjective associations as he listens. Greenberg and Mitchell's plea that we cannot escape our subjectivity (1983) has also been taken up by Renik (1998), who insists we must renounce the false god of neutrality and what he considers the error of the monologue (see also Greenberg, 1995). His focus on "what works" (1996) begs the question of what a specific technical approach does to the observational field, of changes in the nature of the data that emerge as monologue shifts to dialogue. In a more moderate mood, Henry Smith (1994) writes: "when I am most carefully following the patient's subjective experience I tend to lose sight of the larger picture, such as the patterned expression of unconscious fantasy. I believe this is inevitable. . . . a focus on the patient's subjective experience, for example, diverts me from experiencing and seeing the eliciting power of the patient's transference and the self-defeating patterns and repetitive interactions that are driven by the patient's capacity to create his or her own painful experience" (p. 477).

We should recall that Freud and most classical ego psychologists were in fact never as neutral or abstinent as might be inferred from Freud's prescription. After all, Freud fed the Rat Man. Descriptions by Wortis, Kardiner, and the poet H.D. of their analyses with Freud similarly document his intrusion on the analytic monologue. An old saw from philosophy of science is apt: We should attend not only to what scientists write or say, but to what they do. The intersubjective mode was presaged also by self-psychology, as initiated by Kohut (1977), and by Modell's application of data derived from mother-baby researchers (Stern et al. 1998), who necessarily attend to a two-person field.

Perhaps Winnicott's dictum that there is no such thing as a baby (1960) provided a portent of what was to come. Kohut's description of the relatively silent analyst waiting for the patient to experience a break in empathy, requiring an interpretation that includes an admission of responsibility, builds on the idea that an empathic rupture mirrors in one-to-one fashion the earliest experiences with a significant adult or parent. The characterization of changes in equilibrium between patient and analyst as "now moments" (Stern et al. 1998) suggests a homology between adult interaction and mother-infant nonverbal interactions in the service of establishing mutuality and the optimal timing of mutative effect. Even more complexity is added by Ogden (1994), who designated the interpersonal matrix as the "analytic third." The central focus here is interpsychic or intersubjective, according to how we read him. Such theoretical modifications clearly lead us away from closed intra-psychic scrutiny toward dialogical study.

Language and Psychoanalysis

I have sketched the broad trends of twentieth-century psychoanalytic thought and now turn to some aspects of language theory. I will suggest that the progressive change in practice from monologue to dialogue can be informed by a linguistic analysis. This is an extension of my earlier work on the interplay of linguistics and psychoanalysis, begun in the late 1960s. I believe that the application of linguistic parsing clarifies what has happened in psychoanalysis and why we may suffer from category confusions as we seek to achieve our goals. Jacob Arlow (1995), in a paper on stilted conversations in psychoanalysis, has addressed the errors made by those who too rigidly apply the classical frame of analysis. In a paper on neutrality (Shapiro 1994), I noted that there is nothing so austere, nothing so removed or so wooden, as a first-year psychiatry resident's vision of a classical analyst (p. 275). In truth, even in monologue our patients address an imagined partner or interlocutor in inner speech. Although the therapist remains relatively silent, the patient is indeed talking to him or her, making an appeal and awaiting some kind of response, as in conversation. Insisting that the analyst not offer opinions, guidance, or relief, the classical monologue theory assumes that analyst and patient will become acutely aware of the need-state that drives the latter's fantasies. Loewenstein (1951), invoking the communication scheme of Karl Bühler, the early-twentieth-century developmental psychologist, suggested that the patient's utterances move from expressive ("I feel") to appeal ("I want") functions and finally evolve as propositions ("It is") about underlying conflicted wishes. Loewenstein employed a developmental linguistic frame of reference to describe psychoanalytic progression and anticipated a wave of interest in the application of linguistic models to psychoanalysis.

We can study the interchange during the psychoanalytic situation as a distinctive subclass of conversation. Each psychoanalyst behaves in accord with what he or she believes is best for the establishment of this unique process. Although psychoanalysis today tolerates various practices that were anathema during the heyday of classical ego psychology, a set of basic canons continues to prevail across theoretical fault lines.

In the United States in the 1950s, Sullivan's interpersonal school was distinguished from the more formal requirements of the ego psychologists. As time went by, however, the differences became less sharp. Moreover, we are now able to witness firsthand what some analysts do by studying the increasing library of taped analyses available (Thomä and Kächele, 1995).

Language as expressed in speech is a socially derived vehicle; its medium is discourse. Prelinguistic mother-infant dialogues are internalized, and later the infant learns a verbal code capable of describing inner states, as well as outer percepts. While some complain that language expresses these inner states imperfectly, it is, by many measures, the best means that we have. Other modes of communication, such as grunting or hugging, are not appropriate in psychoanalysis, and communion is not communication. Expressive and even vital appeal functions cannot be memorized for future application, in the way that neurotic action is revisited in rational thought via the medium of language. Thus, by default, psychoanalysis is committed to verbal exchange and conversation.

Nonpsychoanalytic studies provide descriptions of conversation in terms of the pragmatic rules of exchange derived from speech-act empirical studies that reveal the various constituents of an exchange. These constituents can be analyzed in common conversations, as well as in special formats, such as psychoanalysis. While Arlow stresses the commonality of the psychoanalytic dialogue with other forms of linguistic exchange, I offer that it is an unusual conversation in many ways. The elements of conversation include turn-taking, topic maintenance, synchrony of theme, sincerity assumptions, proxemics, and an array of related behaviors. These include use of a code as revealed in choice of lexicon and grammatical form; gestural and mimetic accompaniments of speech; prosody, or the music of expression; and, last but not least, eye contact. (A full analysis of Gricean maxims of conversation—quality, quantity, relevance, and manner—will not be attempted here.)

When we consider the psychoanalytic situation, we notice immediately that psychoanalysis is definitely a variant of normal conversation. This deviation from usual conversational form requires that analysands become acculturated to the new format of the interchange or be instructed about what is to happen lest they become frustrated, angry, and nonparticipant. Many analysts demur at explaining and would rather allow the patient to discover the new rules during the analytic experience. They believe that in the process of discovery they will elicit dependency conflicts, frustrations at not having guidance, and the like. Each of these dynamisms can be analyzed. Lichtenberg and Galler (1987) polled analysts concerning the injunction to patients that they speak freely, associate, and not censor, and found that many analysts no longer give this instruction. Often they simply assess ego strength and the adaptability of the analysand with respect to ability to follow the procedural canons.

Turn-Taking

Normal conversation requires frequent turns, sometimes without a complete sentence having been uttered. This is especially so where familiarity is intense. These interruptions can become irritating if there is a dominant speaker who does not permit others to express their thoughts. In an analysis, the turns are undefined and may even seem random to the patient. Long patient soliloquies may dominate a session.

The initial analytic instruction, if given at all, is to "say what comes to mind"; the expectant analysand must then bear the frustration of waiting until the analyst speaks. This is the arena in which a number of analyzable problems may arise, simply because most of us are taught from early on that answering and responding are marks of sociability. Turn-taking has been viewed by developmentalists as a precursor and facilitator of socialization and early attachment. Ninio and Bruner (1978) have described brilliantly the protolinguistic exchanges of nine-month-olds. These childhood experiences stamp our expectations, making an analysis seem anomalous and frustrating. In addition, there is ample evidence that mother and child coconstruct dialogues and story lines. These narratives are then internalized and repeated unilaterally in the analysis. As childhood wishes for earlier interactional formats emerge, the patient may long for the familiarity of those formats and experience regressive wishes from that time that create transferential objects in the analysis. These developmental events create an inner dialogue with a fantasied addressee who is ever present, even in monologue.

In the analytic situation, this entrained conversational form is disrupted. The patient may respond with various forms of explicit or veiled anger to the initial lack of verbal reciprocity. Some patients, narcissistic or not, may enjoy the opportunity to deliver an uninterrupted diatribe or declamation. They may also learn which cues and topics have a switchlike effect on the analyst, allowing them to elicit verbalization from behind the couch. Deeper concerns about contact and attachment may be acted out in the desire to hear an affirmation by verbalization rather than attend to what the analyst actually says. The analysand, searching for such security, can fall into a positive transferential mode simply on the basis of having elicited a repeated response from the analyst as representative of the object. These are but a few of the issues that can arise in the unique form of turn-taking that is required in an analysis.

A young graduate student in his twenties (Shapiro, 1999) presented a unique pattern of pseudostupidity in his remarks entering a session whenever he had experienced a sexually exciting fantasy in my waiting room, sometimes elicited by the presence of a female patient there. Together we came to designate these as "dumb questions." One such utterance occurred when my office carpet had been shampooed and a temporary paper path led from door to couch. The patient entered, looked at the paper, and asked plaintively, "Should I walk on the paper or the carpet?" I knew from past experience with him that this query could be understood as an indirect communication signifying defensiveness. At that point in the analysis, I believed that his attempt to elicit dialogue served as an avoidance of the analytic monologue; it turned out to be a formatted confession of lustful fantasies. Once we both realized this, either of us could follow the diatribe or the "dumb question" with, "What were you thinking on the way in that you'd rather not tell me?" This is clearly dialogical, and responsive to the need to conceal because of anxiety concerning my response. The dumb question was a semiotic sign that required more than a designative parsing of what he said: "Where should I walk?" It was a conversational detour. However, it also indirectly addressed the unconscious fantasy that was to be uncovered later in the analysis by listening to his monologues about fantasies, dreams, and narratives that were better elaborated when the analyst was silent.

Such dialogues directed toward patient behavior bring patient and analyst together as mutually gratifying conversational turn-takers. However, as noted, the topic shift within the dialogue leads the inquiry to a level that has been discovered in the analysis. The parties attend to the query not by parsing it semantically, but by viewing it from the psychoanalytic perspective of defense. Analysts will see that the surface exchange can itself be a satisfying reprise of earlier conversations, interpersonal riffs, and exchanges, the content of which can be irrelevant.

Topic Maintenance

In usual discourse we adapt to our partner and read the intention of an utterance (i.e., its illocutionary force) in the pragmatic situation to determine how long a specific topic is to be maintained. This is a back-and-forth decision that in optimal dialogue is made with some sensitivity between the participants. In an analysis, we permit the patient to determine the topic and how long it is pursued. Indeed, it is the very persistence and redundancy of a theme that alerts us to its drivenness. Freud's remark to Dora that she must love her father very much to spend so much time complaining about him has a paradoxical ring to the uninitiated, but not to the analyst. The use of a single topic can also signal defense against the intrusion of other matters and alert us to defensive and resistive trends in the discourse. The patient who insists on the here-and-now as the sole topic of conversation is surely denying the impact of the past on current life; the reverse may also be the case. A more subtle analytic skill involves the recognition of topic maintenance across thematic jumps. Here the analyst is called upon to find the shadow narrative and expose it as the patient flounders from topic to topic (Makari and Shapiro 1993). Play therapy offers a brilliant opportunity to see how children represent the same theme as they shift from one concrete play object or game to another.

The instruction that the patient should not try to censor sometimes wreaks havoc with topic maintenance, but it also teaches patients to be alert to what up to now they have considered noise; it helps them recognize that thoughts usually ignored are to be taken seriously as potential paths to meaning. Indeed, clinical wisdom suggests that when a patient truly begins to free-associate, the analysis is over. This is merely an aphoristic attempt to note that defensive barriers have crumbled and the patient can now face troubling thoughts and deal with previously unacceptable rumblings in awareness. Nonetheless, we also know that in some hands free association can be used as a defense mechanism, rendering the monologue less than understandable.

In the asymmetric arrangement of an analysis the patient calls the topic, but the analyst can broaden the scope by pointing to defensiveness of behavior, or interpret latent meaning by connecting trains of thought or by exposing the transference significance of a pattern. When interpretations are offered, the exchange may truly sound like a conversation, with description, denial, modification, and affective accompaniment arising as the discourse approaches a new discovery. Once the topic has been established, the turn-taking may expand as each party tries to establish deepening communication and a broadened understanding. Formal disruption of the free-associative stream, which has been encouraged, is now the means by which the analysis proceeds. While this phenomenon has not been systematically studied, I suspect that even the most monological of analysts becomes more of a participant as an analysis is prolonged.

Topics become redundant and familiar, and the work becomes more interactive as the parties become co-observers. Over the years, I have become aware that I frequently stage interpretations. My first intrusion awaits the patient's response and elaborations; I am then in a position to add touches that broaden understanding. The cooperation at the end of such a sequence is often beneficial to the alliance, and the consequent feeling of coconstruction and participation is sometimes a repetition of the sense of satisfaction experienced in earlier dialogues with parents.

Even in a self-psychological framework, where the conversational focus is on the patient's perceptions of slight and injury, the analyst intervenes to clarify the sense of injustice and permit transmuting internalization of the interchange between the offender and the injured patient. In the more classical frame, transference interpretation also disrupts the topical monologue. More important, it directs attention to a topic that has not been considered consciously—the interaction with the analyst. In Gray's technique of attending to the analytic surface (1973), changes in pace, topic, mood, and progression become signals to the analyst that significant unconscious factors are at play that require the patient's defensive action. Interpretation redirects the conversation to what the analyst infers has all along been the "true" topic of conversation, dimly hidden beneath the surface discourse.

Let me revisit the patient who used pseudostupidity to deal with his discomfort regarding lustful fantasies. In his continuing monologue, he was able to elaborate the semiotic clues that permitted us to interpret his unconscious fantasy. From early adolescence he recognized he was sexually aroused by seeing young girls from behind. This heightened desire during early adolescence led to his lying down and rubbing up against a sleeping teenager at a party. The ideas of no resistance, attack from behind, and immature girls as the object of desire were also the components of his fantasy and arousal as an adult. However, during analysis it became clear that he also unconsciously invited the reverse—being taken from behind as a passive feminine victim while asleep. He dreamed of receiving power from the male phallus to compensate for his ineffectual and childlike self-image.

Over time he enacted aspects of this wish within the analysis. He took brief naps on the couch and accused the analyst of masturbating behind him. At other times he fantasied expectations of anal attack. I believe that I could not interpret the unconscious fantasy in a convincing way without convergent evidence derived from his monologues and associations. Continuous dialogue would have diverted him from discovery.

The patient reported a dream in which he was in a tub with a small frog that grew very large. The frog skin was associated with a skin condition on his groin. He guiltily believed the skin lesions marked him as a masturbator. As an adolescent, he had indeed masturbated in the bathtub. This revelation changed his aggressive stance into a piteous one; it made him appear to be a mere child in a tub with a bath toy and not the author of a wish to sexually exploit young girls. Once these defensive fantasies of passivity were interpreted, the patient permitted himself conscious sexual wishes toward adults, specifically his wife's aunt. She possessed traits that he contrasted strongly with those of his aggressive and depriving mother, toward whom he felt only rage and suspicion and with whom he became childlike.

The analyst, too, was now viewed as depriving. The patient's symbolic conflict was re-represented in condensed form in another dream: again, he was behind a woman. She was wearing "little girls' pants" that reminded him of his wife's underclothing, but she had the breasts of an older, more mature woman, his wife's aunt. The setting was a large open area where his mother and grandmother were looking down at him while cooking his favorite childhood food. The analyst's interpretation addressed the exhibitionistic elements of this dream as a regressive wish to be admired and loved for his exploits. The patient's anxiety about castration, as represented in his preference for approaching women from behind, could then also be aired.

The literature on pragmatics and speech acts (Searle, 1969; Austin, 1962) directs us to consider the intentions behind our verbalizations, as well as the semantic and syntactic forms used. Speech-act theorists have directed us to explore meaning in an expanded manner, taking us beyond the semantic categories of reference and signification. In dialogue, we use culturally specific reference and personal intention, as well as context, to decipher meaning. Intentions are inferred from data other than sequence, form, and signification. This is nowhere more true than in psychoanalysis. Indeed, we may credit the inter-subjectivists for their insistence that meaning includes the context of the exchange and is incomplete with a consideration of semantics alone. A nonanalytic example I have used to illustrate the function of context is that of a young man entering a room and his father saying, "It is hot in here." The fact that the son then opens the window is logical only if we know things other than the semantic and syntactic information given in the utterance, which is at first glance merely propositional but in fact is an appeal for action (Shapiro, 1979; Makari and Shapiro, 1993). Patients in analysis frequently use locutions that should alert us to the shadow narrative of intentions other than those expressed in the surface meaning of verbalizations. We have all become acquainted with such pat phrases of defense as "I had a thought," "I had an insignificant dream," "You'll like this one," "I know it's not real," "This is not an analytic issue," "I want to talk business now," "I don't seriously think this," and so on. Stein (1989) recasts these as marks of the redactor patient's editing his script but revealing his hand in the process.

There are numerous other locutions and turns of phrase that permit patients to tell us what they believe they are concealing. The usual rhetorical devices of irony and metaphor occur prominently in analysis and should not be taken at face value, for they, too, can lead us to the unconscious desire of patients to deceive themselves, as well as us.

Gesture, Mimesis, Kinetics

As noted earlier, use of the couch impedes both patient and analyst in availing themselves of channels of communication found in most conversations. The analysand is deprived of the facial cues by which we normally judge the receptivity, the approval or disapproval, of an interlocutor. Using the couch, however, permits us to focus on inner cues and on the projected stream of the flow of ideas. Freud's metaphor of seatmates on a train, one of whom has access to a window, is apt. Lack of eye contact can facilitate monologue but also helps hide the speaker's intentions while prattling on. Only after considerable time did one patient of mine confess that while he recited a grand soliloquy he was visualizing himself doing stunts and somersaults above the office door, thereby revealing his intention to divert me with his nimble talk.

The analytic situation does not often afford us an opportunity to observe the dynamics of proxemics, that is, the spatial relations between the two partners to a conversation: how close or how far from each other they stand, whether they meet each other's gaze, whether they regularly shift position. All of these nonverbal communicative channels are packed with information that some believe to be of paramount importance for interpretation. Research psychoanalysts like Norbert Freedman (1977) have shown the power of messages conveyed by hand movements. Clinicians do well to watch for gestural and affective shifts and paralinguistic prosodic accompaniments to messages from the couch. These add nuance and color to the pragmatic tone of simple semantic analysis (Needles 1959; Shapiro 1979).

Not looking at the analyst can be distressing to the patient. Lack of visual feedback can create anxiety that enhances resistance and delays exposure, while patients with strongly dependent needs may panic at the isolation. By contrast, where the dynamism of shame comes into play, lack of eye contact can be experienced as comforting. These reactions are all grist for the analytic mill, but in individual cases we must take note of the intensity of the disturbance if the analytic process is to proceed. Rigid application of the canons of position and the analyst's silence does not enhance the progression unless some understanding is offered that attests the analyst's grasp of the odd nature of the exchange in comparison to everyday conversation. In the case I have cited, surely the patient's position on the couch and lack of eye contact promoted his fantasy of attacking the helpless sleeping girl, just as his pseudostupidity helped him avoid the aggressive, angry, or lustful intentions that were conditions for his arousal.

I have only briefly discussed the specific features of the unique dialogue we call psychoanalysis—a form of conversation designed to produce a specific result. The classical aim is to bring to light the defensive functions within the discourse that mask the feared emergence of unconscious fantasies. Thus, it is unlike any other conversation. The emergent facts revealed by the psychoanalytic method are not otherwise available. The microscope is necessary to see microbes. The free associative monologue is our technique—our microscope.

If I have established the idea that we follow the canons of a modified conversation, even within the classical analytic framework, and that the yield has been good, why has the shift away from monologue been so insistent in this last quarter century? The shift to more dialogical modes parallels the heightened focus on issues of intersubjectivity and is a move away from unconscious fantasy.

A Linguistic Summary

Linguistic inquiry has changed over the past century, just as the focus in psychoanalysis has changed. This parallelism should at some time be addressed in terms of social milieu and *Zeitgeist*. Within linguistics the shift has been from semantics and semiotics (the theory of signs) to syntax (form and grammar) and now includes a heavy emphasis on pragmatics, or language in use, and an understanding of the contextual frame of meaning and reference.

The interests of linguistics during the nineteenth century and the early twentieth—semantics and semiotics—are also the stuff of Freud's earliest work. He postulated dream work and other tropes and mechanisms of mind in his study of dreams and the transformation of mental conflicts into bodily symptoms in hysteria (Freud, 1900; Breuer and Freud, 1893–1895). Interpretation of unconscious fantasy is central to this form of uncovering. In an attempt to integrate linguistics and psychoanalysis (Shapiro, 1970), I suggested that the therapeutic action of interpretation is similar to naming. In purely semantic terms, the relation between signifier and signified is a conscious enterprise that Lacan extended to unconscious factors. I further cited the developmental proposal that children master their world as they learn to name things—when they can represent their experiences as common condensed symbols with social valence due to their appeal function. Moreover, interpretations in words have the advantage over other forms of mental content because verbal expressions can be carried in memory for later use and applied to a new experience for recognition and mastery. Words thus learned in a social matrix are used adaptively to label inner life and external circumstance.

The developmental advantage of language has been examined by many. Vygotsky (1934) noted that once the knot between prelinguistic thought and language is tied, a social linkage is secured, for speech comes from the culture and inner speech binds preexisting thought. While words sometimes seem inadequate to express all that we feel, they do pretty well. The philosophical movement represented by Davidson (1984) and, closer to psychoanalysis, Cavell (1998) offers the assurance that words are naturally dialogical, having been learned at the mother's knee and bound to pragmatic interchanges. Developmentally, we are supported by a social scaffolding of dialogue and expectancy of reciprocity. Linguistic symbols are our guarantor of contact with others. At the same time, they are linked semantically to fantasy and unconscious thought.

Monologues, in turn, expose in social form the patient's inner dialogues between internalized objects. In a depth-psychological sense, they offer a bridge between the representations of the drives in wishes and the person's adaptive interpretation of what is permissible in the culture. In structural jargon, the id and the ego, in the context of the superego's prohibitions, provide compromised meldings of psychic content. Curiously, modern intersubjectivists no longer seem to refer to the structural theory. I believe this is because they do not often choose to deal with internal idiolectic symbols derived from the interplay of experience (Erlebnis) and psychic structuralization. Sandler (1990) once wrote in a self-critical vein that he had been guilty of some misrepresentation "in not distinguishing between the experiential content of the mental representation—the perceptual and ideational content—and the structural organization behind the content, an organization that lies outside the realm of conscious or unconscious experience" (p. 869). This issue has been brought to a new head as intersubjectivists and similar thinkers ask what in inner life can be represented and, if something can, whether rendering it in words is imitative.

As we signify in words during discourse, we watch for agreement or disagreement. Freud warned that positive responses to interpretation during positive transference are suspect, and he warned also about the power of suggestion during gratification. The interactive states and reciprocity observed between babies and their mothers by Stern and others are surely universal, but in psychoanalysis we seek to know the conditions under which the patient is able to see more clearly and so overcome the defensive distortions necessary for psychological comfort. Verbal representation may be compared to face recognition: "I know that pattern. It is my enemy; it is a pattern derived from repetitive interactions from a time when I was not in control, when I was a child. I now can cast it in words. I can do something about it if I choose." This process of designating the unnamed for future semantic reference is essential to the Freudian concept of interpretation.

Chomsky (1957) directed linguists to focus on syntax. He claimed to have discovered an infinitely generative grammar, a minimal set of rules underlying any possible sentence. Looking to structural unities, he was not interested in real dialogues. Linguistics under his sway was contextless and devoted to a mathematics-like analysis of basic sentence structure, which he assumed was isometric with the mind's inner capacity to format in language. However, when he talked of surface and deep structures he caught the psychoanalytic ear. Edelson (1972) and others seized on his basic tenets to understand the parallels between these formalisms and Freudian topographic theory (Shapiro, 1988). Within this schema the focus is on intraindividual psychology and transformations, not on interactions. I suggested then that our ideas about primary-process thinking must be revised (Shapiro, 1979), because Freud had used the idea of mobility or cathexis to satisfy the workings of a biological, nonrepresentational neural network. These operations may bear some analogy to software slots for grammatical tokens, but unconscious wishes must be structured like a sentence—or else they could not be interpreted. Even Freud's early idea that drives have sources (to be studied biologically), aims, and objects is a syntactic form. The personal "I" is assumed, the vector of the wish describes the aim as passive or active, and the object of the wish is the grammatical object of the verb. This is compatible with an object-relational format, in which an aim can change and the identity of object and subject can oscillate (Kernberg, 1987). Both schemas can be considered slot grammars into which we can insert different nouns and polar verbs.

I can wish to be the active party to do x to you or vice versa. Thus, syntax is a formula with which to represent action schemata. When we make them conscious, we interpret in words—we render sentences. The psychoanalytic contribution is to recognize that the content of our wishes is determined by the maturational circumstance of our long dependency and the capacity to remember.

Neither semantics nor syntax represents a complete description of language as it is used in psychoanalysis. The third area of inquiry, pragmatics, is the study of how use and context extend and change meaning. The British philosopher J. L. Austin (1962), among others, proposed that meaning can be generated by the context of use. "I do" in a wedding ceremony, "I promise," etc. are performative utterances used in social contexts that prescribe their signification.

A pragmatic view of the psychoanalytically modified conversation must admit to the rules that govern this unique arrangement. Renik (1998) and others now strongly argue that we must acknowledge the analyst's subjectivity. This concession is easy, but recent reports from those quarters also prescribe repeated incursion on the patient's monologue. The clinical work described is more of a dialogue than before. What must be asked is where it directs the patient.

Topic maintenance is of course affected by dialogue. Early on, inner dialogue was preferred to interpersonal dialogue as the royal road to the unconscious. Indeed, as I have indicated, the more the analyst joins the dialogue, the less is learned about the patient's response to frustration and the less opportunity is afforded for witnessing the emergence of transference phenomena. In fact, the more two-sided the dialogue, the more we see of patterned behavior and performative enactments that detour us away from the discovery of unconscious fantasy derivatives. I would venture that the more primitive fantasies linked to here-and-now action patterns cannot easily be addressed in an analysis made up only of dialogue.

Had I responded to my patient's dumb remarks, I might have made him aware of their effects on others, of his need to hide something, or of his attempt to appear subservient to cover his anger. But I would not easily have understood the emergent unconscious fantasy linking his sexual practices to his fear of grown women, his castration anxiety, and his wish to be infused magically with my power, through a regressive wish that he incorporate my power from behind. Indeed, had I known earlier about his dynamic organization, I might have interpreted his provocations as wishes for counterattacks from me.

Syntax, semantics, and pragmatics are complementary perspectives, and each describes only its domain, as limited by the tools of study. If we wish to fully examine the language of psychoanalysis, we need convergent data from each perspective.

I recognize that each patient is in dialogue with the analyst. Nonetheless, the analyst must also, in Arlow's words (1995), help the patient "learn about how his mind works." This requires careful study of the patient's habitual expectations, tendencies to disappointment, and tendencies to unconscious enactments, leading to poor adaptations and the repetition of untoward behavior with unhappy results. This is a distinctively intrapsychic perspective. The task set by Arlow requires also a study of symbols (word-representations and interactions) and their origin in early experience. An exclusive focus on either the intrapsychic past or the interpersonal here-and-now leads to an incomplete description of what has happened in the analysis and to an inability to decipher the data in a way that will help the patient. Concepts like "now moments" (Stern et al. 1998) are attempts to describe a nonlinguistic sense of community with others; the suggestion is that verbalization without the right context is insufficient to induce change. Nevertheless, therapeutic action is attendant on verbalizations that codify, as best we can perceive, how our patients distort reality and live anachronistically and unrealistically.

We often make the error that any one modification in technique covers all patients. "Now moments" may simply reinvent the idea of correct timing, tact, or interactive readiness. Kohut's abandonment of Freud's idea that human beings are in conflict within is a judgment call based on his belief in the role of tragic narcissism in all psychopathology. The intersubjectivist school, with its emphasis on the analyst's subjectivity and the impossibility of neutrality, has simply caught us, I believe, in the act of trying to be external observers when we are participant observers—a designation, by the way, that Sullivan borrowed from anthropology, revealing the influence of social psychology within the intersubjective group. Much can be learned from these new perspectives, but we miss the intrapsychic dialogue if all monologue is ignored. Anthropologists in the field learn by participating in the life of the culture being studied, but its rituals, magic, and sexual taboos yield better to a semiotic, depth-psychological approach. So, too, with the psychoanalytic patient.

In conclusion, the essence of psychoanalytic method and study, I believe, is a focus on the intrapsychic meaning of behavior, defenses, wishes, and unconscious fantasy, and on the repercussions of these phenomena in interaction with other people, including, of course, the analyst. We have much to learn from our patients' monologues; when these are complemented by dialogue and by the analyst's self-scrutiny, we gain even more inclusive understanding. Using both perspectives—the monological and the dialogical—we can more completely describe the human mind at work in psychoanalytic conversation.

REFERENCES

Arlow, J. (1995). Stilted listening: Psychoanalysis as discourse. *Psychoanal. Q.* 64:215–233.

Austin, J.L. (1962*). How to Do Things with Words*. New York: Oxford University Press.

Boesky, D. (2000). Affect, language, and communication. *Int. J. Psycho-Anal.* 81:257–262.

Breuer, J., & Freud, S. (1893–1895). Studies on hysteria. *Standard Edition* 2.

Cavell, M. (1998). Triangulation, one's own mind, and objectivity. *Int. J. Psycho-Anal.* 79:449–467.

Chomsky, N. (1957). *Syntactic Structures*. The Hague: Mouton.

Davidson, D. (1984). *Inquiries into Truth and Interpretation*. Oxford: Oxford University Press.

Edelson, M. (1972). Language and dreams: The Interpretation of Dreams revisited. *Psychoanal. St. Child* 27:203–282.

Freedman, N. (1977). Hands, words, and mind: On the structuralization of body movements during discourse and the capacity for verbal representation. In *Communicative Structures and Psychic Structures*. New York: Plenum, pp. 109–132.

Freud, S. (1900). The interpretation of dreams. *Standard Edition* 4/5.

———— (1912). Recommendations to physicians practising psycho-analysis. *Standard Edition* 12:111–120.

———— (1916–1917). Introductory lectures on psycho-analysis. *Standard Edition* 15/16.

Gray, P. (1973). Psychoanalytic techniques and the ego's capacity for viewing intrapsychic conflict. *J. Amer. Psychoanal. Assn.* 21:479–494.

Greenberg, J. (1995). Psychoanalytic technique and the interactive matrix. *Psychoanal. Q.* 64:1–22.

—— & Mitchell, S.A. (1983). *Object Relations in Psychoanalytic Theory*. Cambridge: Harvard University Press.

Jacobs, T. (1986). On countertransference enactments. *J. Amer. Psychoanal. Assn.* 34:289–301.

Kernberg, O. F. (1987). An ego psychology-object relations theory approach to transference. *Psychoanal. Q.* 56:197–220.

Kohut, H. (1977). *Restoration of the Self.* New York: International Universities Press.

Lichtenberg, J.D., & Galler, F.B. (1987). The fundamental rule: A study of current usage. *J. Amer. Psychoanal. Assn.* 35:47–76.

Loewenstein, R.M. (1951). The problem of interpretation. *Psychoanal. Q.* 20:1–14.

Makari, G., & Shapiro, T. (1993). On psychoanalytic listening: Language and unconscious communication. *J. Amer. Psychoanal. Assn.* 41:991–1019.

Needles, W.F. (1959). Gesticulation and speech. *Int. J. Psycho-Anal.* 40:291–294.

Ninio, A., & Bruner, J. (1978). The achievement and antecedents of labelling. *Journal of Child Language* 5:1–15.

Ogden, T. (1994). The analytic third: Working with intersubjective clinical facts. *Int. J. Psycho-Anal.* 75:3–20.

Renik, O. (1998). The analyst's subjectivity and the analyst's objectivity. *Int. J. Psycho-Anal.* 79:487–497.

—— (1996). The perils of neutrality. *Psychoanal. Q.* 65:495–517.

Riesman, D. (1950). *The Lonely Crowd: A Study of the Changing American Character.* New Haven: Yale University Press.

Sandler, J. (1976). Countertransference and role-responsiveness. *Int. Rev. Psycho-Anal.* 3:43–47.

———— (1990). On internal object relations. *J. Amer. Psychoanal. Assn.* 38:859–880.

Schafer, R. (1999). *The Contemporary Kleinians of London.* Madison, CT: International Universities Press.

Searle, J.R. (1969). *Speech Acts: An Essay in the Philosophy of Language.* New York: Cambridge University Press.

Shapiro, T. (1970). Interpretation and naming. *J. Amer. Psychoanal. Assn.* 18:399–421.

———— (1979). *Clinical Psycholinguistics.* New York: Plenum.

———— (1988). Language structure and psychoanalysis. *J. Amer. Psychoanal. Assn.* 36:339–358.

———— (1994). On neutrality. *J. Amer. Psychoanal. Assn.* 32:269–282.

Shapiro, T. (1999). The representational world and the linguistic idiom. In *Psychoanalysis on the Move: The Work of Joseph Sandler,* ed. P. Fonagy, A.M. Cooper, & R.S. Wallerstein. New York: Routledge, pp. 105–117.

Smith, H.F. (1999). Subjective and objective listening. *J. Amer. Psychoanal. Assn.* 47:465–484.

Stein, M. (1989). How dreams are told. *J. Amer. Psychoanal. Assn.* 37:65–88.

Stern, D., Sander, L.W., Nahum, J.P., Harrison, A.M., et al. (1998). Non-interpretive mechanisms in psychoanalytic therapy: The something more than interpretation? *Int. J. Psycho-Anal.* 80:449–464.

Stone, L. (1981). Noninterpretive elements in the psychoanalytic situation. *J. Amer. Psychoanal. Assn.* 29:69–118.

Strachey, J. (1934). The nature of the therapeutic action of psycho-analysis. *Int. J. Psycho-Anal.* 15:127–139.

Thomä H., & Kächele, H. (1995). Process, development and outcome. In *Research in Psychoanalysis*, ed. T. Shapiro & R. Emde. Madison, CT: International Universities Press.

Toffler, A. (1970). *Future Shock*. New York: Random House.

Vygotsky, L.S. (1934). *Thought and Language*. Cambridge: MIT Press, 1962.

Wasserman, M.D. (1999). The impact of psychoanalytic theory and a two-person psychology on the empathizing analyst. *Int. J. Psycho-Anal.* 80:449–464.

Winnicott, W.D. (1960). The theory of the parent-infant relationship. *Int. J. Psycho-Anal.* 41:585–595.

Use Your Words![1]

(2004). *Journal of the American Psychoanalytic Association* 52:331–353.

"Use your words!" is a phrase admonishing preschoolers to divert their action-proneness to thought and language. Freud's injunction against acting out had a similar aim, placing control over drives in the domain of "inner language." The twenty-first-century psychoanalyst continues to employ models that depend on mentalization viewed from two angles—neural inhibition and social discourse. Psychoanalysts bolster their position by borrowing from the basic scientific work in each area. The recent focus on enactments, intersubjectivity, and social constructivism is reconsidered from an historical vantage point, as is the work that seeks to reconcile recent findings in neuroimaging and cognitive neuroscience. Freud's vision included a holistic hope that a comprehensive science of human beings might be achieved

---

1 This paper was presented in a briefer form as a plenary address to the American Psychoanalytic Association, Boston, June 2003. Submitted for publication September 24, 2003.

by understanding derived from biological inquiry and the artifacts of social and cultural narratives. The author's experience in both domains is recounted, and a new reconciliation of disparate approaches is offered in linguistic complementarity.

Use your words! is a demand often heard in preschools. It is a cry used by teachers trying to divert the hasty and impulsive action of motor-prone three-and four-year-olds as they interact with one another. When I hear this admonition, I am reminded of an early Freudian injunction curtailing hasty action while in analysis. The intent of this restraint on acting out is born of the same central tenet as "use your words" in toddlerhood. It is an attempt to delay action and modulate impulses (both conscious and unconscious) and fantasied wishes. Thus, impulse and action are to become matters of contemplation and, in analysis, reflection and understanding. The latter proposal is merely a paraphrase of Heinz Werner's idea that development carries us from the apprehension of "things of action" to "things of contemplation" with the accretion of memories and psychological control mechanisms during maturation (Werner and Kaplan, 1963). Freud (1893a) carried the notion to the social domain in quoting the words of an unknown English writer: "The man who first flung a word of abuse at his enemy instead of a stone was the founder of civilization" (p. 36).

While analysts no longer ask patients to defer major life choices, we still encourage mentalization and thought prior to action (see Fonagy, 1999). Indeed, even those who espouse a two-person psychology analyze enactments. In analysis, we seek to represent actions and reactions in verbal descriptions that serve the patient. Together patient and analyst can appreciate the neurotic constellations and unconsciously patterned interactions that stir the patient to repetitive behavior.

This parallel prompt toward words, both in the nursery and on the couch, encourages me to consider two significant trends in psychoanalytic thought from the developmental viewpoint. The two trends include, first, a renewed interest in the link between mind and brain and a revival of the drive concept in a new form. The second trend is the two-person psychology movement, which takes as its theoretical source an extension of object-relations theory and translates into interactive cocreation of narratives and the social determination of meaning.

The first, the neurocognitive trend, is evinced by the emergence of the journal *Neuro-Psychoanalysis* and a surge of papers in other journals concerning the neural basis of our practice and theory-building (see, e.g., Westen and Gabbard 2002a, b); indeed, in July 2003 the Fourth International Neuropsychoanalytic Congress will abut the biennial IPA Congress. The second trend, toward a two-person psychology, calls attention to our social interactions, in which mental miseries are viewed via action patterns cast in dyads. Some believe that the patterns that emerge in interactive form in transference-counter-transference enactments and social discourse are derivative of infantile experience. Others hold us to the study of the dyad as an empirical constraint of the psychoanalytic situation and make no claims about continuities with childhood.

Both domains of inquiry have their roots in Freud's inclusive theory, which encompassed both biological and social proposals. His initial focus on the neuroscience of his day is exemplified by his interest in the aphasias (Freud 1891) and in the mysterious leap between mind and body in hysteria (Breuer and Freud 1895). The biological basis of his inquiries into the origins of thought and wishes and his continuing demand that we consider the drives as the work the body causes the mind to do (Freud 1915) are central features of his model of mind. In addition, he offered the notion of thought as trial action as a key to understanding the intrapsychic representation of reality.

Even when Freud diverted his topographic thinking to consider the mind in terms of structure and signals for anxiety derived from the appreciation of danger (1923, 1926a), he sought to describe conflict between bodily based drive and ego factors. It was only later in our history that George Klein (1976) reminded us that Freud actually proposed two theories: one steeped in biology and the other a psychology of mental defense responsive to signals of danger and, perforce, to social demands. Klein's interpretation was historically prescient, as psychoanalysts in the decades to follow all but discarded Freudian economics and the concepts of drive and libido. Subsequent theorists concentrated on object relations, self-psychology, and the two-person psychology associated with social constructivism. Now we struggle with the idea that we are inextricably contained by subjectivity (Renik 1993) and attempt to determine the inner life of our patients via a web of intersubjectivity and interpersonal expectations carved from inborn and experiential impressions (Greenberg and Mitchell 1983). How intersubjectivity is achieved is our new mystery.

These two areas of inquiry, however—the neurocognitive and the social-psychological—are not unique to our discipline. They mirror the twenty-first century's specialized and segmented scientific views. New technology permits us to examine the brain in relation to thought, on the one hand, while, on the other, social scientists can now model social systems and interactive matrices in complex formulae. We now can image the brain in action and even vex the brain itself with cognitive probes to alter the blood oxygen level in various areas as neuronal activity is enhanced—the BOLD effect (Posner and Rothbart, 2000). This represents but one avenue of inquiry into the nervous system as it interacts with thought, perception, and social provocation. Within psychoanalysis itself we have developed theoretical propositions that represent a form of social-systems theory, using constructs such as "analytic space" and the "analytic third" (Ogden 1994). We also extend understanding of the dyad by suggesting that there is no such thing as a patient, a take on Winnicott's developmental dictum (1960) that there is no such thing as an infant. I will argue that these seemingly disparate sectors of inquiry (neuroscience and drives vs. intersubjectivist and social constructivist approaches) are inevitable and complementary. They even enrich our science if considered from the perspective of the meaning and cogency of the nursery school injunction "Use your words!"

It may come as no surprise to those who have attended to what I write and know my interests that I introduce language as a way to understand our divergent theories (see Shapiro, 1970a, b). I believe it can be the key to unlocking our recent analytic history, as well as our current analytic disjuncture. The most recent interest in language in its pragmatic sense concerns the ability to get things done with words. However, this use of words reaches in both directions, as neural dis-charges and modulators and as a series of trial actions that permit contemplation and symbolization. Symbolization in turn allows for a stay on action and confines personal urgency in civil propriety.

The obvious proposal that there are no minds without brains was recast recently in the conundrum that in the middle of the last century we were working with a brainless mind and now, as we enter a new century, there is a frantic push toward knowledge in a science that features a mindless brain. In this climate, many in psychoanalysis have shifted away from drive theory and the brain toward a more socially derived psychoanalysis, mired in the specifics of finely examined interactions and case study. They leave the brain to those who can better read the dials of technically advanced instruments. This new psychoanalytic empiricism of studying the intersubjective and the dyad has focused on the particular (i.e., the case) as a hermeneutic text—in technical terms, it favors the idiographic over the nomothetic.

There are those in both the neuroscientific and the social-psychological camps who believe that the psychoanalytic model has gone as far as it can go and has outworn its usefulness. They reach out to adjacent sciences and border theories to justify and gain support for one or the other of these apparently polar views. The argument offered is: "We will again attain ascendancy if we find ties to sciences that are currently productive and vibrant." These ventures, of course, are in many ways imitations of Freud (1895, 1919, 1923), who also reached out to the biology and sociology of his time to provide questions and underpinnings for his new science of mind. However, in his case he tried also to show how psychoanalysis enriched the broth of understanding from its unique stance; he worked to expand the understanding of the sociology and biology he examined.

Freud never fully relinquished any area of inquiry—the brain, the body, the mind, or the social surround as represented by cultural products.

Although throughout his career all of these areas remained in his purview, at various times he emphasized one over the others. Initially his model was clearly an extension of *On Aphasia* (1891) and his unpublished 1895 Project; in his *Dream Book* (1900), he used the language of energetics and charge [charge, or change?]. Later, in *The Ego and the Id* (1923) and in "Inhibitions, Symptoms and Anxiety" (1926), psychological and social concerns became prominent. In his work on group psychology (1921) and in "The Antithetical Meaning of Primal Words" (1910) and *Civilization and Its Discontents* (1930), he borrowed from the sociology and linguistics of his time.

I will selectively examine the two recent paths of psychoanalysis from the standpoint of the new knowledge gleaned from neuroscience and the social sciences, insofar as they seem relevant to our field. "Use your words!" offers an entrée, as well, to seeing how the developmental view of language bridges body, mind, and society and enriches both our practice and our theory. Bonnie Litowitz (2002) in a recent paper, "Sexuality and Textuality," offers a more epigrammatic link of body and mind: "the Freudian body was always a semiotic entity and therefore deeply contingent..." (p. 187).

Neuroscience and Psychoanalysis

A number of reviews have appeared recently that cheer us on in semi-technical language concerning the idea that Freud was right, and that modern neuroscience has added to our understanding of how the brain interacts with thought and language and how patterns of memory are written into the substrate (Westen, 1999; Solms, 1998; Kaplan-Solms and Solms, 2000). My purpose in the exploration of this side of the duality is not to praise Freud. Rather, I would like to enable us to determine if new data from the neurosciences can show us if and how words indeed mediate our derivative wishes and representations. I will also show how various neurotic symptoms and inhibitions limit our "range of motion" because they are based on anachronistic mental constellations that may have parallel inscription in the very structure of the CNS.

I will report from three bodies of work about how the cortex of the CNS modulates motor discharges from deeper structures appreciated as drives and impulses. As developmental competencies known as controls from within take over for external modulators known as parents and caretakers, an internal voice of control and modulation is established. Indeed, Winnicott's oft-quoted phrase "There is no such thing as an infant" is elaborated in the original text as meaning that wherever one finds an infant one finds maternal care (1960). This explanation is but a paraphrase of Darwin's dictum from the standpoint of biology that small broods require long caretaking. To this I would add that long caretaking makes for neurosis, because early wishes become fantasied relationships with others and live on as unconscious fantasies.

The biological unfolding of the human infant can be viewed as the gradual accretion of various ego and superego functions that are directed to replacing the parental roles. Freud borrowed the J. Hughlings Jackson idea that, as the outer mantle of the brain matures, it inhibits and modulates the discharges from the deep brain structures. This brain model lives on in the structural theory, as well as in the topographic model highlighting the conflict to be explained by positing two mental agencies.

I direct the reader's attention to a portion of work in the neurosciences that shows that behavior is modulated by words; that the disposition of attentional mechanisms is now within reach and can be mapped by brain imaging; that inbuilt fear responses can be conditioned by experience, permitting a conjecture that this is the basis for irrational phobias. Finally, I would like to mention a brief series of experiments I was privileged to participate in at the laboratory of Homer Smith at NYU and with Amir Raz and Michael Posner at the Sackler Institute for Developmental Psychobiology at the Weill Medical College of Cornell. These experiments clearly indicate that words can interrupt the usual tendencies of the CNS through hypnosis and suggestion and that words not only change behavior but also penetrate to the substrate. Thus, Kandell's experiments (1999) with Aplysia (sea slugs), in which conditioned reflexes derived from external contrived environments actually led to changes in the biochemistry at the nerve endings, find their partial demonstration in humans at the level of localized brain activation. Each example will emphasize brain-mind interaction. However, I will not argue for a simple reductionism, but rather will maintain that brain and behavior are each constructed within the confines of their own complexity, requiring a complementary inquiry into individual behavior in the social domain, as well as in the brain. The transduction from one form to the other has yet to be worked out.

I will first reintroduce the work of Alexander Luria (1961), the Soviet scientist and heir to Vygotsky. In a classic work, Luria sat three-, four-, and five-year-olds in front of an inflated rubber ball attached to a recording device and simply instructed them to squeeze when the light went on. The three-year-olds were much less able to bring their motor response under control for the delayed signal than were the older children. Once directed, they squeezed slowly in anticipation of the light. They were not able to wait for the instruction. More important, the four-and five-year-olds were progressively able to delay and also modify their responses when given more complex verbal instructions such as "Only press when the red light is on." Luria thus demonstrated the developmental sequential acquisition of the capacity to respond differentially to verbal instructions to modulate and modify behavior. By five, children were able to respond to "go" and "stop" commands, and they could deflect their impulses in accord with more complex verbal instruction.

These simple observations led to an array of later experiments under the rubric of go/no-go paradigms carried out while children are tested in an fMRI apparatus (Casey et al. 1997). Using such techniques, neuroscientists are now able to demonstrate out-of-awareness learning and patterning of behavioral dispositions. Most interesting for us, newly learned patterns become fixed in working memory and speed up response times when the task is repeated. These findings suggest that prior experience readies children for new challenges and creates patterned restraints during development. In addition, the localization of patterned behaviors in the brain can direct investigators to which neuro-transmitters and their receptors are likely to be operative. In turn, the differentially localized receptor density can be used to discover which controlling genes may be implicated as future studies are completed.

Parallel to these findings is the now well-established fact that early exposure and experiences have a direct effect on neuronal growth, axonal migration and proliferation, and dendritic spread (Huttenlocker 1994). As children approach latency and pass through early adolescence, the very same dendrites are pruned in accord with relative disuse. The new circuits that are associated to affective and emotional pathways of repeated expression are preserved. These data all point to the basic idea that motor pathways and our most primary emotional responsiveness are modulated and redirected under the sway of neuroanatomical patterned circuits shaped by experience. Thus, while the general pathways of neuronal growth are predetermined by genetic maturation, the strength of the signals and the capacity to delay discharge into selective motor channels, at first uniquely fashioned by inborn stimulus barriers, are then influenced by early experiences and relationships.

Note that I have shifted to the language of Freud. I do so to again reinforce the point that whatever we mean by object-relations constellations, or by prepotent genetic and learned behavioral complexes, there is now ample evidence that these patterns are represented by the circuitry of the brain itself. Some may complain, "But that is a neurally based cognitive unconscious and not a dynamic proposal pertaining to defending against loving and hating one's father. The tension between the systems is not in an equilibrium in terms of defense." This is true; nonetheless, the model points to further anatomically based patterns of brain activation that now can be characterized and elicited developmentally. Moreover, the behavior and the brain act in parallel in real time to modify responses in relation to a verbal order. We also have reason to believe that cognitive and dynamic phenomenology may share similar brain pathways.

Neuroimagers (Karama et al. 2002) have also made preliminary inroads in studying sexual arousal and have verified the storied lore that men are differently aroused sexually by visual stimuli than are women. The researchers imaged both sexes while watching so-called erotic tapes and found that there were different reports as to arousal and that different areas of the brain showed BOLD (blood oxygen) effects. More important to our task, when men were verbally instructed to constrain their arousal, the areas of the brain that had formerly showed activation were now diminished or absent (Beauregard, Levesque, and Bourgouin, 2001).

To return to Freud's admonition that we speak in analysis, and not act, he suggested that thought was trial action using little psychic energy in the service of delay followed by understanding. This proposal is based on the prescient idea that from the flow of relatively uncensored talk the patterns of wish and defense would emerge. While he used the language of neuronal discharge and drive inhibition, he also gave us hope that behavior, including words, would reveal unconscious patterned behavioral dispositions such as the preprogrammed oedipus complex and primal scene constellation. What modern neuroscience is elaborating is that the social animal who uses language does indeed respond with preset patterns on the basis of genetic disposition, but also yields to experiential patterning that can be measured by new techniques that probe the CNS.

Freud's interest in anxiety as a crucial emotion was surely as zealous as his interest in sexuality. Modern neuroscientists have studied fear responses in rats as a biological analogue to anxiety. LeDoux (1998) established that the amygdala, a deep brain structure, is activated in response to danger recognition. The same activation is present in primates and humans. However, this inbuilt response can be influenced by conditioning. A second loop from cortex to the hippocampus (LeDoux, 1998) is the anatomical parallel of this form of conditioned memory. Without belaboring the neuroanatomy, I offer that the role of memory and storage of images is enhanced by connections to a selective pathway, known as the Fusiform Face Area (FFA), that guarantees that facial configurations are discriminated from nonfacial patterns and then interact with the amygdala, which is sensitive to facial emotion. The mechanism of anxiety and phobia may be dormant in such brain pathways as mediated by the prefrontal cortex (Thomas et al. 2001; Tottenham et al. 2003).

Also relevant to my argument are findings about what neuroscientists call top-down modulation via the use of language, as employed during hypnosis (Raz and Shapiro, 2001; Raz et al.

2002). As we know, Freud's prepsychoanalytic endeavors included the use of hypnosis. This was so because the trance was a state of mind that hysterics seemed to enter easily or spontaneously. Anna O.'s designation of the talking cure is relevant (Breuer and Freud, 1895). The mysterious leap from mind to body is no more mysterious than the leap from words to behavior, or than the question of how we influence each other interpersonally by words. Each question requires an explanation of how ideas are generated and stored, and each requires understanding of how communication is possible. Hypnosis may be looked at as an enhanced means of communicational influence through verbal suggestion. However, we must strip the process of its aura of mystery and view it as a tool in asking and studying the questions I have touched on.

Early in my career I joined a research group under Homer Smith (Hulet et al. 1963), the renal physiologist and philosopher, in which an hypothesis was to be tested concerning whether urine flow could be increased by conditioning, as had been demonstrated in dogs. More interesting, since we could not talk directly to the glomeruli and the renal tubules, was the problem of what verbal instruction would affect urine flow. We would, as in the case of the hysteric, have to craft a suggestion in language that would influence the physiology via the logic of the mind. We thus instructed subjects under hypnosis that they were drinking numerous cups of water. While controlling for all the physiological variables, we were able to induce a fivefold increase in urine flow, even though the subjects were conserving water because of a twelve-hour prohibition against drinking. Words penetrate to the substrate—in this experiment, to the kidney itself via the cerebral cortex, the hypothalamus, and the pituitary.

Yet another triumph of words' penetrating to the substrate is to be described in experiments done in collaboration with Raz, Posner, and others. There is a well-known and robust experimental finding known as the Stroop Interference Effect (SIE). In this paradigm the subject is asked to name the color of the ink in which a word representation is displayed. This is a task dictated by a verbal instruction. However, if the word *blue* is presented in red ink there is a cognitive conflict and a consequent delay in response time. There are innumerable fMRI studies to show that the anterior cingulate gyrus of the brain is activated when such a conflict is operative. We thus have two ways of demonstrating the Stroop effect, first in the delayed reaction time, and second in the fMRI BOLD effect. Our research team offered subjects the post-hypnotic suggestion that they cannot read the presented word, as if the letters were from a foreign alphabet. The subjects no longer suffered the usual delay in reaction time (SIE) and the fMRI BOLD effect activation in the anterior cingulate gyrus of the cerebral cortex was absent (Raz 2004).

These experiments probing brain and mind suggest some basic tenets that can be used by psychoanalysts. For example, experimental manipulation by cognitive probes can now be observed in parallel with the substrate in real time. These experiments show that we can localize more or less fixed circuits that correspond to patterned units of meaning. We know that dynamically conflictual bodily symptoms, which we translate into wish and defense, can be rendered as words. Personal fears and societal constraints that are clinically evident are worded as prohibitions that were internalized in the form of inhibited, delayed, or modulated action (i.e., superego constraints). The injunction in childhood to use words does indeed make sense if we are to grow up and become part of a civilized community. But the injunction against acting out also offers the analyst a closer look at the cost to the individual who is unconsciously striving to enact unconscious fantasies within the transference and outside it. It lets us see how this action or enactment serves as a protection against the exposure of shameful derivatives in the analysis.

In summary, recent neuroscientific advances permit analysts to again consider the body as a substrate for the generation of wishes and drive derivatives, and the work it causes the mind to do. Moreover, we have new evidence to assert that there are structural parallels between psychic constellations in memory and language and complementary neural circuits. Top-down modulation of relatively fixed brain circuitry is possible. Verbal instruction has now been shown to penetrate the mental apparatus to the brain, and to change physiology.

Psychoanalysis and the Social Surround

The second trend in recent psychoanalytic thought that has been significant for both theory and clinical practice is the interpersonal and intersubjective, or two-person, model. Adherents of the two-person psychology warn us not to go beyond the empirical purview of the clinic; we should simply attend to what happens in the here-and-now, in the transference- countertransference dyadic relationship. The rubric of social constructivism has generally been applied to encompass this now popular point of view. What can be learned from the phenomenological observation of the dyad in interaction, and the meaning evoked between the parties within the psychoanalytic process?

In "Constructions in Analysis," Freud (1937) hinted that the uncovered past was *about* the past, but not *from* the past, permitting the idea that conviction can be a product of analytic suggestion or transference love, rather than a demonstration of the reality of remembered past events. Current psychoanalytic observers seek to establish how mutual intention is shaped, and how narratives are constructed within the dyad. The speculative aspects of the drives, their source in the body, and their effect on mental derivatives have been left to the neurosciences. Careful scrutiny of the interaction and the hermeneutic approach was articulated early by Ricoeur (1970), and finding oneself "in the other" was surely the keystone of Sullivan's ideas (1953). The latter is quoted by Mitchell and Aron (1999) as saying that "mind always emerges and develops contextually in interpersonal fields" (p. xv).

Sullivan and his followers were initially shunned by the more orthodox psychoanalytic community, because of their focus on the interpersonal or social context, which was less relevant to the drive- and conflict-focused ego psychoanalysts. Sullivan paid tribute to the work of G. H. Mead (1934), the American social psychologist, and the linguist Edward Sapir (1921), but he and these thinkers are barely acknowledged by many of the current two-person psychologists. Nonetheless, we now hear the reverberations of interpersonalism in the very terms *two-person psychology* and *intersubjectivity*. We hear similar echoes in self psychology and object-relations theory, insofar as they objectify the object and the self as direct replicas of past interactions, rather than using the earlier Freudian proposal that the drives direct the nature of the relationship. (We owe to self psychology and object-relations theory, however, the renewed interest in affects, the means to their modulation, and the close clinical scrutiny of narcissism.)

While some who work within social constructivism seek continuity with the ontogenetic past, others declare their independence and announce a paradigm shift. For example, in a recent panel on enactment and acting out (Levinson 2003), Maria

Ponsi "noted that with a radical paradigm shift based on a relational two-person perspective, the concepts of enactment and acting out have grown apart in meaning" (p. 151). This statement, mimicking many others, exposes the shift away from Freud's earlier views of acting out unconscious fantasies. In the introduction to their book, Mitchell and Aron (1999) write the following: "We favor a form of constructivism that grants some weight to the materiality of the body and its attributes, while at the same time we recognize that any ways in which those attributes are described are themselves social structures"; they note further that relationalists are "a set of theorists who had rejected drive theory and who instead placed relationships at the center of the theoretical system" (p. xvi). Later they lay claim to the rubrics of two-person psychology, the analytic third, and intersubjectivity.

I intimated earlier that infancy research has been treated ambivalently by the two-person psychologists. Thus, there is a split within this somewhat varied camp that I am treating as a unit. There are also many psychoanalysts who emphasize the ego and compromise formation, such as Brenner, who deny that infant investigation is useful to us in understanding the analytic process. André Green, as well, from his Gallic stance and secular devotion to the early Freud, rejects the relevance of such study (see Kohon 1999). By contrast, the Kohutians have been well-rewarded by Daniel Stern (1985), whose research supports the self-psychological propositions that guide their theoretical position (see Kohut, 1977).

Nonetheless, the hermeneuticists, new Kleinians, and inter-subjectivists all attend carefully to the observation of analysand and analyst in enactments, and concepts such as projective identification color their clinical work and remain their dominant theoretical explanation. If I were to designate a social scientist who best describes their approach to data, it would be Clifford Geertz (1983), who embraces "thick description" as a basis from which theory can be elaborated to designate underlying trajectories and intent. A correspondingly thick intra-psychic infrastructure seems unnecessary.

The two-person psychologists, devoted or not to the formative impact of infancy, are centrally focused on detailed descriptions of specific clinical interactions. There is a recent trend toward long, exquisite recounting of meetings between patient and analysand that are sometimes admired as virtuoso performances. The tendency is to elaborate the meaning of the interactions in a search for the mutative influence of the new relationship. The Now-Moment Boston Study Group (Stern, Sander, and Nahum, 1998) surely observes the waxing and waning closeness of the interaction between patient and analyst and maintains a devotion to modeling derived from infant-watching. Are these simply variants of the corrective emotional experience of the Alexandrian past? I think only partly so. However, in each case there is a search for the seeds of change within the dyadic interchange that attracts interest.

The analytic third (Ogden, 1994) is another shibboleth that borrows from the field theory of social psychologists, who map social interactions as if forces and behaviors obey predictive rules and organismic models. An earlier version that was offered by Serge Viderman (1979), a French analyst, but did not receive much notice in the U.S. Social constructivists, according to Donnel Stern (1983), seek to understand the interaction and claim that the "enemy of their theory is essentialism under the banner of nature" (Mitchell and Aron 1999, p. xv). They thus turn away from biological determinants and are less interested in intrapersonal meanings and intrapsychic systems.

The rejection of such theoretical positions leads to a distinctly idiographic analysis of single pairs and discourages the nomothetic generalization and theory-building across patients that was Freud's trenchant original hope. Moreover, viewing the new focus on enactment, some (e.g., Busch, 2001) have protested that we may be fostering a distinctive neglect of the intrapsychic and of unconscious fantasy, because the notion of enactment implies a two-sided partnership that can ignore the root of the patterning in the patient's unconscious preference for such repetitive encounters.

In the panel noted earlier, Maria Ponsi added that "the term 'enactment' theoretically referred to a two-person interpersonal episode and reflected the analyst's inevitable subjectivity and participation" (Levinson 2003, p. 151). We see in this assertion the sharpest demurral from the idea that the fantasies of the patient in the dyad are singularly relevant. Thus, there is a conundrum in the two-person approach to understanding, because the intersubjectivity to be understood tacitly equalizes patient and analyst as independent units, each with the unwitting intent to influence. Nor is the patient to be considered a carrier of prepatterned behavior based on a past that must be articulated as a means of understanding the present response patterns in the dyad. How, then, can I offer some new slant on this trend as construed from the vantage point of "Use your words"? That is my task here. I hope I can convince others that it is worthwhile.

Remember that the injunction "Use your words!" is one of the earliest constraints on action in the service of socialization. It is Freud's equivalent of don't act, but speak and free-associate. According to Vygotsky (1934), the first pragmatic social incursion curtailing action is what leads to speech acts' becoming internal speech. Language use then modifies behavior and the expression of impulse. Observations of children at solitary play reveal subvocalizing, which has been construed as a step toward internal speech serving to regulate behavior. As we develop, we speak and encourage thought and internal speech, formulating ideas and waiting, rather than acting mechanically. We learn to share and take turns.

I had a recent interaction with a six-year-old in consultation. When asked what he does when angry, he answered, using his kindergarten mantra, "I use my words, but when I am really frustrated I use my hands! I push my sister." He added, "But I don't do that anymore because I know when I am done she will bite me." A child's Hobbesian social contract was thus born, but the interdiction of action preceded it. Ana-Maria Rizzuto (2002) has written about the process of dyadic talk as a direct replica of early speech acts between mother and child. In 1970 I offered the idea that the naming of unconscious constellations mimics an earlier sense of mastery, as children learn to comprehend the world by naming and symbolizing (Shapiro, 1970a, b) The dramatic accompaniment of speech by prosody, mimesis, and gesture embellishes our words and lends potency and valence to messages. But we do not assault or hit or push or murder or rape. By using words we permit the other to recognize where we come from, how serious we are, and how cutting or soothing we wish to be by our growling or purring. It was not by chance that the medieval university taught rhetoric and that our serious communicators are interested in their audience. Words are capable of inciting, calming, placating, diverting, exciting, eliciting understanding, etc.

In the dyad of the analysis, in the matrix, an interaction unfolds that permits the parties to understand the intentions of each, and the analysis of the resistances in classical terms becomes the whole effort. The interaction is itself an exemplar of the patient's limited repertoire of action. We now have been directed to analyze who the patient is by virtue of how he or she acts in a conversation. The content of speech is also an action. For some, the two-person theory may be taken to endorse the earlier psychoanalytic aim of uncovering unconscious fantasy, but that is often omitted as an intended aim.

Words modulate affects and the tendency to action, strife, and sexual expression. Words also reveal intent as a parallel message, or shadow narrative, to be distinguished from the explicit narrative. The pragmatics of the circumstance within dyads dictates the usage, and the semantics are referential only in the simplest designative sense. Makari and I (1993) used the concept of shadow narrative to delineate the rules of the interaction and how words are selected distinctively in dyads according to the stature, rank, kinship, and assumed role of each party. For example, a grandson entering a room where his grandfather sits may respond to the latter's utterance "It's hot in here!" by turning on the air conditioning, even though semantically the message is merely a declaration and not a request. Thus, the response is not determined by the meaning of the words alone. If the two people were a married couple, the response might be otherwise, or if a child said it was hot, the mother might act to cool the room. We need additional, socially determined information to see how an interaction will unfold, rather than simply depending on what has been said.

Indeed, the nature of the dyadic analytic arrangement is itself embedded in social convention. The professional training of the analyst, the respect for titles, and the manner in which someone accepts or rejects the idea of being a patient are all socially determined. The parties each become an arm of the dyad, to be explicitly described from the perspective of their interactions and statements, as well as by the cultural constraints that define social behavior. An analysis of this dyadic situation requires exquisite observation and is well within the empirical tradition of "*N*-of-one clinical experiments."

In summary, I have just reprised the George Kleinian idea of Freud's two theories. Modern analysts seem to have allied themselves with the brain and its drive derivatives, on one hand, or with the socially defined dyad, on the other. However, I do not believe that we can prosper as a discipline that claims an inclusive theory if we reject either arm of the current polarity. In each arm of our polar description, our search for understanding and our quest for better theories have contributed to the classical psychoanalytic edifice. I will now present a reconciliation aimed at a pragmatic appreciation of the virtues of work in each area.

Reconciliation

Psychoanalysis in the twenty-first century is beset by pluralism, despite the efforts of many espousing integration. Wallerstein's leadership of the International Psychoanalytical Association represents but one of many attempts to find a common ground (1990). While the intellectual world abounds in various Freudian proposals for understanding every human enterprise, Freud himself warned that many would warm their feet at the hearth of our discipline. But he also fiercely sought to preserve "the pure gold" of analysis as he systematically ejected and defrocked followers who had strayed too far. Currently, some again call for unity in diversity. The language of our new theories calls for wholeness, unbroken by hypothetical agencies of the mind. The new theorists shun analytic substructures that fragment the "experience-near" person. We seek wholeness in selfhood, and in local and international politics as well. Our organizations now include many who once were outsiders. The polylogue has been welcome and smacks more of an open community of scholars—a University of Psychoanalysts without gates. At the same time, how can we encompass such wholeness in a world that has the technology to analyze not only the brain, but also the functional aspects of mind, into operationally segmented agencies? Most important for many is the question of how we hold mind and body together, even as our new theories and technologies study them separately.

My answer is implicit in my title. We do it by understanding, at every level of the organism and the person, how we use our evolutionary and biologically given words both as internalized speech and as a way of naming things and actions in the social surround. We even name unconscious fantasies and dispositions in order to designate maladaptive action patterns. In so doing, I have suggested, we penetrate right down to the brain itself, to the cingulate gyrus and from there to the renal tubules. All levels function together, even though we segment horrifically in order to study the person and the organism separately (Rubinstein 1965).

Psychoanalysts' recent quest for "experience-near" theories that appeal to common sense includes an agenda to designate the obvious effect of emotions (with their roots in our bodies) on behavior. To repeat what I said earlier, words are made salient by their meanings—and their meanings are most fully appreciated by their affective valence, which reflects both personal significance and interpersonal impact. Some have argued that psychoanalysis is even more holistic than anthropology, because it seeks to grasp the totality of meaning systems developmentally and culturally; intrapsychically and biologically; interpersonally and in light of developmentally induced intrapsychic conflict. As I have noted, we attend to both person and organism. Our explanatory modules must not contradict each other, or, if they do, there is a reason to seek reconciliation. I have often thought about the physicist Sir Arthur Eddington's paradox that the table of physics is largely intermolecular space, while the table we eat on is quite solid. Certainly Bohr's complementarity is also cogent. Data from different perspectives are to be considered within the limits of the methods used to create the new information. We should not dismiss what doesn't suit us. Instead we should ask, "How can that be?"

I am not ready to give up Freud's dream of a science of the mind that awaits new probes into attention, consciousness, intention, repetition, drivenness, and the experiences of satisfaction and closure. All these strongly implicate important brain-based components. I am more willing to give up nihilism, cast in the light of buzzwords such as postmodernism or interpretive relativism. Psychoanalytic hermeneutics, derived from principles appropriate to the study of texts rather than from the study of dynamic minds in open systems of flux, seems now to be a false path.

We are just at the threshold of understanding language competence in evolutionary terms, its rhetorical power and descriptive cogency, and its function in the control and modulation of action and affect. It even seems that Freud was right again that verbal invective is more civilized than smart missiles. Indeed, smart missiles exist because of our linguistic competence. Language study is the anthropology of everything we do that leads to systematic knowledge, and the task of transforming passion leads to a new semiotic whose cipher we must learn about. We need more study of how psychoanalysis in its dyadic format works the slow magic of insight and change by any means in individuals (Whitebook, 2002).

Freud's encompassing psychological musings dipped into what he knew of the brain from the aphasias and the tendencies toward discharge and action as studied in reflexes. He learned from patients

424

that hysterical paralysis follows the logic of the mind and of fantasy, not of neuronal dermatomes and pathways. And he asked, *How is that leap possible?* To learn more, he gave up the study of the mind's substrate in the brain. Instead he listened to his patients talk in and out of altered states of consciousness. The exchange in words became the medium in which he could learn about unconscious fantasies and inhibition of action and infer the developmental influences operating at a distance in transference.

We modern psychoanalysts deal no longer with hysterical conversion, but with patients who suffer aberrant proclivities leading to loneliness, isolation, untoward anger, and narcissistic hurt. Our techniques seem to have switched to adapt to treatments in which the two-person model is more evocative. A long-range vision makes the trend reasonable, but to split our understanding of human beings in such a way that social behavior and biology are separated from each other does not make sense in a clinical science.

I have suggested that the injunction "Use your words!" can be a powerful means of keeping us metaphorically whole. It has been applied potently from early toddlerhood to senescence as an emotional and social modulator, as well as an internal means of maintaining compromise formation. Moreover, I have tried to show that the penetration of linguistic forms into the substrate is a fact of evolutionary biology. Our common-sense ideas about the social communicative value of language makes it a logical instrument that aids in mediation between people. Language is an inborn capacity in average expectable biological conditions, as well as a means of modulating and regulating social exchanges and systems.

We reach within via words, not to the level of primary process (which better describes neuronal discharge patterns), but to patterned unconscious fantasies that can be rendered verbally. Lacan's formulation that the unconscious is structured like a language (1953) is amenable to me. We reach out to others by using a common tongue that links human beings by communication. This function supersedes mother-infant immediacy and communion. Thus, language is the bridge between body and mind and between persons. Language is a function of the mind's propensity to modulate the reflex arc of stimulus-response. The mediation process is what psychoanalysts study in the form of personally construed meaning units. The coding of meaning is perforce in language—and it is via words that we interpret meanings to our patients, even in the throes of irreducible subjectivity.

As we seek to plumb our patients' minds and therefore also to appreciate their feelings, we invoke other new methodological shibboleths, such as empathy, intersubjectivity, and unconscious communication. But we dare not use these designations as explain-alls or empty fillers for ideas lacking theoretical power. They should rather be translated into meaningful new mechanisms for processes, as yet unknown, that guide thought and action. Their mere invocation is not consonant with what constitutes a psychoanalytic explanation. As Geertz (1983), writing about understanding people of other cultures, wisely notes,

> In short, accounts of other peoples' subjectivities can be built up without recourse to pretensions to more-than-normal capacity for ego effacement and fellow feeling.... Whatever accurate or half-accurate sense one gets of what one's informants are, as the phrase goes, "really like" does not come from the experience of that acceptance as such, which is part of one's own biography, not of theirs. It comes from the ability to construe their modes of expression, what

I would call their symbol systems…. Understanding the form and pressure of, to use a dangerous word one more time, natives' inner lives is more like grasping a proverb, catching an allusion, seeing a joke—or as I have suggested, reading a poem—than it is like achieving communion [p. 70].

Here then is my point. All variants of experience, immediate or mediated, can come under scrutiny and be reconsidered under the light of reason translated into verbal form (Shapiro, 2002, 2003). The data or raw experiences must be recast in an approachable manner, using our new techniques for observing both the person and the organism—the two-person social exchange and studies of the biological substrate. I will not praise or fault those who say the understanding and new knowledge will never replace the experience. The latter will not, I hope, be diminished by our study. However, I advise that we should be less mystical and romantic in our vision and apply the technology we have in the service of better understanding.

"Use your words!" rings out from the nursery to the couch as a means to mediate interpersonal experience. From that, inner language develops to mediate intrapsychic affects and impulses, and even mentally creative narratives. All this is further evidence that the human condition is, in its most civilized form, language-based. Each level of inquiry and exploration offers different data. We seek convergence when possible, not isomorphism or reduction. Love will never be reduced to its chemical co-occurrences or its neural discharge or its BOLD effect, just as the word is not the thing or the experience itself. In the absence of any other possibility, human communication and internal monologue and dialogue (Shapiro, 2002) require that we "Use our words!"

REFERENCES

Beauregard, M., Levesque, J., & Bourgouin, P. (2001). Neural correlates of self-regulation of emotions. *Journal of Neuroscience* RC165:1–6.

Breuer, J., & Freud S. (1895). Studies on hysteria. *Standard Edition* 2.

Busch, F. (2001). Are we losing our mind? *J. Amer. Psychoanal. Assn.* 49:739–767.

Casey, B.J., Trainer, R., Orendi, J.L., Et Al. (1997). A developmental functional MRI study of prefrontal activation during performance of a go-no-go task. *Journal of Cognitive Neuroscience* 9:935–947.

Fonagy P. (1999). Memory and therapeutic action. Three essays on the theory of sexuality. *Standard Edition* 7:130–243.

Freud, S. (1891). *On Aphasia*, transl. E. Stengel. New York: International Universities Press, 1953.

——— (1893). On the psychical mechanisms of hysterical phenomena. *Standard Edition* 3:27–39.

——— (1895). Project for a scientific psychology. *Standard Edition* 1:295–397.

——— (1900). The interpretation of dreams. *Standard Edition* 4/5. (1905). Three essays on the theory of sexuality. *Standard Edition* 7:130–243.

———(1910). The antithetical meaning of primal words. *Standard Edition* 11:155–161.

——— (1915). Instincts and their vicissitudes *Standard Edition* 14:117–140.

——— (1919). The "uncanny." *Standard Edition* 9:219–256.

——— (1920). Beyond the pleasure principle. *Standard Edition* 18:7–64.

————— (1921). Group psychology and the analysis of the ego. *Standard Edition* 18:69–143.

————— (1923). The ego and the id. *Standard Edition* 19:12–66.

————— (1926). Inhibitions, symptoms and anxiety. *Standard Edition* 20:87–174.

————— (1930). Civilizations and its discontents. *Standard Edition* 21:64–145.

————— (1937). Constructions in analysis. *Standard Edition* 23:257–269.

Geertz, C. (1983). *Local Knowledge: Further Essays in Interpretive Anthropology*. New York: Basic Books.

Greenberg, J., & Mitchell, S.A., (1983). *Object Relations in Psychoanalytic Theory*. Cambridge: Harvard University Press.

Hulet, W.H., Shapiro, T., Schwarz, B.E., & Smith, H.W. (1963). Water diuresis after hypnotic suggestion in hydropenic subjects. *Journal of Applied Physiology* 18:186–189.

Huttenlocker, P. (1994). Synaptogenesis, synapse elimination, and neural plasticity in human cerebral cortex. In *Threats to Optimal Development: Integrating Biological, Psychological and Social Risk Factors*: Vol. 27, ed. C. Nelson. Hillsdale, NJ: Erlbaum, pp. 35–54.

Kandell, E.R. (1999). Biology and the future of psychoanalysis. *American Journal of Psychiatry* 156:505–524.

Kaplan-Solms, K.E., & Solms, M. (2000). *Clinical Studies in Neuro-psychoanalysis*. Madison, CT: International Universities Press.

Karama, S., Leroux, J., Bourgouin, P., Beaudoin, G., Joubert, S., & Beauregard, M. (2002). Areas of brain activation in males and females during viewing of erotic film excerpts. *Human Brain Mapping* 26:1–13.

Klein, G. (1976). *Psychoanalytic Theory: An Exploration of Essentials.* New York: International Universities Press.

Kohon, G. (1999). *The Dead Mother: The Work of André Green.* New York: Routledge.

Kohut, H. (1977). *The Restoration of the Self.* New York: International Universities Press.

Lacan, J. (1953). The function of the field of speech and languages in psycho-analysis. In *Ecrits: A Selection*, transl. A. Sheridan. London: Tavistock, 1977, pp. 30–113.

Ledoux, J. (1998). *The Emotional Brain: The Mysterious Underpinnings of Emotional Life*. New York: Touchstone Books.

Levinson, N. (2003). Panel on "acting out" and/or enactments." *Int. J. Psycho-Anal.* 84:51–154.

Litowitz, B. (2002). Sexuality and textuality. *J. Amer. Psychoanal. Assn.* 50:171–198.

Luria, A.R. (1961). *The Role of Speech in the Regulation of Normal and Abnormal Behavior*. New York: Liveright.

Makari, G., & Shapiro, T. (1993). On psychoanalytic listening: Language and unconscious communication. *J. Amer. Psychoanal. Assn.* 41:991–1019.

Mead, G.H. (1934). *Mind, Self, and Society*. Chicago: University of Chicago Press.

Mitchell, S.A., & Aron, L. (1999). Introduction. *Relational Psychoanalysis: The Emergence of a Tradition*, ed. S. Mitchell & L. Aron. Hillsdale, NJ: Analytic Press, pp. ix–xx.

Ogden, T.H. (1994). The analytic third: Working with intersubjective clinical facts. *Int. J. Psycho-Anal.* 75:3–19.

Posner, M., & Rothbart, M.K. (2000). Developing mechanisms of self-regulation. *Developmental Psychopathology.* 12:427–441.

Raz, A. (in press). Atypical attention: Hypnosis and conflict reduction. In *The Cognitive Neurosciences of Attention*, ed. M. Posner. New York: Guilford Press.

———— & Shapiro, T. (2001). Hypnosis and neuroscience: A crosstalk between clinical and cognitive research. *Arch. Gen. Psychiat.* 59:89–92.

———— ————Fan, J., & Posner, M.I. (2002). Hypnotic suggestion and the modulation of the Stroop interference. *Arch. Gen. Psychiat.* 59:1155–1161.

Renik, O. (1993). Analytic interaction: Conceptualizing technique in light of the analyst's irreducible subjectivity. *Psychoanal. Q.* 63:553–571.

Ricoeur, P. (1970). *Freud and Philosophy: An Essay on Interpretation.* New Haven: Yale University Press.

Rizzuto, A.-M. (2002). Speech events, language development and the clinical situation. *Int. J. Psycho-Anal.* 83:1325–1343.

Rubinstein, B.B. (1965). Psychoanalytic theory and the mind-body problem. In *Psychoanalysis and Current Biological Thought*, ed. N.S. Greenfield & W.C. Lewis. Madison: University of Wisconsin Press, pp. 35–56.

Sapir, E. (1921). *Language: An Introduction to the Study of Speech.* New York: Harcourt, Brace, 1955.

Shapiro, T. (1970a). *Clinical Psycholinguistics.* New York: Plenum.

————(1970b). Interpretation and naming. *J. Amer. Psychoanal. Assn.* 18:399–421.

———— (2002). From monologue to dialogue: A transition in psychoanalytic practice. *J. Amer. Psychoanal. Assn.* 50:199–219.

———— (2003). Whatever happened to meaning? Paper presented to the Western New England Psychoanalytic Society, May.

Solms, M. (1998). Preliminaries for an integration of psychoanalysis with neurosciences. *Bulletin of the British Psychoanalytic Society* 34:23–38.

Stern, D. (1985). *The Interpersonal World of the Infant.* New York: Basic Books.

——— Sander, L., & Nahum, J. (1998). Non-interpretative mechanisms in psychoanalytic therapy. *Int. J. Psycho-Anal.* 79:903–921.

Stern, D.B. (1983). Unformulated experience: From familiar chaos to creative disorder. *Contemp. Psychoanal.* 19:71–99.

Sullivan, H.S. (1953). *The Interpersonal Theory of Psychiatry.* New York: Norton.

Thomas, K.M., Drevets, W.C., Whalen, P.J., Eccard, C.H., Dahl, R.E., Ryan, N.D., & Casey, B.J. (2001). Amygdala responses to facial expressions in children and adults. *Biological Psychiatry* 49:309–316.

Tottenham, N., Haxby, J., Casey, B.J., Whalen, P., & Worden, M. (2003). Establishing age-appropriate times for masked faces. Poster presentation, Cognitive Neuroscience Society.

Viderman, S. (1979). The analytic space: Meaning and problems. *Psycho-analytic Quarterly* 4:257–291.

Vygotsky, L.S. (1934). *Thought and Language.* Cambridge: MIT Press, 1962.

Wallerstein, R. (1990). Psychoanalysis: The common ground. *Int. J. Psycho-Anal.* 71:3–20.

Werner, H.E., & Kaplan, B. (1963). *Symbol Formation.* New York: Wiley.

Westen, D. (1999). The scientific studies of unconscious processes: Is Freud really dead? *J. Amer. Psychoanal. Assn.* 47:1061–1105.

—— & Gabbard, G. (2002a). Developments in cognitive neuroscience: I. Conflict, compromise, and connectionism. *J. Amer. Psychoanal. Assn.* 50:53–98.

—— &—— (2002b). Developments in cognitive neuroscience: Implications for theories of transference. *J. Amer. Psychoanal. Assn.* 50:99–134.

Whitebook, J. (2002). Slow magic and psychoanalysis. *J. Amer. Psychoanal. Assn.* 50: 1197–1217.

Winnicott, D.W. (1960). The theory of the parent-infant relationship. In *The Maturational Processes and the Facilitating Environment.* New York: International Universities Press, 1965, pp. 37–55.

PART IV.

FROM SILENCE TO COMPLEXITY (DEVELOPMENTAL CONTEXT OF SYMBOLIC COMPETENCE)

This group of papers concerns the role of development on emerging competence in the use of words and stories. The papers describe a broad swathe of inquiry that derives from my role as an academic Child and Adolescent psychiatrist and investigator, focused on developmentally disordered children, as well as a psychoanalyst. I devoted research and clinical time to studying young children with serious disorders who routinely presented with delayed and deviant language landmarks, often diagnosed as autistic or intellectually challenged. This population, encountered as toddlers, could be approached from the standpoint of their language behavior.

I applied the principles of development, derived from study of academic and psychoanalytic proposals concerning emergent symbolic function, to various queries that were designed to better understand salient questions: What is the difference between variation and deviance; how should we characterize the alterations in linguistic capacity and cognition during maturation? Can we use normative tools of measurement to study disturbed and deviant children? The normal and pathological variables discovered in symbolic function, and the laws of reorganization that accompanies maturation, became the focus of this body of empirical research, as we sought to follow the development of fantasies as well as social communication in its rich variation.

The first paper is a systematic study of a mixed population of toddlers with early disturbances in social communication (PDD; ASD, etc.,). We adapted data from normal developmental studies and applied the techniques of language measurement to children who were autistic (at the time at Bellevue we used the term schizophrenia, childhood type). It was before DSM III, and before the introduction of PDD and autism and then ASD were standardized for better reliability across institutions. We proceeded from the most prominent feature of the disorder, Autism, to study social communication as language behavior. One of the first tasks was to query whether echoing and poorly contextualized speech in this population reflected deviance in comparison to the imitation in normal language learning. We explored further the context of echoing to determine if it was reflexive, without consideration of meaning in a thoughtful, mediated manner. This was but another demonstration that these children were deviant. They were not on a linear maturational path. Their echoing was not imitation as usual: it was not generative of more flexible forms that could be applied for future use.

Another issue that we were eager to understand was the contextual relevance or the pragmatics of language, i.e. its use as a communicative tool, and how deviant children coded their inner world. Most important, we discovered that the most productive sector of measurement concerned the pragmatics and the use of language in communication, rather than the structure and form of their units of communication. Indeed, autistic children display a paucity of fantasy and their capacity to play differs from that of normals. This opened the way to study turn-taking and topic maintenance in discourse as a means of better describing the variables that contribute to poor or deviant social communication and, later, poor adaptation. (I would here like to note my appreciation to my academic colleagues at NYU and Cornell Medical Colleges, Margaret Hertzig, Margaret Snow, and Miriam Sherman for their hard work and brilliant contributions)

The next paper augments Freud's idea of latency as a universal maturational landmark. The academic postulate that development may be understood as a series of hierarchic reorganizations during the early years was introduced to integrate a large corpus of data from neurodevelopment, cognitive studies, and social landmarks, both historically and synchronically. It was a neat correlate to the analytic inference of infantile repression and subsequent primacy of the Oedipal resolution as a nuclear concept incorporating and superceding prior stages. "Latency Revisited," (coauthored with Richard Perry, 1976) proved to become one of my most cited integrative essays, and it was later applied to a GAP Publication *How Old is Old Enough?* that I also helped shepherd to publication.

Moving on to adolescence in 1985, I wrote an essay on Adolescent language and its use in individuation, diagnosis, and definition of the changing idiolects of the post-pubertal period. The use of secret or selective group understanding of a linguistic variant is a way of balkanizing the teen group designed to separate from the family as the prior linguistic community (we start our linguistic life using the mother tongue). This new argot is redesigned in each generation for a community of peers.

"Preschool Children's Concept of Ghosts" (1980) is an offshoot of a replication of an earlier paper on the newly acquired skill of figure drawing of 2-and 3-year olds, as well as a study of how ghosts are perceived by children. It applies a systematic empirical approach to developmental issues concerning the origin of symbolic thought and the early representation of our bodies and the bodies of others. The growing ability to think in ideas and in images and the constraining role of nominalization and culture on these images becomes the stuff of adult communication. The developmental inquiry was impeded by a social artifact of a popularly disseminated contamination—Casper the Friendly Ghost.

The final contribution to this section concerns normalization in adolescence, as the inner life of middle childhood fantasies must be adapted to the pubertal demands of a changing body and the new biologic capacity for adult sexuality during the teen years. The role of masturbation and the specifics of masturbation fantasies in adult sexual life are explored, as they provide the unique personal conditions for arousal derived from the dim past of childhood rumination. These unique inner stories are explored as influences on and deterrents to socializing, because they have not been revealed in open discourse and are surrounded by secret prohibitions espoused by the culture. It is one of Erikson's crucial steps in adaptation, requiring the integration of intimacy and sexual procreative aims and thus permitting species survival. This paper remains a further justification for analysts to consider the early Freudian focus on fantasy and depth psychology.

These papers are derived from empirical observation of deviant toddlers and multidisciplinary efforts. They complement earlier papers, from clinical and theoretical musings during psychoanalytic practice. Each area employs thinking developmentally and using the humanistic approach to meaning.

The Speech Act:
A Linguistic Framework of Reference to Study Ego Adaptation of a Psychotic Child

(1977). In *Communicative Strategies and Communicational Structures* (ed. N. Freedman). New York: Plenum Press.

I n recent years, infant research and early childhood studies have focused on the interaction between mother and child as the relevant unit to be explored in the march of developmental adaptation. This is the vantage point of many psychoanalyst-trained infant investigators (Sander, 1975; Stern, 1971), as well as of a number of animal behaviorists (Schneirla, 1960). Mahler's (1975) view of the separation-individuation process likewise focuses on interactional matrices and postulates "psychic hatching" along with biological maturation. This dominant psychoanalytic view of the problems of infancy also derives in part from Hartmann's concept of "average expectable biological equipment in an average expectable environment" that also focuses attention on interaction.

While these propositions have yielded rich information about the psychology of functioning individuals, this psychology tends to omit the effects of the "limitations of the flesh" upon the mental apparatus. Freud himself emphasized these other factors in his early formulations of actual neuroses (1895) hypnoid tendencies (1895), constitutional factors in libidinal fixation (1905), the molding effect of body ego on maturing ego function (1905), and narcissistic ego distortions (1914) Greenacre's (1952) later insistence on the predisposing effects of intrauterine experiences on later manifestations of anxiety in the borderline state is an extension of theseideas. Similarly, the recent deluge of writing by analysts on narcissistic development is an attempt to deal with the fact that patients who roughly correspond to these descriptions are seen more frequently in practice.

The specific solution in theorizing about object-splitting, I believe, originates in the simple methodological fact that psychoanalysis is an interactional process. The transference is its major tool, enabling practitioners to best explore the distortions in object relations of their patients. However, as a general psychology, psychoanalysts should not be content with an exclusively object-relations theory of development. That route has been traveled before by Sullivan (1953). M. Klein (1932), and other classical analysts have always felt these positions to be too fragmentary as a general approach. While it is plausible that object-relations theory refers to one of the most aspects of our functioning, it is also the case that a developmentally holistic view requires that human relations, among other behaviors, rests upon background distortions and limitations of cognitive and other autonomous ego apparatuses.

Reading the literature, with the hope of finding the reasons for pathology in faulty mothering, has led to as many distortions as postulating intrinsic ego defects. Moreover, many psychoanalysts cover themselves for these distortions by shifting from intrapsychicto interactional causal statements, and back again as needed. Too few adopt Winnicott's caution that there is such a thing as "good enough mothering," and we are not certain as yet which are the "limiting" factors that encroach upon the "experience of mothering" versus "actual mothering." Dyadic studies remain plausible if the hypotheses generated do not automatically exclude nature-and-nurture weightings. The research to be described attempts such a task. The framework is semi-naturalistic and not analytic.

BACKGROUND

I have selected the most deviant children, seen by child psychiatrists, who are without known structural defects of the central nervous system for study. Autistic or early-childhood schizophrenic children provide a model of severe early behavioral deviance—in which inadequate or "damaged" ego structures may be inferred. However, the interactional matrix is also affected, and careful analysis of the structure of their interaction may generate the best hypotheses, studying language, via the actually deviant speech development of these children. As practicing psychoanalysts, we usually emphasize the potent effect of conflict upon autonomous functions. Such childrenprovide us not only with instrumentality for observing an aspect of ego functioning, but also offer clues to the elements necessary for normal development that are not observable when speech develops smoothly. In the latter instance, we may not see the discontinuities or hierarchic stepwise progression of development because the steps are slurred over. Former work by the author has shown that autistic and schizophrenic children have a number of disturbances in linguistic processing and coding (such as echoing) so that their production appears deviant from the standpoint not only of content, but of structure and context orientation (Shapiro et al., 1975). This paper will focus upon utilizing a framework of "speech acts" (Searle, 1969) in order to examine and understand the communicational significance of echoing in psychotic children, and from that offer suggestions regarding its developmental role in normals.

Shapiro, Roberts, and Fish (1970), showed that psychotic children at age four echoed more rigidly than normal compeers at ages two, three, and four. It was even found that a large number of responses of two-year-olds were newly recoded creative imitations rather than recorder-like replays, When psychotic children were studied for grammatical contrast of negation (Shapiro & Kapit, in press), they proved to "be most competent imitators compared to three-year-old normal controls, who insisted on changing grammatical form even after being instructed not to." Normal five-year-olds were also good imitators because they were compliant, but were fully able to produce the most varied grammatical forms when free to do so.

Studying normals, Nelson (1973) showed that children do not invariably learn nouns-for-things as their first words, as formerly thought . Rather, there seem to be what she calls "referential" children whose early corpus (first 50 words) contains a predominance of nouns, and "expressive" children who do not build their early vocabulary in that way. The former are more likely to imitate. Bloom (1974) similarly showed in a naturalistic longitudinal study of four children, that two were imitators and two were not. She went on to show that the imitators were as likely to have the same grammatical forms in their imitative utterances as in their nonimitative ones, suggesting that imitation was "progressive," i.e., even when echoing was a significant behavior, it was a sign of cognitive or grammatical readiness. This view is in line with Piagetian developmental studies

(Sinclair de Zwart, 1969), and contrary to the view that imitation precedes comprehension and production, as indicated by Fraser, Bellug L, and Brown (1963). Propositions endorsing reinforcement and generalization have been criticized before this latter work as not fully explaining the rapid onset of creative syntactic forms in small children (Lenneberg, 1967; Bloom, 1970; McNeill, 1970). Fay and Butler (1968) have studied the echoing of non-psychotic, retarded children, and discussed the function of echoing.

One of these suggestions will be expanded in the current paper, and explored, to understand something about the distorted speech function of psychotic children. Careful experiments by Hermelin and O'Connor (1970) show that autistic children have an intact auditory span, but that decoding and association processes are impaired. They coined the term "echo-box memory" to characterize the performance of these children. Extending this notion, Aurnhammer-Frith (1969) found the effects of phonological structure to be equal for a group of eight autistic and a group of eight normal children, but autistic children were deficient in their appreciation of syntax as presented in the sequential structure of language. Others (Bartolucci & Albers 1974; Bartok & Rutter 1974) have similarly showed the inabilities of these children in syntactic understanding in the specific area of development of deixis.

Our observations have led us to understand, and the current paper tests further, the propositions that echoes in young psychotic children represent a device for social closure in a child whose limited cognitive capacities permit a limited repertoire of other responses. The index child seems to be saying, "I understand that I am expected to speak in this social situation, but I neither understand what is appropriate nor have the wit. to do so. However, I can say something, and that seems to stop you, the interlocutor, from making the

445

same sounds to me." Parenthetically, I believe it is for this reason that behaviorist techniques, as utilized by Lovaas (1974), Hewett (1965), etc., have been grabbed up so readily by many "therapist-investigators" not because they produce greater fluency in language, but because the increment in productivity of pat imitative phrases pleases investigators, who count any advance as significant in what seems to be an uphill battle,

The notion of a speech event as a "speech act" utilizes the interactional or communicative frame of reference and goes beyond the simply structural view which has been taken in prior studies. It suggests an illocutionary intent in an interchange, and a perlocutionary response which says to the initiator of the communication, "I have heard you; I understand you; and I intend to answer relevantly or irrelevantly in whatever way I am able." While this interactional model again stresses a two-party system for linguistic understanding, it leaves open the possibility that the nature of the response could be analyzed from the standpoint of its functional pragmatism in a communicative situation.

This framework, in conjunction with prior structural models, suggests a number of expectations that can be tested empirically. These expectations will be explored in the speech sample of a single autistic child of five years, six months, at the time of interviewing. If echoes were but device for social closure, the following ought to be demonstrated:

1. The total number of responses per unit time of such a child ought to be greater than the number of responses of a comparable child at a similar age. A subhypothesis of this notion is that if the increased number of responses within the time sample were due to the "social closure strategy" of echoing,

then echoes would have a more rapid reaction time. Thus, we could compare the reaction-time for echoes versus non-echoes, as well as the uniformity within each subsector of utterances to infer the degree of processing time necessary.

2. Mean length of utterance (MLU) of echoes should be somewhat longer than the mean length of utterance (MLU) of other responses of the same child, because intrinsic grammatical coding devices would be bypassed for echoes and not constrained as much as when the child is trying to code his or her own response on the basis of restructuring and matching processes.

3. The echoing ought to occur at points in the interview where the question asked taxes the child's comprehension, i.e., echoing ought to follow demands which are more complex than those that elicit appropriate acceptable responses.

4. It would be expected that when an echo chain is set into motion that echoes might cluster, as though the child falls into a perlocutionary mode that satisfies the interaction, and this becomes a "sticky set" used beyond the necessity of the moment.

5. The remainder of the corpus of responses of the child ought to be limited in its variety, suggesting the functional need for so simple a device as echoing as an intermittent response type when cognitive-linguistic capacities are stretched beyond available resources.

If we can demonstrate these five points in a sample of speech of an autistic child, we will have satisfied the hypothesis that viewing echoing as a speech act offers a sufficient frame of reference to understand an aspect of the limited ego-functions of this psychotic child. This interpretation, then, may be used to suggest parallel deficits in object relations leading to distorted "child-mother" or "child-other" interactions. Both of these functional problems would need be secondary to the limitation of cognitive substructure, and neither would have priority in this child, but viewed as typical of a group. It also would be instructive to compare the speech act of this child to the child with average biological equipment, to see how normal language learning facilitates object relations as well as the reciprocal proposition.

BRIEF HISTORY

Evan was first seen at 4 years, 6 months, after a speech and hearing evaluation at four. His mother's chief complaint was that he was withdrawn and had not developed language adequately. He screeched and spent much of his time at the television set, panicking when it was turned off, but was not "really" watching it. He was interested in mechanical things, and took a can of coffee or oil to bed rather than a soft object. He had recently been destructive. He was coordinated, but seemed unaware of dangerous temper tantrums, in which he threw himself on the floor, undressed, and threw things, and which were elicited at the slightest provocation, He grimaced, played with his fingers, and occasionally covered his ears and walked on his toes.

He was the first child of an 18-year-old black mother and a German-born white father. Both were teachers. Evan was full-term (birthweight of 7.7 pounds) and aside from an occipital hematoma, no birth defects were noted. The hematoma subsided in two months. The infant was hypotonic but irritable until nine months. He was described as "colicky, had difficulty falling asleep at night unless he was held and rocked," which his mother did. Bedtime rocking continued until he was 2.6. Evan was breast-fed and began drinking from a cup at nine months without a transitional bottle.

He began to feed himself at three years of age. He was not yet trained at time of admission.

No significant medical history was elicited. He sat unaided at six months, stood at seven months, and walked at 11 months. He smiled at six weeks, and is described as having made good eye contact until about 1.6 when he withdrew. However, he was never considered an affectionate child. He would sit in a corner when people, other than his parents, were present, and avoideye contact.

At 2.6, Evan was enrolled in a day-care program but was dropped after three months because he was "not interested." At home, he was hyperactive but withdrawn and quiet in the nursery. His mother stopped working to care for Evan and her second child, born when Evan was 2.10.

Evan's language development included vowel sounds between three to five months, but no babbling. At 18 months he said a few single words, e.g. "cookie,"and "juice," and responded variably to his name. At two, he pointed at words that his mother was reading to him, and learned the alphabet and numbers "within a week." His production was exclusively designations. His vocabulary expanded little between two to three. years, and he did not combine words. At three, he echoed entire sentences, and identified pictures "if he wished to." While he understood a few simple directions at four, his parents still thought he might be deaf.

On admission, Evan was described as a handsome, neatly dressed, tall, well-developed, light -kinned Negro boy. His facial expression was bland except for grimacing. His responses were delayed, and his attention was fleeting, He made no overt social overtures and cried only briefly when his mother left him. When she returned

1-1/2 hours later, he did not look at her, but ran out of the nursery. At first he would not sit at the examining table, but was soon able to be engaged in testing. He adapted to the reversal of the Gesell formboard (36 months level) and played with the. non-animate toys, ignoring the family dolls, He only scribbled at pencil and paper tasks, he did not pay attention when his mother encouraged him to make an "o" and responded, "No" when she asked him to draw a pumpkin, which he apparently had been capable of doing.

He sat in the examiner's rotary chair saying, "Take it off, I get off" and turned around on it. He named items such as "zipper" and "egg," but would not name "letters." He named his mother's mouth, but. no other parts of her body. He added a few words out of context, with no apparent relevance to the current setting. He comprehended minimally. Some of his speech was unintelligible, he did not respond to his name, and he ignored many questions and commands.

He was diagnosed as having an early-onset psychosis corresponding, in varying nomenclatures, to early infantile autism or childhood schizophrenia, autistic type. He improved at the Bellevue Nursery with milieu, educational, and drug therapy. He made some attachments to nursery personnel and sought them out on occasion to verbalize his wishes and aims. While he continued to spend much of his time alone, some interaction and eye contact was tolerated; his attention span increased, and he could persist at assembling a picture puzzle for up to 30 minutes. His affect broadened with better modulation and less irritability. His language production and comprehension improved. At discharge, his speech was largely intelligible and more spontaneous, but stilted. Much of what he said was as though speaking out loud to himself, but he also used speech to communicate needs. His productions usually referred to the current circumstance, and his vocabulary remained limited. He was discharged to a specialized treatment center and his mother continues to work with him.

METHOD

1. Evan was seen between the ages of four years, nine months and seven years, six months. During the three years, he was audiotaped ten times for ten-minute stimulated sessions. In addition, special linguistic testing was instituted from time to time. The examiner stimulated the child's productive speech by asking simple questions about objects, picture books, and other play material. A transcript of the recording was prepared and correlated with an observer's context notes of the interview. The utterances were classified according to a two- dimensional scale of morphological complexity and communicative value (Shapiro, Fish, 1969). Communicativeness included distinction between non-communicative and communicative speech. The latter encompasses such utterances as simple social greetings, appeal, or wish-oriented speech, as well as complex symbolic speech. Noncommunicative speech includes isolated expressive speech, echoes, and utterances with little or no contextual reference. The present study contrasts the echoic and nonechoic responses in terms of MLU, stimulus conditions, and latency of the child's echoing of the examiner's speech, compared to the mean latency of all other functional categories of the child's speech. Response latency, for our purposes, is defined as the time intervening between the examiner's model sentence or query and the child's utterance.

A duplicate tape of the original recording was made, and a ten-second gap was introduced at the end of each of the child's utterances to facilitate analysis with reaction-time equipment. The duplicate tape was played on a Tapesonic deck, the signal from which was fully rectified and demodulated, and then sent to a Bechman Offner polygraph. The tape was also monitored auditorily. The polygraph produced a paper recording which was advanced at a rate of 50 mm. per second. The modified signal caused a pen on the polygraph to produce a peak corresponding to each syllable of recorded speech. The response latencies were obtained by measuring the interval on the polygraph recording between the last peak of the examiner's speech and the first peak of the child's utterance. (The error of the circuitry and polygraph was 1/100 of a second. The intervals on the polygraph recording could be measured to within a millimeter so the error from this source was two hundredths of a second. Presumably these two sources of error often canceled each other. In any case, all response latencies are accurate to three hundredths of a second). Evan progressed in his language development from a MLU of 1.1 to a MLU approximating 2. He always remained highly deviant and echoed frequently. When he was 5.6 years, he had a of MLU of .78, indicating that many of his utterances were above two words in length, and that he was beginning some syntactic structuring, This sample was selected for study.

RESULTS

Evan produced 139 utterances in the ten-minute period with MLU result 1.78, consisting of 58 echoes (41.7%) and 81 nonechoes (58.3%). See Table 1. There were ten prespeech utterances among his nonechoes that were not used to calculate the mean length of utterance. There were 12 poorly contextualized utterances, B [?] appeal utterances, 48 designations, and 3 answers to questions.

Table 1
Ten Minute Speech Sample
Evan (5 years 6 months)

	Echoes	Nonechoes	Total
Number of Utterances	58	81	139
Percent of Utterances	41.7	58.3	100%
MLU	1.95	1.67	1.78
Reaction Time Variance(s)	603.54*		

* 53 Echoes used for reaction time
** Omitting noncommunicative responses
+ Mann–Whitney U p < .00011

1. Evan's 139 responses in ten minutes were compared to the average frequencies of children formerly studied for echoing behavior during similar ten-minute examinations (Shapiro, Roberts, & Fish, 1970). A sample of eight hospitalized psychotic children produced a mean total number of utterances of 84.6 (range. 62C123; only two of these subjects had more than 100 responses). A combined sample of 18 normal children between the ages of 2.0 and 4.9 had a mean number of utterances of 93 (range 72C113). The group of four-year-olds more closely comparable to Evan's chronological age showed a mean total number of utterances of 90.1. Thus, Evan produced more utterances during the. examination time than his comparison groups of psychotic children and clearly more than normal The overall impression was that Evan's high frequency of

echoes accounted for the increased number of responses, because it appeared that he responded to the examiner with shorter latency. To test this hypothesis, the reaction times of echoic and nonechoic responses were measured separately. The hypothesis was further extended that echoic responses would be more uniform in their latency because varied processing times might be necessary for other responses as compared to echoes. The variance of the echoic was then studied in terms of the four dimensions previously outlined:

(1) Speed of response and total number of responses within the examination period, and

(2) MLU of echoes was contrasted to nonechoes

(3) Analysis was made of which of the interviewer's questions elicited echoes and whether they clustered.

(4) Finally, the nonechoic responses were analyzed for complexity of syntactic structure and appropriateness of reference. The sample was S=603.54, while the nonechoes variance was S=18467.94, verifying the greater uniformity of the latency of echoic response in this sample, Because of the difference in variance, a [?]test was not used to test the significance of the difference between means. The nonparametric Mann Whitney U Test was employed. The difference between the echoic and nonechoic responses was highly significant (p >.00011) . (Because of difficulties in the time sample, 53 of the 58 echoes were used for study or 44.570 of the entire sample.)

2. The mean length of utterance: It was hypothesized that if the echoes were not processed by the usual encoding, but only subject to a more general constraint on length, that the echoes

should be longer than coded utterances . The WU of echoes was 1.95, and the nonechoes, 1. 67. However, since MLU does not take into account syntactic structure or the context in which they are produced, further hypotheses were tested.

3. Echoes were elicited a total of 58 times during the interview, However, a number of the echoes occurred in bursts ranging from two to 11 consecutive responses so that 27 of the 58 echoic responses initiated a group of echoes. That is, there were nine bursts of echoing that were more than two echoes long, some ranging as high as 8 to 11 times. This observation suggests than when a child begins echoing, this becomes a temporarily preferred strategy.

For structural analysis, we included some responses which were not completely congruent echoes, because we wanted to test the range of all imitative responsiveness. Consequently, some productions had inflectional changes, telegraphic selection, and grammatical transformations which suggested that, at the least, he was on the verge of grammatical development (Table 2, B) .

Structural alterations, however, accounted for a small percentage of the corpus of echoes (13 of 58) . The single perseveration does not require presumed grammatical knowledge or new words. Correct naming, associated with pointing, was ambiguous as to function because he was simply repeating what the examiner has said, though it was associated with a concrete environmental object. Again, no restructuring was required. The mitigation [?] was a response to "count fingers." He repeated verbatim, and proceeded "one, two, three, four, five." This was an often-heard rote sequence for Evan. The only two utterances classified as echoes that comfortably can be considered as being at the threshold of new grammatical forms were the inflected plural change and a negative transformation. When the examiner said, "Show me and touch it." He responded "Don't touch it." However, this also may not be a true negative transformation because he had often heard the prohibition in just that form. The positive phrase may have triggered the more-often-heard negative. At best, we may say he showed knowledge of the relationship between the two phrases.

Table 2
Analysis of Echo (Variants) and Nonechoes
Evan (5 years 6 months)

Nonechoes	Utterances
A. Prespeech	1
Designations	0
Wish/Command	4
	0
Answers	3
Phatic	6
PoorContext	1
	2
B. Structurally Altered Imitations	
Perseverative	1
Telegraphic (omits article)	1
Telegraphic (omits clause, object pronoun, preposition)	1
Names as points	1
Inflectional change (pluralizes final S)	
Mitigated echo (adds rote counting)	1
Mitigated phatic	1
Negative transformation	1

Turning now to the variety of questions that elicited echoes, aside from those where he responded in a phatic way or continued a burst of echoing that had begun, it was evident from the relative complexity of the queries chat that he may not have comprehended the question. For example, when the examiner asked, "Where is the boar[bear?] blue? Show me," he said, "Blue" and pointed to the yellow. At another point, the examiner asked, "What kind of book? He responded, "Book." After he named a ball, he was asked, "What can you do with the ball?" He answered telegraphically "Do ball." Then the examiner asked, "Can you throw a ball ?" Evan answered, "Throw a ball." Continuing, the examiner then asked, "Can you bounce a ball?" The child ignored the query, turned the page, looked at another picture, and named a brush. He could then comply when the examiner asked what else was shown and said "comb" clearly, indicating that he could readily name things. Indeed, some 48 of his nonechoic, communicative utterances were designations (Table 2, A).

Further verification for this proposition comes from a burst of echoing that was initiated after he had named an orange. The examiner asked, "What do you do with an orange?" He repeated "Orange." The examiner again asked, "What can you do with an orange?" The child said, "Do orange" The examiner then offered a semi-nonsense query, "Do you throw it?" Evan responded, "Throw it." Examiner, "Or eat it?" He responded, "Eat it." Similarly, later on, when the examiner suggested "Let's talk about something else," the child responded, "Talk something else." These responses suggest that there is limitation in comprehension which, in turn, severely limits the appropriate productive output of this child, and at such junctures, he resorts to echoic behavior.

CONCLUSION

A speech-act framework permits us to stress the dyadic nature of early-language learning rather than the emergence of facility with the code. In that sense, it corresponds to what psychoanalysts have recently emphasized in their developmental hypotheses that lean on interactive matrices to study the individuation processes. Jerome Bruner (1974) makes the point that "Grammar originates as a set of rules abstracted from jointly regulated activity which has been codified in the culture of the linguistic community"' (p. 7) . Bruner sees grammar's emergence, even if naturally latent, as paralleling prior perceptual and attention structures, each of which enables the development of prediction and sentence closure. Action structures usually carried out with the mother'saction toward or away from the self leads to "case grammar forms (agent, action, object) and ultimately in its most sophisticated form to deixis! (the changing referent for a single object where in one instance it is here, and then there, or regarding persons at once I, you, and he)." The question that our data asks is, why did Evan not emerge with a normal repertoire, if potentials for grammatical and cognitive structures are part of average biological equipment in humans? Are we to turn to schizophrenogenicity in mothering for explanation? Our exploration of the structure of his interactions does not include his early interactions with his mother. However, even with adequate environmental exposure in the nursery, he did not show adequately progressive language development. By contrast, even neglected children in postmarasmic states learn to speak. While institutionalized children may, at times, emerge as affectionless criminals, they seem to know noun from verb, etc. Could one argue for a specific "quality of mothering as yet undefined" to account for autistic language as described? We think not. The deficits seem to penetrate deeply into cognitive structures themselves. A recent report by Simon (1975) goes so far as to localize a substrate deficit in the brain itself .

The interactive developmental view should not force us to propose that all that evolves as a result of that interaction. Rather, the interaction also describes the species of capability of each of the parties. We are not simply as we are acted upon. That would satisfy a behaviorist's paradigm in which all that emerges was once in the environment. Parenthetically, autistic children are much studied by behaviorists because there seems to be so little in the way of intervening variables in the black box. On the other hand, preformist postulates do not tell us how and when language and speech emerge or the limits of the environment that any given organism will tolerate.

Freud has been attacked from both sides, as a biological maturational 1st[?] on the one hand, and an overzealous environmentalist on the other. However, in actuality. Freud echoed the classicist' s epigram that all of behavior is a combination of "necessity and accident," thus leaving the way open to examine the contribution of each. Hartmann's adaptational view, likewise, demands study of the contribution from both sides. Let us see how behavior revealing contributions from both sides of our postulated dyad.

Evan can form few grammatical constructions. He has turned toward the most concrete environment reflected in his limited, largely nominal vocabulary, but is stymied in understanding and producing creative grammatical forms, as even normal 30-month old children can. He echoes when in doubt and that he does with a uniform reaction time suggests limitations in integrating and encoding for such a response. He avoids the human environment because he cannot process what is offered, so he backs off. His echoing is an adaptation to some dimly recognized need to speak even though he does not understand. A mentally deficient child functions differently. He is retarded across the board, can tolerate close contact and affection, and use his deficient intelligence to its limits, but the autistic child has learned to make short shrift of the world because it confuses him. The inability is not outside, but at the experiential level. Perhaps, mimicking Bruner, his attentional and perceptual apparatuses are timed differently and are too variable to be a reliable guide to later grammatical development: i.e., the neuroperceptual background of action schemata which are said to underlie grammatical form may be awry. This still leaves room for etiological hedging, but not for hedging in adequate description of structure of behavior. This careful description of behavioral structure within the framework described permits greater clarity with respect to designating the direction for our interest, while not disrupting the human context in which development takes place.

Object-relations theory and theories of environmental determination are as incomplete a description of the scope of human adaptation as is Behaviorism. Psychoanalysts who emphasize only these parameters should remember that they represent but one sector of a possible bevy of functions and interactions that create *homo communicandis.*

REFERENCES

Aurnhammer-Frith, U. (1969). Emphasis and meaning in recall in normal and autistic children. *Language and Speech* 12:29–38.

Bartak, L & Rutter, M. (1974). The use of person pronouns for autistic children. *Journal of Autism and Childhood Schizophrenia* 4:217–222.

Bartoluccii G. & Albers, R. (1974). Deictic categories in the language of autistic children. *Journal of Autism and Childhood Schizophrenia,* 4:2.

Bloom, L (1970). *Language Development: Form and Function in Emerging Grammars.* Cambridge, MA; MIT Press,

Bloom, L, Hood, L, & Lightbovn, P. (1974). Imitation In language development : If, when, and why. *Cognitive Psychology* 96:380-420.

Bruner, J.S. (1974). The ontogenesis of speech acts. *Journal of Child Language,* 2:1–19, Great Britain.

Fay, W. Ho, & Butler, B.V. (1968). Echolalia, IQ and the developmental dichotomy of speech and language-systems. *Hearing Research,* 1:365–371.

Fraser, C., Bellugi, U., & Brown, R. (1963). Control of grammar in imitation, comprehension and production. *Journal of Verbal Learning and Verbal Behavior* 2:121–135.

Freud, S. (1895b). On the ground for detaching a particular syndrome from neurasthenia under the description anxiety neurosis. *Standard Edition* 3:87.

——— (1905). Three essays on the theory of sexuality. *Standard Edition* 7:125–245.

——— (1914c). On narcissism: An introduction. *Standard Edition* 4:73–102.

——— & Breuer, (1893-5). Studies on hysteria. *Standard Edition* 2. Greenacre, P. (1952). The predisposition to anxiety. Part I. In: *Trauma, growth and personality.* New York: Norton.

Hermelin, B. & Connor, N. (1970) *Psychological experiments with autistic children.* Oxford, England: Pergamon Press,

Hewett, F.M. (1965). Teaching speech to an autistic child through operant conditioning. *American Journal of Orthopsychiatry,* 35:927–936.

Klein, M. (1932*). The psychoanalysis of children.* London: Hogarth Press.

Lenneburg, E.H. (1967). *Biological foundations of language,* New York: Wiley,

Lovaass, D.T., Schrefdman, L., & Koegel, R.L. (1974). A behavior modification approach to the treatment of autistic children. *Journal of Autism and Childhood Schizophrenia,* Vol. 4, p. 131.

Mahler, M. Pine, F, & Bergman, A. (1975). *The psychological birth of the human infant.* New York: Basic Books.

.McNeill, D. (1970). *The acquisition of language: The study of developmental psycholinguistic.* New York: Harper and Row,

Nelson, K. (1973). Structure and strategy in learning to talk. *Monographs of the Society for Research in Child Development* 38 (1–2 Serial #149) .

Sander, L.W. Some determinants of temporal organization in the ecological niche of the newborn. Read at the Annual Meeting of the. American Academy of Child Psychiatry, St. Louis.

Searle, J, (1969). *Speech acts: An essay of language* . London: Cambridge University Press,

Schneirla, T.C. (1960). Instinctive behavior. maturation, experience and development. In B. Kaplan & S. Wapner (Eds.) *Perspectives in psychological theory.* New York; International Universities Press.

Shapiro, T. (1975). Language and ego function of young psychotic children, In E. J. Anthony (Ed.), *Explorations in child psychology.* New York: Plenum.

———— & Fish, B. (1969). A method to study language deviation as an aspect of ego organization in young schizophrenic children. *Journal of the American Academy of the Academy of Child Psychiatry.* vol. 9, No. 3.

———— Roberts, A., Fish, B. (1970), Imitation and echoing in young schizophrenic children. *Journal of the American Academy of Child Psychiatry* vol. 9, No. 3.

———— & Kapit, R. Negation in young schizophrenic children. *Journal of Psycholinguistic Research* in press.

Simon, N. (1975). Echolalic speech in childhood autism. *American Journal of General Psychiatry* 32:1439–1446.

Sinclair de Zwart, H. (1969). Developmental psycholinguistic In D. Elk, & J.H. Flavell (Eds.) *Studies in honor of Jean Piaget.* New York: International Universities Press,

Stern, D. (1971). A microanalysis of mother-infant interaction: Behavior regulating social contact between a mother and her 3 1/2-month old twins. *Journal of the American Academy of Psychiatry* 10:501–517 .

Sullivan, H.S. (1953). *The interpersonal theory of psychiatry.* New York: Norton.

Latency Revisited—*The Age 7 Plus or Minus 1*[1]

(1976). *Psychoanalytic Study of the Child* 31:79–105.

Scientific investigation generally proceeds within disciplinary lines. Chemists do chemistry and biologists do biology. However, there is also an interpenetration of individual scientific approaches when data derived from one method seem relevant to the theories and constructs of another. Psychoanalysis is not exempt from this interpenetration or the revisions in theory made necessary by advances in other sciences. Indeed, awareness of such changes is sometimes salutary, in that they elaborate or better define ideas derived from the psychoanalytic method alone. While Freud (1950,1919) sought to keep analysis methodologically free of encroachment by other therapeutic modalities, he frequently borrowed from data of biologists of his time and often modified his theory to bring it into relation with current clinical practice

---

1   The title of this paper is offered with considered respect to George A. Miller (1956), who wrote of a "Magical Number Seven, Plus or Minus Two," which concerns limits in the capacity for processing information. Partial support for this project derives from NIMH Training Grant #MH07331.

and data from other sciences. Among Freud's more controversial concepts was the idea of a biological basis for the latency period, an idea which was both supported and criticized during his lifetime and since his death. He seemed ever expectant that biological and chemical studies would provide the evidence that clinical science could not provide regarding the source of drives and their postulated quantitative alterations during development. His hope revealed a tacit belief in the complementarity of all science.

This paper will reexamine Freud's changing thoughts on the latency period and survey the reformulations of subsequent psychoanalytic writers. The concept of latency will then be examined in the light of recent research gathered from methods outside of psychoanalysis. We shall argue that these new data tend to support Freud's initial surmise that latency has a biological basis, but not for the reasons he proposed. We will suggest that (1) the functional changes in the child's neurobiological, perceptual, and cognitive development that cluster about the 7th year of life are probably functionally associated with the dissolution of the Oedipus complex; (2) these functional changes in the organization of mental life and their dynamic concomitants provide latency with the behaviors which characterize this stage; (3) these assertions will be supported by correlative evidence gleaned from other sciences which, while discontinuous in their method and vantage point, provide a remarkable concordance of new information useful to clinical psychoanalysts.

Among the data we present, we place special emphasis on the remarkable fact that the chronological age of 7^2 is referred to so frequently as to suggest a milestone marking discontinuous

---

2 Nursery school and kindergarten do of course also prepare for learning; some continuous educational aim is exploited at these earlier stages, *but* these remain pre-first-grade groups and have appeared somewhat late on the historical scene.

development. Had Freud never alerted us to latency in the first instance, we would have been compelled to discover it anew. Indeed, the longer view of history and sociology of childhood antedating Freud's work indicates that empirically many cultures had already discovered the unique competence of 7-year-olds that permitted them to assume new roles not available when they were younger.

Society seemed to know empirically when to begin its push on the child toward greater autonomy. During the Middle Ages, children were sent away from home to become pages at Court at age 7 (Pinchbeck and Hewitt, 1969), and later, at the time of the Guilds, children were apprenticed at 7. In modern society children are considered to be ready for learning in school at age 7: grade school begins at 6 in the US, at 7 in the USSR. Kohlberg and Gilligan (1971) state that there is an implicit recognition by almost all cultures of "two great stages, or transformations of development" (p. 1056). These are the years of 5 to 7 and adolescence, which respectively usher in and end the period of compulsory education. The Roman Church considers age 7 "the age of reason" in that only then can the child differentiate between the bread of everyday life and the "Host." Therefore, First Communion also coincides with latency. Moreover, in English Common Law, children under 7 are deemed incapable of criminal intent.

Among the post-Freudian authors, Erikson (1950) refers to latency as an "era of industry," accentuating the positive step in ego-formation rather than the suppression of sexuality. Prior to Erikson, Sullivan (1940) focused on the interpersonal shift to peer relations and talked of a "juvenile era" which has lasting portent for future human interactions. Longitudinal observations of urban children led Thomas and Chess (1972) to opt for abandoning the term as misleading because they found that not much was "latent" during this period of childhood. Even their "interactionist" point of view, which places great stress on the temperamental continuities evolving within a social milieu, suggests to them that during what they prefer to call "middle childhood" a number of different patterns are available that need to be distinguished from earlier periods. Any view of development that is "simply biological" necessarily omits the crucial influence of culture, but the converse is also true. In this essay we are attempting to tease out just which, if any, biological alterations underlie the observable behaviors which Freud designated as latency. When Freud wrote about the concept of latency, he could not yet draw on the broad array of facts which recent scientific advances have provided. These facts constitute the basis of our argument for biological maturation as the most important variable in determining the changes we call latency.

Psychoanalytic Literature

In 1905, Freud stated that development is in part "organically determined and fixed by heredity" and indicates that there are mental forces, such as shame, disgust, and moral ideas, that "impede the course of the sexual instinct and, like dams, restrict its flow" (p. 177). He further stresses that education "will not be trespassing beyond its appropriate domain if it limits itself to following the lines which have already been laid down organically" (p. 178). With these statements, Freud laid the groundwork for our view that latency is biological in origin and relatively immutable in the march of development.

While continuing his testimony to its biological basis, Freud later assigned more importance to the environmental contributions to latency, as well as to the effects of castration anxiety. In a footnote added to his autobiography (1925) in 1935, he states, "The period of latency is a physiological phenomenon. It can, however, only give rise to a complete interruption of sexual life in cultural organizations which have made the suppression of infantile sexuality a part of their system. This is not the case with the majority of primitive peoples" (p. 37). Thus, throughout his life, Freud maintained the assertion of biological determinism.

Among the factors associated with the psychological manifestations of latency were the vicissitudes of the incestuous object choice, the resolution of the Oedipus complex, and superego formation. In 1919 Freud wrote, "Most probably [incestuous loves] pass away because their time is over, because the children have entered upon a new phase of development in which they are compelled to recapitulate from the history of mankind the repression of an incestuous object-choice, just as at an earlier stage they were obliged to effect an object-choice of that very sort" (p. 188). Then in 1924, while noting the necessary disappointments associated with the dissolution of the Oedipus complex, Freud reaffirmed his deterministic biological stance: "the Oedipus complex must collapse because the time has come for its disintegration, just as the milk-teeth fall out when the permanent ones begin to grow" (p. 173).

Freud's view of libidinal development was influenced by Abraham's early training as an embryologist. It was probably he who suggested a formal timetable of ontogeny of stages culminating in the Oedipal phase, followed by the latency period. However, when forced to explain the apparent sexual inhibition that characterized latency, Freud was not content with epigenesis, borrowed available data from outside of psychoanalysis, and yielded to biological analogy. At that time, research in the development of sexual tissue revealed changes in growth patterns that seemed to coincide with his sexual theories. While the first peak of growth was intrauterine and not coincident with the development of infantile sexuality, the diphasic growth of these tissues was significant to Freud. In a footnote added in 1920 to the *Three Essays on Sexuality* (1905), he said, "There is, of course, no need to expect that anatomical growth and psychical development must be exactly simultaneous... Since a period of latency in the psychological sense does not occur in animals, it would be very interesting to know whether the anatomical findings which have led these writers to assume the occurrence of two peaks in sexual development are also demonstrable in the higher animals" (p. 177). The "interest" in phyletic discontinuity indicates Freud's own caution in analogizing to animal studies, but also shows his willingness to extend his theory by building on the basis of a speculative extension.

Turning to the vicissitudes of the quantitative aspects of sexual drive during latency, Freud offered two possible explanations. On the one hand, he spoke of the impulses' being diverted into sublimations without a quantitative decrease (1905, p.178). At this point in theorizing, however, the drives were the only source of energy, and productive activity as well as drive-ridden behavior were viewed as having the same source, subject to hydraulic like laws. On the other hand, in 1926, Freud said that during latency "the sexual urges diminish in strength" (p. 210).

The post-Freudian writers on latency may be divided into theoretical speculators, who reason by analogy to other scientific observations, and a second group who base their conclusions on direct child observation. Another group that cannot be ignored, but will not be stressed, derives from Kardiner's early opposition to Freud's strict biological maturational scheme. The so-called culturalists, who took up this banner, denied latency as nothing more than a cultural imposition of certain Western societies and an artifact of rearing practices.

Among the theoretical speculators, Ferenczi (1913) was perhaps the most imaginative. He "surmised" that the geological changes in the surface of the earth had catastrophic consequences for primitive man, who was compelled to repress his favorite habits in order to survive. Neurosis was thus an outgrowth of catastrophes suffered over generations. Within this model, "the great step in individual repression, the latency period [is brought] into connection with the last and greatest catastrophe that smote our primitive ancestors, ... i.e. with the misery of the glacial period, which we still faithfully recapitulate in our individual life" (p. 237). These ideas should not be criticized out of the context of Ferenczi's *Zeitgeist*. He and others of his time were steeped in the new Darwinism, which attempted to deal with human characteristics as complex adaptations to changing requirements for survival over long time spans.

Hans Lampl (1953) incorporated Ferenczi's idea into a phylogenetic program that considered the latency period an inherited recapitulation of the glacial period within the individual. Indeed, the fluctuating manifestations of instinctual drives are the consequence of hormonal changes during latency. Lampl, like Freud, cites the work of Bolk and Lipschütz concerning the observed changes in anatomy and physiology of the sexual organs. Lampl's strict adherence to tissue-psychology parallelism is so extreme that he concludes: "We would be justified to speak of the absence of a latency period only after we have established the existence of a continuous development of the genital organs from birth to sexual maturity" (p. 386).[3]

---

3 Current knowledge of the growth of the genital organ and hormonal secretions is actually in opposition to this view. Scammon (1930) found that the prostate, testes, epididymis, and seminal vesicles in the male, as well as the ovaries, follow a typical

As late as 1967, Yazmajian attempted to explain latency on the grounds of embryological, genetic, and evolutionary concepts. He views latency as the maturation of organ systems, said to follow the sequence of infantile sexual development espoused by Abraham and Freud. He points to Abraham's views, according to which psychosexual development lags behind somatic development, inasmuch as the oral, anal, and urogenital embryological sequence precedes the oral, anal, and phallic psychological progression. When latency is reached, Yazmajian asserts, the "more uniform redistribution of libidinal energies throughout the body would result in a relative decrease of the libidinal investment of the erotogenic zones" (p. 226). Clearly, Yazmajian continues to reason by analogy of biological systems to psychological processes and provides no further explanation of what biological processes may underlie latency as a period with specific behavioral characteristics.

We now turn to analytic investigators who observed children directly and did not rely on reconstructions or reexperiences in the analyses of adults.

On the basis of observations of "thousands of children over a ten-year period," Alpert (1941) stated that "the seven-year-olds represent the closest approximation of the sexual quiescence supposedly characteristic of the period from five to puberty." Even though the 7-year-olds' impulses and conflicts are held to be only disguised,

---

"genital type of growth." In the growth of these organs there is little change from the end of the first year to the latter part of the child's first decade of life. Physiologically, the secretion of estrogens (Nelson et al., 1969) in both boys and girls is fairly constant to the age of 7 years, when it begins to increase slightly until the age of 11. At this age, there is a large rise in production in the female as compared to a slight one in the male. Similarly, 17-ketosteroids show a gradual rise in both sexes to the age of 7. Then until the age of 18, there is a greater rate of increase in both sexes, with the male's ultimately secreting more androgens than the female.

there is a relative calm as compared to the 6-year-olds, who show an "active frank sexual curiosity," and the 8- to 11-year-olds, who show an "active, homosexual and heterosexual curiosity and interest, often of an aggressive and sadistic sort" (p. 127). Berta Bornstein (1951) divided latency into two periods, the first extending from 5½ to 8 years, the second from 8 until 10. In the first, "The ego, still buffeted by the surging impulses, is threatened by the new superego which is not only harsh and rigid but still a foreign body" (p. 280). Moreover, in this first phase, defenses are directed against both genital and pregenital impulses. In the second phase, the ego is exposed to fewer conflicts, because of lesser sexual demands as well as a less rigid superego.

Two more recent investigators have arrived at similar conclusions on the basis of neurological and physiological findings, as well as the personalities of latency children. Kaplan (1965), following Bornstein, also divides latency into two periods, while Williams (1972) prefers a triphasic division into early latency (5–7), latency proper (7–9), and late latency (9–11). The children in latency proper as compared to those in the early phase "pursue their activities with greater concentration. Their elaboration of a theme, while playing or drawing, shows more cohesion and permits easier access to their defenses, functioning, and interests" (p. 601). Late-latency children are more balanced in functioning, but prepubertal phenomena begin to encroach on the earlier quiescence.

The papers summarized initially in this section suggest that the views concerning the biological origins of the latency period are based on evolutionary speculation, anatomic-psychological analogy, and reconstructions derived from the analyses of adult patients, most of whom belonged to the middle class. Moreover, those authors who work essentially within the psychoanalytic framework and who observe children directly agree on the subdivisions of the latency period. Kaplan went beyond clinical observation to cite recent neurological and physiological data that she felt supported her subdivision. Similarly, our own review of the recent literature from disciplines which lie adjacent to analysis suggests that we may have arrived at a point of scientific convergence where we can outline the biological and/or cognitive substrate for the preservation of latency. In our discussion, we maintain the "levels concept" and suggest that there may not be a one-to-one parallelism between behavior and mind and body data, and that any linkage implied should be seen as supportive, converging, and compatible rather than confirming. Each discipline proceeds within its methodological confines, applying its skills at specific levels of biological organization. We do not yet have the tools or the theory to make clean linkages. We therefore state consistencies and convergences.

In accord with Hartmann et al.'s (1951) distinction, we will first look at maturational growth processes which "are relatively independent of environmental conditions" and then at developmental growth processes that are "more dependent on environmental conditions." While keeping to this plan, we shall highlight the compelling concatenation of discontinuities in development at age 7 within the data of each scientific discipline.

Brain-Behavior Correlations and Maturation

Brain-behavior correlations may not hold any more hope than sexual-tissue-hormone-behavior correlation if one were concerned only with one-to-one intercorrelation between substrate and function. However, at this point in scientific knowledge, the brain is clearly the material basis of significant higher integrative functions, and there does seem to be a striking correspondence of timetables in brain anatomy, physiology, and chemistry with changes at perceptual and cognitive levels. This section should not be taken as a plea for reductionism, any more than we accept the earlier analogizing to changes in sexual-tissue substrate. However, it is another sector of work to notice where the age of 7 intrudes on awareness. Moreover, the changes described may be enabling for the cognitive shift of latency. At the same time, we have no adequate understanding of the mechanism of interaction between levels of organization. We do, however, note simultaneity.

The anatomical growth of the brain follows what Scammon (1930) calls the "neural type of growth." The "growth pattern" which typifies height and weight and most of the other organ systems is more linear. By contrast, at the age of 7 the brain has attained about 90 percent of the total weight gain from birth to 20 years. Microscopic structure and differentiation also change in the frontal lobes at 6 and 7, according to Blinkov and Glezer (1964). The rate of growth of pyramidal cells throughout the frontal lobe decreases with age, with intermittent critical stages of pyramidal cell growth at about 3 months, 2 to 3 years, and about 6 to 7 years. The dimensions of pyramidal cells also vary and "the maximal values of the coefficients of variation are observed synchronously in all areas and they coincide with the above-mentioned critical growth of the dimensions of the cells" (p. 190). Blinkov and Glezer (1964) have verified this proposition by cross-sectional study.

Data concerning longitudinal and cross-sectional changes in material substrate are but one source of information regarding neurological development. Neural scientists have traditionally learned much of brain-function relations from the study of lesions

475

and ablations as well. Loss of function late in life also may point to a critical age for the establishment of functions, which may not be developed adequately if lesions occur early in life.

The frontal lobe comprises about one third of the hemispheric surface; it includes the primary motor areas, premotor areas, and frontal eye fields, and "represents a relatively late phylogenetic acquisition which is well-developed only in primates, especially in Man" (Truex and Carpenter, 1969, p. 587). Russell (1948) stresses the importance of the frontal lobes in maturation, stating that in children with frontal lesions, behavior is disinhibited and they are consequently less educable. However, following frontal lobotomy, adults sometimes show little change in behavior. Russell feels that "the frontal mechanism during mental development impresses the pattern of behavior" (p. 359) in such a way that its influence may persist after the prefrontal lobes have been severed from the lower centers, thus suggesting that experience "writes" on a maturing brain at levels lower than the cortex itself.

The frontal lobe also plays a role in the verbal regulation of behavior. Teuber (1962) describes patients who had undergone *frontal* lobectomies, which included the superior frontal regions, for relief of focal seizures. They were given a card-sorting task by Milner (1962), who found that they would perseverate in sorting the cards following a certain criterion, e.g., color, even after that ceased to be appropriate. "They thus show a curious *dissociation* between the ability to verbalize the requirements of the test and the ability to *use this verbalization* (and other verbal cues) as a guide to action" (p. 322f.; italics added). In maze learning she found that the patients with frontal lobectomies disregarded the maze that was outlined on the floor, but they went directly from start to finish without regard for the one permissible route.

In their experience with patients who have massive frontal lobe tumors, Luria and Homskaya (1962) found that behaviors formerly controlled by verbal instruction were no longer amenable to this mode of regulation. These authors also state that, whereas the behavior of a small child can be initiated by a verbal instruction, it cannot be arrested or reprogrammed by instructions until after 5. They further cite workers in the Soviet Union who document the efficacy of verbal regulation only after 5 years, which seems to parallel frontal obe maturation.

Such a relationship of the frontal lobes to self-regulation, particularly verbal self-regulation, is of central importance to psychoanalytic concepts of superego and ego controls, which are expected following the resolution of the Oedipus complex.

Among those authors who seek brain-behavior correlations in their work, Kaplan (1965) alone based her subdivision of latency on neurological and physiological data, as well as behavioral observation. She supports her argument for this division with the following maturational data: "By eight years, myelinization of the tracts from the cortex to the thalamus is completed. Around the same age, the alpha-wave pattern on the EEG stabilizes" (p. 227). These data are attributed to the unpublished work of Madow and Silverman (1956). However, Dustman and Beck (1969), studying the visually evoked responses of 215 normal subjects, found that there was a rapid increase in responses recorded from the occiput, reaching a maximum in the 5- to 6-year-old level followed by a decline in amplitude. At 13 to 14, an abrupt increase in amplitude appeared and stabilized at about age 16. They suggest that it is reasonable to infer that behavioral changes seen during latency may be related to these neurophysiological alterations.

At yet another level of observation of substrate changes Bogoch (1957) found that children of 6 or below had low values of CSF neuraminic acid, whereas the children age 7 to 16 had higher levels. He hypothesized a "barrier antibody system" designed to isolate the brain from substances which pass readily from the blood to other tissues and noted that the low level of CSF neuraminic acid in children under 7 may reflect a chemical immaturity. No other significant data on biochemical alterations have been discovered, but many recent studies of severely disturbed children are seeking disturbances at this level of organization.

Biochemical and histological discontinuity in development is far removed from psychological and behavioral processes, but we include data from such disparate methods to indicate the significant convergence on the age-7 landmark.

Higher Level Changes at 7

The changes in brain substrate occurring at 7 do not stand alone. A number of measures of perceptual and neurological development and cognitive organization also show significant discontinuities. To facilitate our presentation, we divide these advances into several groups. The first deals with perception and integration of external stimuli; the second with temporospatial orientation; and the third covers cognitive processes.

1. *Perceptual-postural maturation* which is said to underlie the development of body image (Schilder, 1935) has been studied by simple tests that rest on general laws of development such as *cephalocaudal maturation* and *intersensory integration*. Each

of these processes provides the neural and perceptual base for sensory input and screening. The data derived from the senses are ultimately integrated centrally. Such integrations must perforce influence mental organization and strikingly can be shown to reveal discontinuities at 7 years. M. Bender (1952), studying two-point, face-hand discrimination in the maturing child, showed that only about one-sixth of a group of 3- to 6-year-olds reported two stimuli, whereas in a group of 7- to 12-year-olds, half made both responses and thus approximated the performance of the adults studied.

Pollack and Goldfarb (1957a) and Pollack and Gordon (1959–60) showed that children having a mental age of 7 years or more on a standard IQ test made very few errors on the face-hand test. In a normal 6-year-old group, 41 percent made errors, whereas only 6 percent of the 7-year-olds did so. In a longitudinal study of 59 children of ages 5 to 7, Kraft (1968) similarly found that 78 percent of the 7-year-old group made mature responses, whereas 54 percent of the 6-year-olds and only 14 percent of the 5-year-olds did so. These findings represent nonlinear progressions in maturation and are dramatic discontinuities in neuroperceptual appreciation.

Studying intersensory integration, Birch et al. (1964), (1965) likewise demonstrate that children between the ages of 5 and 7 change rapidly. Birch and Belmont (1965) state that "it is of interest that the rapid period of integrative growth in auditory-visual functioning coincided with those ages ... [of] the most rapid emergence of visual-haptic, visual-kinesthetic and haptic-kinesthetic integrative competence" (p. 303). While these integrations are proceeding, the authors stress, the child is moving from a stage where visceral and skin sensations appear to be predominant in directing behavior to a stage where vision and audition are paramount. Such work echoes Sherrington's proposition that organisms move from proximal to distal receptor preference, as well as Freud's and Mahler's notion of splanchnic to peripheral cathexis.

1. Bender (1938) borrowed Wertheimer's figures, which were used to demonstrate the basic laws of Gestalt perception, and adapted them to the study of the maturing visual-motor functions of children and brain-damaged adults. The age of 7 again receives special notice, in that 70 percent of the figures are drawn correctly at this point. Moreover, Fabian (1955) noted a peculiar tendency in children at 7 to verticalize angled figures and then to return to the slanted position. Koppitz (1964) elaborates that "for children 7 years and younger the Bender test is useful for the identification of both immature and bright youngsters; for children 8 years or older, the Bender test can only screen out those with immature or malfunctioning visual motor perception" (p. 35). In her studies of figure drawings Koppitz (1968) found poor integration of parts of a figure in both brain-injured and nonbrain-injured boys at age 6. However, while 44 percent of the drawings of the brain-injured boys aged 7 to 12 were poorly integrated, only 5 percent of the human figure drawings of the healthy control subjects showed poor integration. These investigations again assign special significance to age 7.

2. *Temporospatial orientation* also matures at approximately the same time. The child can discriminate his own right from left at about the age of 6. Then after one or two years, he can also

make these discriminations in an examiner sitting across from him.

Ames (1946) studied time concepts in a group aged 2½ to 8 years and found that "as to general divisions of time, the child first knows whether it is morning or afternoon (4 years), then what day it is (5 years), then what time it is (7 years),... what year (8 years), and what day of the month (8 years). Days of the week are named correctly by 5 years, months of the year not until 8 years" (p. 123).

Pollack and Goldfarb (1957b) demonstrated that in normal children between the ages 5 to 8, "it was not until seven years that a majority of the children attained correct knowledge of time of day and calendar organization" (p. 540). Furthermore, they found that responses of the majority of 7-year-olds were in terms of specific measurements, whereas those of 5- and 6-year-olds were relativistic or approximate. They suggested that this reflects a "conspicuous improvement in orientation between the fifth and seventh years" (p. 549).

Piaget (1947) found that by the age of about 7 or 8, the child is capable of temporospatial operations. At the age of about 7 or 8 there are constituted "the qualitative operations that structure space: the spatial order of succession and the joining together of intervals or distances; conservation of lengths, areas, etc." (p. 145). At about the age of 8 the relations of *temporal order* (before and after) are coordinated with *duration* (longer or shorter length of time).

While this presentation will not accentuate Piaget's contributions, recent work by Laurendeau and Pinard (1970) must be mentioned. These authors studied five tests of spatial representation (stereognostic recognition, construction of projected straight line, topographic localization, left-right distinctions, and appreciation of perspectives) in order to assess whether there is a topological level that precedes a later period when projective and Euclidian relations become possible in spatial orientation. They found that the use of configuration of object and its environs that characterizes topological organizations had an upper limit of 7.2 years. They also offered evidence of the relationship of their findings to concepts of egocentrism, which tends to drop off during the same period, as a correlative organizer of the spatiotemporal world.

Elkind et al. (1964) also have shown that there is rapid advance in children's abilities to perceive both parts and wholes in drawings at 7 and 8. They state that their work, in general agreement with Piaget's study of the decentering of perception, has also shown "that the 7- to 8-year level is the point of abrupt perceptual improvement" (p. 86). Other studies by Elkind et al. (1962), (1967) appear to support this finding.

3. *Cognitive changes at 7.* We do not argue here that neuro-maturational and integrative advances underlie cognitive progression and new skills; rather, we continue to present the data from cognitive studies which also suggest a discontinuity of function at 7.

Kendler and Kendler (1962b) examined problem-solving by using a simple learning task that involves presentation of two abstract forms that differ in one of two qualities—color and size (a white and a colored square of two sizes). The child is asked to discover or explicate a rule of organization that unifies the forms. Significant differences were found in the responses of children younger than 6 or 7 from those of older ones (12 percent of 6- to 7-year-olds gave direct integrative responses versus 67 percent of the 8- to 10-year-olds). The authors suggest that the direct integrative response reflects reasoning, insight, and inferential behavior, whereas the indirect, nonintegrated response that predominates in the younger children is based on trial-and-error learning. Studying children's performing a task that again permitted two ways of responding, the Kendlers (1962a) found that, with age, children develop a tendency to respond in a mediational manner.

In an experiment examining a similar problem, Kuenne (1946) found that 100 percent of children with the mental age of 6 were capable of far transposition, as compared to 50 percent of those children with the mental age of 3. This is attributed to the older child's ability to use verbal cues in making discriminations. Kuenne suggests that younger children tend to transpose in a manner similar to infrahuman primates.

In more recent work concerning the importance of verbal mediators in transposition tasks, Marshall (1966) showed that children aged 4½ to 5½ who had verbal knowledge of the concept of middle-sizedness did better on a middle-size transposition task than children of the same age who had either a nonverbal knowledge of the concept or no knowledge of it at all. Among the older children studied, including some up to 6½ years, there were more children with verbal knowledge of the concept than those in the older two groups.

Whereas the above procedures report on specific aspects of the child's cognitive development, White (1965) and the work of Piaget bring such work into a broader scope for generalized application.

White reviewed current developmental research extensively to support his thesis of a "hierarchical arrangement of learning processes." Focusing on the behavioral changes in children of age 5 to 7, he argues that they reflect a transition between two levels of mental functioning. The first level, which he calls *associative* functioning, is present before the age of 5 and is inhibited by a new "higher" cognitive level of function after the age of 7. The transitions in cognitive strategies are geared toward (1) the change in use of language representation as a "pure stimulus act," to second-order cues evoking behavior that the stimuli themselves would not call forth; (2) the ability to maintain orientation toward invariant dimensions in a surround of variance; (3) the ability to string together internal representations of stimulus-response-consequence into sequences that can be projected into the future to allow planning and projected into the past to allow inference; (4) increased sensitivity to distance-receptors of vision and audition and decreased sensitivity to near-receptors.

Corsini and Berg (1973) followed White's suggestion and explored the performance of children aged 4, 6, and 8 on three tasks that White had said required the subject to maintain "orientation (toward invariant dimensions) in a surround of variance" and support his observation that the "5–7 year age period is one of great transition" (p. 473).

It may strike the reader as odd that Piaget's work has not yet been explored, especially in a review directed toward cognitive functions. We have neglected to do so not because we believe his work to be insignificant, but only because we assume that analysts are familiar with it. He, too, found the child of 5 to 8 years to be capable of temporal and spatial operations, which undergo transition in strategy. The ability to carry out certain tasks differentially at this stage reflects the passage from the preoperational level of cognitive functioning to the level of concrete operations. Piaget (1947) describes the thought of the preoperational child as intuitive, egocentric, subjective; children at this stage are incapable of social cooperation. "Oscillating between distorting egocentricity and passive acceptance of intellectual suggestion, the child is, therefore, not yet subject to a socialization of intelligence which could profoundly modify its mechanism" (p. 162). The "essential characteristic of logical thought is that it is operational" (p.

36) and it succeeds preoperational thought at about the ages of 7 and 8. Operationality, whether at the concrete or abstract level, demands a stability of mental structure, a frame to apply to experience, rendering events less heterologous.

The relevance of Piaget's work to the views proposed in this paper is best exemplified in research involving the development of moral thinking and socialization by theorists heavily influenced by his cognitive theories.

Kohlberg (1964) indicates that the development of moral thinking is a stepwise process, in which he discerned six sequential stages. His data support the fact that moral character is dependent on ego strength and the ability to make decisions. In 1971, Kohlberg and Gilligan clearly point to the relation between cognition and morality, stating that cognitive maturity is a necessary, but not a sufficient condition for moral-judgment maturity (p. 1071).

Damon (1975) also investigated the relation between cognitive development and the development of the concept of positive justice and found that "logical and moral reasoning inform and support each other in the course of ontogenesis" (p. 312). The children who had arrived at the last two of six substages of positive justice were 8 years old and had also passed from the cognitive preoperational stage to that of concrete operation. Rubin and Schneider (1973), also following Piaget, contend that egocentric thought and immature moral judgment in the preoperational child is determined by the inability to decenter. Fifty-five 7-year-old children were tested and their results "provide clear support for the hypothesis that among 7-year-olds there is a positive relationship between decentration skills, as indicated by scores on measures of communicative egocentrism, and moral judgment and the incidence of altruism" (p. 664).

Zigler (1971) highlights the importance of cognitive development for socialization, and offers an explanation for differences in social-class behavior as an alternative to the simply sociogenic explanations. He posits an ontogenetic, "developmentally changing hierarchy of reinforcers" that serve to regulate social behavior. Self-cuing, the possibility of "turning against the self" and guilt accompany increasing cognitive development; i.e., these phenomena represent a movement away from action and toward thought and therefore increased mediation. Studies of lower- and middle-class 7-year-olds showed that the former were more responsive to verbal reinforcers such as "good and fine," while the latter did better with "right and correct" (Zigler and Kanzer, 1962). Zigler uses these and other data to suggest that cognitive capacity alone does not make manifest behavior, but capacity in interaction with social milieu helps to ensconce preferred reinforcers.

To conclude this section we again must return to the practical implications which the capacity for cognitive strategies has on the carrying out of life tasks. Moreover, one might wonder if there is a minimal neural maturation which is required to achieve new cognitive levels. While we have kept the data from investigations of substrate separate from data of higher-level functions in this review, some authors study two or more levels simultaneously and confound our intention, but stimulate our integrative interest. Cohn (1961) studied children with reading and writing disabilities. Both of these skills are practical in our world and require the integrity of a number of functions. He examined the neurological competence of both impaired and normal children by "all tests that potentially could be correlated with structural lesions of the brain" (p. 153). Four categories of test were used—language, somatic receiving and expressive systems, personal spatial organization, and social adaptation. A composite of test results served as an index of neurological deficit. In the group of 130 control children, those of ages 7 to 10 had the lowest index of neurological deficit and the change approached its limit at the age of 8. Thus, again the phenomenon is repeated that curves of functional development in many sectors level off at 7.1 years.

Discussion

What light does the research on maturation and development gathered from diverse scientific investigations shed on the psychoanalytic concept of the latency period? Although Freud assumes that the emergence of the latency period follows some biological timetable, it appears that a biphasic growth of the sexual drive is not the significant substratum on which this timetable is based. We would argue that processes within the central nervous system and cognitive strategies derived from maturation may provide latency with its biological clock.

The normal child of 7.1 has reached a level of maturation and development that permits autonomy. He is emotionally less dependent on his family, has at his disposal a neuromuscular apparatus that is ready for the challenge of environmental mastery; and he has a new set of cognitive strategies to outwit and control his environment. This we view as a discontinuity in behavioral development.

The greater stability and invariance of mental process and the new cognitive structure at 7 also permit the *inhibition and control of drives* and the postponement of action. The intrusive animism of the preOedipal child, which is based on associative thinking, is no longer seen as intrusive. Stable structures have replaced earlier instabilities and can now be used in the service of new cognitive skills, while keeping sexual-drive components in greater isolation. What we call repression may rest upon the splitting and reorganization of archaic and more integrated forms of thinking, which complement each other and are simultaneously present in different organizational frames within the same psychic apparatus. Lipin (1969) suggests that maturation provides the possibility of two such organizations and elaborates the conditions under which the archaic levels may irrupt into consciousness as sensory elements, rather than thoughts within and outside of the analytic situation.

Psychoanalytic theory has defined a number of factors that facilitate the socialization characteristic of the latency child's functioning. Among these are the transition from primary to secondary process modes of discharge; the cognitive basis for the structuralization of the mental apparatus, which includes the possibility of resolving the Oedipus complex; infantile amnesia; and the establishment of an invariant, internalized superego to direct and modulate behavior without the constant need for external controls. We recognize that man in conflict is the essential datum of the psychoanalytic clinical practice, *but* man in conflict depends upon opposing internalized structures, which in turn are a feature of the new abilities of the 7-year-old.

We note that although our researches have led us to conclusions that differ from Freud's as to just what the biological basis of latency is, it is a tribute to Freud that several of his ideas regarding the cognitive basis of latency were prescient.

In 1911, Freud dealt with the transition from the pleasure principle to the reality principle. The latter is established as a result of the inevitable inadequacies of drive satisfaction. This transition implies that secondary processes evolved because drive satisfaction was not achieved by rapid discharge. Because hallucinatory wish fulfillment does not suffice, "the psychical apparatus had to decide to form a conception of the real circumstances in the external world and to endeavour to make a real alteration in them ... the new demands [of the reality principle] made a succession of adaptations necessary in the psychical apparatus" (p. 219f.). The adaptations Freud discussed are: the greater importance and *consciousness* of sense organs; the function of attention necessary to search the external world when a need arises; a system of notation which is a part of memory; an impartial passing of judgment which has to decide the truth or falseness of ideas; and the process of thinking which allows for the restraint of motor discharge and its conversion into action.

These "adaptations," by and large, would now fall under the category of autonomous ego functions (Hartmann, 1938). Their relevance to the concept of latency is evident, because they are a feature of the maturational and developmental changes that are documented in this review. It therefore appears that the 7-year- old has made the greatest step in his utilization of secondary-process modes of discharge to achieve the gratifications dictated by the pleasure principle under the adaptive guidance of what is possible in reality.

The last "adaptation" referred to above, that of thinking, deserves more attention, particularly in its relationship to motor discharge and Freud's ideas concerning the "binding of energy," which remains the central factor in distinguishing primary and secondary processes. First elaborated in 1895, this idea was next taken up in 1900 when Freud spoke of two *psi* systems in which the activity of the first *psi* system is directed toward securing the free discharge of the quantities of excitation, while the second system succeeds in inhibiting the discharge and in transforming the cathexis into a quiescent one, with a simultaneous elevation of its excitation level. When the second system has concluded its exploratory thought activity, it releases the inhibition and allows discharge as movement. This inhibitory mechanism—its relationship to thought and its importance in Freud's explanation of the transition from primary to secondary process—is again emphasized in the 1911 paper where Freud states that under the direction of the secondary process,

> Motor discharge was not employed in the appropriate alteration of reality; it was converted into *action*. Restraint upon motor discharge (upon action), which then becomes necessary, was provided by means of the process of *thinking*, which was developed from the presentation of ideas. Thinking... is essentially an experimental kind of acting, accompanied by displacement of relatively small quantities of cathexis together with less expenditure (discharge) of them.

For this purpose the conversion of freely displaceable cathexis into 'bound' cathexes was necessary [p. 221].

The relationship of "the binding of energies," thought, and the alteration of reality can perhaps be reconciled with the work cited by the Kendlers, White, and Piaget. According to these investigators, children of 7 to 8 respond more frequently in "a mediational manner," and are capable of operational thought. One might say that the thought processes at this stage are more structured, inasmuch as the energies underlying them are relatively bound; whereas at earlier stages they are closer to the primary process, inasmuch as there is a freer discharge of energies. The *pars pro toto* nature of associational thinking is one datum to suggest this, and the academic psychologists' claim that the original associational thinking is replaced by the mediated processes is another way of stating the same proposition. Indeed, recent work suggests that, prior to 7 years of age, children tested on word- association tasks use attributive *has* and syntagmatic connections, and after 7 they use copulate *is* connections for their associations. For example, prior to 7, the word "table" is more likely to elicit "eat" or "legs," while after 7 "furniture" might be the response.

One could further argue that memory traces organized according to the associational form of thinking become less available to consciousness once the second mode is established; when ideas organized in the first mode are raised to consciousness, they may appear in more archaic forms as percepts (Lipin, 1968), or according to categorical lines more appropriate to early childhood. The concepts of repression and infantile amnesia might find their organizational base in this two-system arrangement, which is conveniently ordered in a developmental hierarchy.

Significantly, the resolution of the Oedipus complex and the structuralization of the mental apparatus into its three functional agencies also depend upon the newly established mediational thinking, which brings about a new organization of thought and invariant cuing from within. The superego, in its function as a guiding pilot, seems to utilize internalized verbal prohibitions. The development of such capacities has also been noted in the work of the Soviet neurodevelopmentalists. Nass (1966) argues that Piaget's findings on moral development, which are based on levels of cognitive organization, correspond with the psychoanalytic timetable, which is derived from the stages of libidinal development, object relations, levels of ego functioning, and the formation of psychic structures. The replacement of outer control by inner control and organization, and the consequent propensity toward conflict, may then have a material base in the establishment of neurodevelopmental structure. *We would argue that these confluences in development are not fortuitous, but are part of the design feature of the human organism; and this design feature permits higher level organization and, therefore, latency.*

By now, it must be clear we believe that what separate the data from the varied sectors examined are method and vantage point. One would hardly expect a neurophysiologist to arrive at conclusions regarding cognitive organization. Similarly, the psychoanalytic method is an exquisite tool for investigating the meaning of experience and internalized conflict, but it cannot say much about the growth limits of neurons. The limits of each method require complementarity of findings to round out our knowledge. However, these limitations also require that the data from one scientific method not be contradicted by data from another. This excursion through many disciplines converged on a crucial age in the child's development, no matter which sector of behavior or level of organization was studied, and this coincidence, we believe, is worth noting.

In the course of this review, one problem had to be put aside and now will be reconsidered. The central tenets of psychoanalysis rest upon the concept of a "dynamic" unconscious, which, in turn, is based on data derived from the couch. These data attest to the pressure of wishes and the countercathectic powers of the ego and its defensive operations. The explorations of cognitive psychologists and neural developmentalists say little about such dynamic matters and their affective components. Yet, these dynamic features are the motivational core of man and constitute the *raison d'être* of psychoanalysis as a separate branch of investigation.

We believe that the dynamic core of psychoanalytic theory can utilize the mass of data accumulated as corroborative information rather than as an antagonistic system. Freud's dynamic principles did not falter, though he argued for and surmised biological timetables. He went so far as to suggest that latency was as inevitable as the loss of deciduous teeth. Hartmann's demands that ego psychology be expanded to include academic psychological findings did not relinquish a dynamic point of view. In short, the dynamic reasons for the resolution of the oedipus complex and repression, as well as the specific genetic reasons for a specific variety of superego organization, depend upon the meaning of experience, which is what the psychoanalyst studies. To refer to the fact that the organization of meaning rests on species-specific neuronal substrates, which mature according to biological timetables and provide specific cognitive propensities, is merely to restate the "levels" principle. We study what we study with the tools we have, and each tool excludes the possibility of other kinds of knowledge. On the other hand, the psychoanalyst's grasp of the whys of behavior must include the limits and tendencies of the substrate, lest he ascribe dynamic significance to behaviors which are not determined by conflict. Moreover, knowledge about latency arose from psychoanalytic speculations and postulations about the maturation of libidinal energic organization and the ontogenetic sequence in the ebb-and-flow of fantasies which are part of being human. Latency was postulated as universal, because it seemed to transcend particular fantasy constellations and was less idiosyncratic in its essential form than other mental events.

The data presented here represent an attempt to look at the concept of latency in the light of new data from other disciplines. We assert the clinical utility of this concept. However, finding one's way through the evidence presented requires that psychoanalysis can burn some old foundations based on older biological analogy and accept some supports from newer findings by the other sciences.

REFERENCES

Alpert, A. (1941). The Latency Period *Amer. J. Orthopsychiat.* 11:126–133.

Ames, L.B. (1946). The Development of the Sense of Time in the Young Child *J. Genet. Psychol.* 68:97–125.

Bender, L. (1938). A Visual-Motor Gestalt Test and Its Clinical Use. *Research Monograph #3*. New York: American Orthopsychiatric Association.

Bender, M. (1952). *Disorders in Perception, with Particular Reference to the Phenomena of Extinction and Displacement.* Springfield, Ill.: Thomas.

Birch, H. & Belmont, L. (1965). Auditory-Visual Integration. *Percept. Mot. Skills* 20:295–305.

Birch, H. & Lefford, A. (1964). Two Strategies for Studying Perception in "Brain-Damaged" Children In: Brain Damage in Children ed. H. G. Birch. Baltimore: Williams & Wilkins.

Blinkov, S.M. & Glezer, I. (1964). The Human Brain in Figures and Tables. New York: Basic Books, 1968.

Bogoch, S. (1957). Cerebrospinal Fluid Neuraminic Acid Deficiency in Schizophrenia. *Amer. J. Psychiat.* 11: 172.

Bornstein, B. (1951). On Latency. *Psychoanal. Study Child* 6:279–285.

Cohn, R. (1961). Delayed Acquisition of Reading and Writing Abilities in Children. *Arch. Neurol.* 4:153–164.

Coppoletta, J. & Wolbach, S.B. (1933). Body Length and Organ Weights of Infants and Children. *Amer. J. Pathol.* 9:55–70.

Corsini, D.A. & Berg, A.J.(1973). Intertask Correspondence in the Five to Seven Shift. *Child Develpm.* 44:467–475

Damon, W. (1975). Early Conceptions of Positive Justice as Related to the Development of Logical Operations. *Child Develpm.* 46:301–312.

Dustman, R. & Beck, E. (1969). The Effects of Maturation and Aging on the Wave Form of Visually Evoked Potentials. *EEG & Clin. Neurophysiol.* 26:2–11.

Elkind, D., Koegler, R.R., & Go, E. (1964). Studies in Perceptual Development: II. Part-Whole Perception. *Child Develpm.* 35:81–90.

Elkind, D., & Scott, L. (1962). Studies in Perceptual Development: The Decentering of Perception. *Child Develpm.* 33:619–630.

Elkind, D., & Weiss, J. (1967). Studies in Perceptual Development: III. Perceptual Exploration. *Child Develpm. 38:53–561.*

Epstein, H.T. (1974). Phrenoblysis: Special Brain and Mind Growth Periods. *Dev. Psychobiol.* 7:207–216.

Erikson, E.H. (1950). *Childhood and Society.* New York: Norton.

Fabian, A.A. (1955). Reading Disability: An Index of Pathology. *Amer. J. Orthopsychiat.* 25:319–329.

Ferenczi, S. (1913). Stages in the Development of the Sense of Reality. In: *Sex in Psychoanalysis* New York: Basic Books, 1950 pp. 213–239.

Freud, S. (1900). Primary and Secondary Processes. *Standard Edition* 5:588–609.

———— (1905). Three Essays on the Theory of Sexuality. *Standard Edition* 7:125–243.

———— (1911). Formulations on the Two Principles of Mental Functioning. *Standard Edition* 12 213–226.

———— (1919). 'A Child Is Being Beaten. *Standard Edition.* 17:177–204.

———— (1924). The Dissolution of the Oedipus Complex. *Standard Edition* 19:173–179.

———— (1925). An Autobiographical Study. *Standard Edition* 20:3–74.

———— (1926). The Question of Lay Analysis. *Standard Edition* 20:179–258.

———— (1950 [1895] Project for a Scientific Psychology. *Standard Edition.* 1:283–397.

Hartmann, H. (1939). *Ego Psychology and the Problem of Adaptation* New York: Int. Univ. Press, 1958.

———— Kris, E., & Loewenstein, R.M. 1951 Some Psychoanalytic Comments on "Culture and Personality." *Psychological Issues* 14:86–116 New York: Int. Univ. Press, 1964.

Kaplan, E.B. (1965). Reflections regarding Psychomotor Activities during the Latency Period. *Psychoanal. Study Child* 20:220–238.

Kendler, H.H. & Kendler, T.S. (1962a). Vertical and Horizontal Processes in Problem Solving. *Psychol. Rev.* 69:1–16.

Kendler, T.S. & Kendler, H.H. (1962b). Inferential Behavior in Children as a Function of Age and Subgoal Constancy. *J. Exp. Psychol.* 64:460–466.

Kohlberg, L. (1964). Development of Moral Character and Moral Ideology In: *Review of Child Development Research* ed. M. L. Hoffman & L. W. Hoffman. New York: Russell Sage Foundation, pp. 383–432.

——— & GILLIGAN, C. (1971). The Adolescent as a Philosopher. *Daedalus* 100:1051–1086.

Koppitz, E M. (1964). *The Bender Gestalt Test for Young Children.* New York: Grune & Stratton.

———. (1968). *Psychological Evaluation of Children's Human Figure Drawings.* New York: Grune & Stratton.

Kraft, M.B. (1968). The Face-Hand Test. *Dev. Med. & Child Neurol.* 10:214–219.

Kuenne, M.R. (1946). Experimental Investigation of the Relation of Language to Transposition Behavior in Young Children. *J. Exp. Psychol.* 36:471–490.

Lampl, H. (1953). The Influence of Biological and Psychological Factors upon the Development of the Latency Period. In: *Drives, Affects, Behavior* ed. R. M. Loewenstein. New York: Int. Univ. Press, pp. 380–387.

Laurendeau, M. & Pinard, A. (1970). *The Development of the Concept of Space in the Child.* New York: Int. Univ. Press.

Lipin, T. (1969). Sensory Irruptions and Mental Organization. *J. Am. Psychoanal. Assoc.* 17:1055–1073.

Luria, A.R. & Homskaya, E.D. (1962). Disturbances in the Regulative Role of Speech with Frontal Lobe Lesions. In: *The*

Frontal Granular Cortex and Behavior, ed. J.M. Warren & K. Akert. New York: McGraw-Hill, pp. 353–371.

Marshall, H.R. (1966). Transposition in Children as a Function of Age and Knowledge. *J. Genet. Psychol.* 108:65–69.

Miller, G.A. (1956). The Magical Number Seven, Plus or Minus Two. *Psychol. Rev.* 63:81–97.

Milner, B. (1962). Some Effects of Frontal Lobectomy in Man. In: *The Frontal Granular Cortex and Behavior,* ed. J.M. Warren & K. Akert. New York: McGraw-Hill, pp. 313–334.

Nass, M.L. (1966). The Superego and Moral Development in the Theories of Freud and Piaget. *Psychoanal. Study Child* 21:51–68.

Nelson, W., Vaughan, V., & Mckay, P. (1969). *Textbook of Pediatrics 9th ed.* Philadelphia: Saunders.

Piaget, J. (1947). *The Psychology of Intelligence.* London: Routledge & Kegan Paul, 1950.

———— (1973). The Affective Unconscious and the Cognitive Unconscious. *J. Am. Psychoanal. Assoc.* 21:249–261

Pinchbeck, I. & Hewitt, M. (1969). *Children in English Society Vol 1. London*: Routledge & Kegan Paul.

Pollack, M. & Goldfarb, W. (1957a). The Face-Hand Test in Schizophrenic Children. *AMA Arch. Neurol. & Psychiat.* 77:635–642.

————. & Goldfarb, W. (1957b). Patterns of Orientation in Children in Residential Treatment for Severe Behavior Disorders. *Amer. J. Orthopsychiat.* 27:538–552.

———— & Gordon, E. (1959–60). The Face-Hand Test in Retarded and Nonretarded Emotionally Disturbed Children. *Amer. J. Ment. Def.* 64:758–760.

Rubin, K. & Schneider, F. (1973). The Relationship between Moral Judgment, Egocentrism, and Altruistic Behavior. *Child Develpm.* 44:661–665.

Russell, W.R. (1948). Functions of the Frontal Lobes. *Lancet* 254:356–360.

Scammon, R. (1930). The Measurement of the Body in Childhood In: *The Measurement of Man* by J. A. Harris et al. Minneapolis: Univ. Minnesota Press, pp. 173–215.

Schilder, P. (1935). *The Image and Appearance of the Human Body* New York: Int. Univ. Press, 1950.

Sullivan, H.S. (1940). Conceptions of Modern Psychiatry. *Psychiatry* 3:1–117.

Teuber, H.L. (1962). The Riddle of Frontal Lobe Function in Man. In: *The Frontal Granular Cortex and Behavior.* Ed J.M. Warren & K. Akert. New York: McGraw-Hill. pp. 410–444.

Thomas, A. & Chess, S. (1972). Development in Middle Childhood Seminars in Psychiatry 4:331–341.

Truex, R. & Carpenter, M. (1969). *Human Neuroanatomy 6th ed.* Baltimore: Williams & Wilkins.

Warren, J.M. & Akert, K., eds. (1964). *The Frontal Granular Cortex and Behavior.* New York: McGraw-Hill.

White, S.H. (1965). Evidence for a Hierarchical Arrangement of Learning Processes. *Adv. Child Develpm. & Behav.* 2:187–220.

Williams, M. (1972). Problems of Technique during Latency. *Psychoanal. Study Child* 26:598–617.

Yazmajian, R.V. (1967). Biological Aspects of Infantile Sexuality and the Latency Period. *Psychoanal. Q.* 36:203–229.

Zigler, E. (1971). Social Class and the Socialization Process In: *Annual Progress in Child Psychiatry and Child Development,* ed. S. Chess & A. Thomas. New York: Brunner/Mazel, pp. 185–210.

———— & KANZER, P. (1962). The Effectiveness of Two Classes of Verbal Reinforcers on the Performance of Middle and Lower Class Children *J. Pers.* 30:157–163.

.

Preschool Children's
Conception of Ghosts

with Miriam Sherman, M.D., and Irving Osowsky, M.D.[1]

(1980). *Journal of the American Academy
of Child Psychiatry* 19:41–55.

Abstract:

This investigation attempts to clarify 3- and 4-year-old children's perceptions of ghosts and their relation to the hypothesis of the "floating ghost" as an early infantile remembrance. It appears to confirm the notion that young children's representation of ghosts results from an admixture of learned conscious ideas regarding ghosts and an ill-defined part which is based upon primitive unconscious

---

1   [Footnote from original publication] The authors are all at the Cornell University Medical College Payne Whitney Clinic, 525 East 68th Street, New York, N.Y. 10021. Drs. Sherman and Osowsky worked on this study while they were Second Year Fellows in Child Psychiatry. Dr. Shapiro is Professor of Psychiatry, and Dr. Sherman is Assistant Professor of Psychiatry at CUMC. Dr. Osowsky is currently at Kaiser-Pennanente in Los Angeles. Our thanks to Dr. John Frosch for his original idea that provided impetus for this study. The authors were supported in part by NIMH Education Branch Grant Number TOI-MH15244-02. 0002-7138/80/1901-0041 $01.30 c 1980 Academy of Child Psychiatry

ideas about the unknown stranger and the mysterious images of earlier nightly visits from mother and father.

The popular adult conception of ghosts involves an amorphous figure without clear delineation of body parts or apparent lower extremities that moves about by flying or floating.

Freud (1900) said that ghosts in dreams represented the parents: "Robbers, burglars and ghosts, of whom some people feel frightened before going to bed, all originate from one and the same class of infantile reminiscence. They are nocturnal visitors who rouse children and take them up to prevent their wetting their beds, or who lift the bed-clothes to make sure where they put their hands in their sleep" (p. 403f.). Analysis of these anxiety dreams led him to conclude that robbers stood for the father, whereas the ghosts correspond to female figures in white nightgowns.

Frosch (1977) suggests that the perception of these blurred figures' "floating" around the room might persist in later consciousness in the form of the floating ghost. However, by the time the child is verbal and able to represent graphically what he conceives of as a ghost, he is also in contact with the culture and its popular representations of these figures; thus, their relation to the past is uncertain. Moreover, as children move into their fourth and fifth years of life, a series of other frightening monsters, such as Dracula or Frankenstein, begin to dominate their anxieties. Unfortunately, research into the nature and characteristics of ghosts as conceptualized by children at the verbal and graphic stage must rely on empirical cataloging of body parts and cannot directly verify Freud's findings by statistical probability. Such studies may, however, provide suggestive data that link the preverbal past with the verbal years.

Although much has been written regarding the presence and meaning of children's fears at different stages of development (Jersild,

1946; Jersild and Holmes, 1935; Marks, 1969; Nagy, 1948), no investigation has attempted specifically to clarify 3- and 4-year-old children's perceptions of ghosts and the relationship between ghosts and a child's developing body image.

Working directly with infants and children differs from the psychoanalytic retrospective study. From a prospective vantage point, Spitz and Wolf (1946) wrote that the human face is a privileged visual percept. Stern (1974), too, has demonstrated the central role of gaze accommodation in early socialization. The first human gestalt of social significance, then, is the human face; knowledge of lower extremities as a means of motility is acquired later. For the past 50 years, figure drawings have attested to the primacy of the head, and these drawings have been a valuable clinical tool in the study of the developing body image. Goodenough (1926) demonstrated the significance of figure drawing in estimating IQ levels of young children. Analysis of figure drawings also provides information on neurological maturation and integration (Bender, 1946; Cohen, 1953) and on interpersonal preoccupations (Machover, 1949). Schilder (1935) pointed out that the body image is a functional composite that involves layering and integration of numerous body experiences. Therefore, the sequential development of the figure drawings of children should offer a means of exploring an aspect of the formation of the body image.

Shapiro and Stine (1965), reporting on the figure drawings of 61 three- and four-year-old children, found that the mouth (as well as other facial features) was "prominently absent in the earliest spontaneous figure drawings" (p. 305). This finding was somewhat startling in view of the analytic significance of the oral zone in early mutual contact between mother and infant. However, Shapiro and Stine postulated that in the youngest children's drawings, the figure represented is not "the self," as the projective hypothesis would suggest, but is the "visualized other." Shapiro and Stine found, as did others, that there is a linear progression in the inclusion of other body parts, beginning with the head, in such a manner that young children's drawings appear as "tadpole people" (Freeman, 1973). Arms were added later, after the feet. Freeman's (1975) idea about end-anchoring suggests that the child adds later features of the figure only after he establishes the two ends of the tadpole. Freeman's observations suggest that the arms become affixed at those sites which are the largest, so that if a predrawn empty figure is offered, the arms will be placed at the sides of the body and not the head if the body is bulkier. However, since spontaneous drawings usually show body omission in this age group, arms are most frequently attached to the head.

It became apparent that in order to discover the child's conception of the ghost and his means of locomotion, we would have to include a concomitant task of establishing the nature of the child's stage of body representation. We saw in this an opportunity to replicate the Shapiro and Stine (1965) study and to investigate the representation of ghosts. In order to carry out our inquiry, we developed a series of questions, a drawing task, and a serial ordering task, allowing children to select ghostlike from nonghostlike drawings. It became clear, however, that our approach to this task would not address Freud's original question, but that we might discover whether there are remnants of this postulated relationship between floating figures and ghosts and the early recognition of mother, which remain residual in the manifest content of children's conceptions of ghosts.

Method

Forty boys and girls enrolled in two "normal" preschool nursery programs were studied. Twenty-one subjects (9 boys, 12 girls) were 3 years old. Nineteen subjects were between 4 and 5 years old (11 boys, 8 girls). Most were children of medical personnel, and therefore the offspring of upper-middle-class professionals living in a large urban area and exposed to a high degree of social input. The children's parents provided written consent to do this study.

An examiner interviewed each child individually. Interviews were semistructured and consisted of asking a series of questions relating to ghosts (table 1). After the children drew pictures of a person (FD) and a ghost (GD) on different sheets of paper, they were then shown a group of 8 "ghost cards"—pictures of ghosts that differed in number of body parts drawn (fig. 1) and were asked to rank-order them in terms of which looked most and least like a ghost.

Table 1
Interview Questions

1.   Draw me a picture of a person. (Then have child identify all parts drawn)
2.   How does this person get around?
3.   Does this person have legs?
4.   What is a ghost?
5.   What does a ghost look like?
6.   Draw mc a ghost.
7.   How does a ghost get around?
8.   Does a ghost have legs?
9.   Does a ghost have arms?

10. Is the ghost a man or a lady (Boy or girl?)

11. Is the ghost friendly?

12. 1Did you ever dream of a ghost?

13. Story: Once a little boy (girl) saw a ghost. What did he (she) see? What happened?

14. Ghost cards: Which picture looks most like a ghost? (Eliminate this card and ask of the remaining cards: which picture looks most like a ghost?)

The children's drawings of people were first examined for the presence or absence of particular body parts, in order to test Shapiro and Stine's earlier findings. Each child's figure drawing was then compared with his ghost drawing in order to study children's graphic representations of this frightening percept in relation to parts represented in both. Methods of locomotion of ghosts as well as other qualities of ghosts (e.g., gender, friendliness) were tabulated. To ascertain trends in nongraphic psychic projective factors, we asked children to tell stories and describe dreams of ghosts. Themes in stories told by the children and reports of their dreams that included ghosts were gathered to provide clues to their possible anxieties and defenses regarding such figures.

Results

Our results (table 2) showed that unlike Shapiro and Stine's earlier study, mouths appear in a majority (13/16, 81%) of the FD of our group of children below 3; 10 years, which corresponds to Shapiro and Stine's earlier cut-off point. There was no significant difference between the younger children and the older ones (older than 3; 10 years) in their tendency to include mouths.

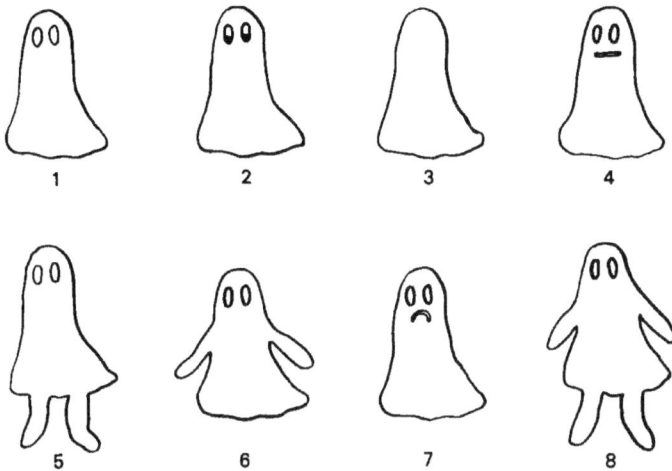

Figure 1. Ghost pictures (8 separate cards) shown to the subjects

Eyes, nose, and mouth all appear significantly more frequently in FD than GD in the 3-year-old group (Table 3). In the older group there is no longer a significant difference. Body, arms, and legs appear more frequently in the FD of the 3-year-olds, but the differences are not significant. However, 4-year-olds drew arms and legs significantly more frequently in the FD than in the GD. The greater frequency of arms and legs in the FDs of older children is to be expected, but the GDS of the older children tend to omit these parts. In short, despite increased maturity's leading to the ability to draw arms and legs, these body parts were deleted from GDS in the older group. In verbalizing the method of locomotion of ghosts, the older subjects' responses ranged from "flies," "walks," "floats," "walks under and over," "moves in circles by ghost power, tippy toes," and "jumps." (See Tables 2 and 3 below.)

Table 2

Subject	Age	Eyes		Nose		Mouth		Body		Arms		Legs	
		F	G	F	G	F	G	F	G	F	G	F	G
1	3.0	−	−	−	−	−	−	+	+	−	−	+	+
2	3.0	−	−	−	−	+	−	−	−	+	−	+	−
3	3.0					Scribble							
4	3.1					Scribble							
5	3.2	+	+	−	−	−	−	+	+	−	+	+	+
6	3.2	+		−		+	−	+		−	−(1)	+	−
7	3.4	+	+	+	−	+	+	+	−	+	+	+	+
8	3.5	+	−	+	−	+	−	+	−	−	−	−	−(2)
9	3.5	+	+	−	−	−	−	+	+	−	−(1)	−	−(2)
10	3.6	+	+	−	−	+	−	+	+	−	−(1)	−	+
11	3.7	+	+	−	−	+	+	+	−	+	+	+	+
12	3.7	+	−	−		+	−	−		−	−	−	−
13	3.8	+	−	−	−	+	−	+	+	−	−	−	−
14	3.8					No drawings							
15	3.8	+	−	−	−	+	−	−	+	+	−	+	−
16	3.9	+	−	+	−	+	+	−	−	−	+	+	+
17	3.9	+	+	+	+	+	+	−	−	−	−	+	−(2)
18	3.9	+	−	+	−	+	−	−	+	+	−	+	−(2)
19	3.9	+	+	+	−	+	+	+	+	−	−(1)	−	−(2)
20	3.10	+	+	+	+	+	−	+	+	−	−(1)	+	+
21	3.10	+	+	+	−	+	−	+	+	−	−	+	−
22	4.1	+	+	+	+	+	+	−	−	+	+	+	−
23	4.1	+	+	−	−	−	−	−	−	−	−	+	−
24	4.1	+	+	+	+	+	+	−	−	−	−	+	+(2)
25	4.1	+	+	+	+	+	+	+	+	+	−	+	+
26	4.6					No drawings							
27	4.6	+	+	+	+	+	+	+	+	+	+	+	+
28	4.6	+	−	+	−	+	−	+	+	−	−	+	−(2)
29	4.8	+	+	+	+	+	+	+	+	+	−(1)	+	−(2)
30	4.8	+	+	+	+	+	−	+	+	+	−	+	−
31	4.8	+	+	+	+	+	−	+	+	+	−(1)	+	−
32	4.10	+	−	−	−	−	−	+	+	−	−(1)	+	+
33	5.0	+	+	+	+	+	+	+	+	−	−	+	−
34	5.1	+	−	+	−	+	−	+	+	−	−	+	−
35	5.1	+	+	+	−	+	+	+	+	+	+	+	−(2)
36	5.2	−	+	+	+	+	+	+	+	−	−	+	−
37	5.3	+	+	+	−	+	−	+	+	+	−(1)	+	+
38	5.3	+	+	+	+	+	+	+	+	+	−	+	−(2)
39	5.3	+	+	+	+	+	+	+	+	+	−	+	−
40	5.5	+	+	+	+	+	+	+	+	+	−	+	−

(1) Verbal response contrary to drawing re: arms of ghosts
(2) Verbal response contrary to drawing re: legs of ghosts

Key: F = Figure Drawing G = Ghost Drawing
  + = Presence of body part − = Absence of body part

Table 3

Frequency of Appearance of Body Parts in Drawings of People and Ghosts Made by 18 3-Year Old Children (A) and 18 4- and 5-Year-Old Children (B)

| | FD | | GD | | | |
	#+	%+	#+	%+	X2	Probability
(A) N=18						
Eyes	16	89	9	50	6.41	<.02a
Nose	8	44	2	11	4.98	<.05a
Moth	15	83	5	28	11.25	<.001a
Body	12	67	10	56	0.46	NS
Arms	5	28	4	55	0.16	NS
Legs	12	67	7	39	2.78	NS
(B) N=18						
Eyes	17	94	15	83	1.12	NS
Nose	16	89	12	67	2.57	NS
Moth	16	89	11	61	3.70	NS
Body	15	83	15	83	0.00	NS
Arms	12	67	3	17	9.25	<.005a
Legs	18	100	5	28	20.34	<.001a

Statistically significant differences between frequency of appearance of each part of body in drawings of people and of ghosts. Chi-square test was used to determine statistical significance.

Most subjects, regardless of age, showed a concordance between their verbal responses and their drawings with respect to the presence or absence of arms or legs on ghosts. In almost all subjects who showed discordance between their verbal answers and their drawings, the children stated that ghosts had arms or legs but failed to draw these body parts.

Of the 29 children who assigned a gender to ghosts, 44% felt that ghosts could be either male or female, 38% felt that ghosts were exclusively male, 12% felt that ghosts were exclusively female.

The assignment of gender to ghosts was unrelated to the sex of the subjects making the assignments. Of the 13 children who felt ghosts could be either sex, 6 were girls, as were 6 of them who described ghosts as males. Three of the 5 children who described ghosts as females were girls. Thus, there were no differences between male and female subjects in their view of the gender of ghosts.

The majority of children (64%) felt that ghost figures were unfriendly or "scary." A smaller number (14%) found that the ghost could be either friendly or unfriendly, and 22% reported that ghosts were friendly creatures. Fifty percent of the children reported that they dreamed about a ghost. For most of these children, the ghost was a frightening figure in the dream.

Wilcoxon's rank sum test (Sokal and Rohlf, 1969) was used to analyze the subjects' ranking of the 8 ghost cards from the cards that were most like a ghost to the cards that were least like a ghost. The 3-year-olds found ghost 3 (outline + no features) and 5 (eyes + legs) least ghostly, while cards 2 (outline + eyes) and 7 (outline + eyes + mouth) were most ghostly. These results contrasting least ghostly and most ghostly were statistically significant. The older group also found ghost 5 least ghostly; but this finding fell just short of achieving statistical significance ($p < .08$). There was no outstanding candidate for the most ghostly figure shown the older children. They tended to choose among the various floating figures.

In reviewing the drawings that the children made, we found a relative fixity of visual motor patterns in each drawing, i.e., the child tended to go through the same motions in both the person and ghost drawings. There were stylistic differences in the graphic representation of a frightening idea. Some ghost drawings were remarkably sparse, while others included irrelevant "static" (see figs. 2 to 5).

The subjects verbally elaborated their individual anxieties and preoccupations with the concept of a ghost. These individual and highly personalized trends were manifested in stories and dreams and varied with each child. Most frequently, they included fears of being physically harmed by a large, unpredictable object, and fears of death. One child, preoccupied with the recent death of a grandfather, told a story of a man who had died. When the child was asked to draw a ghost, she prefaced her drawing with the statement that she would draw a "dead ghost." Stories and dreams frequently were elaborated upon, so that the ghost would be changed into a friendly and less threatening figure. For example, one child said, "He [a ghost] is white and scares people, but I'll draw a baby ghost. It's not big and it's not scary." Another child reported that "A ghost is an animal who bites. His face is mean and it has lots of hair. I once saw a ghost wearing some clothes like mine. It had red ribbons in its hair and it wasn't scary."

Discussion

In order to discuss the results of this study, a number of basic principles will be reasserted. First, the latent content of any production, whether it be graphic or verbal, is not easily available to consciousness or inference by observers unless specific techniques are used to elicit it. Second, as much as we thirst for the concept of body-image as put forth by Schilder (1935) and others, its full significance in development cannot be tapped by the use of a single technique such as a figure drawing, which offers a sample manifest content in a specific medium at a specific developmental phase. Third, in attempting to establish the infantile roots of a later unconscious constellation, examination of children provides us with childhood data, not data congruent with the effect of primary process or the latent content of surface structures. These general principles will enable us to approach the data of this study with greater clarity.

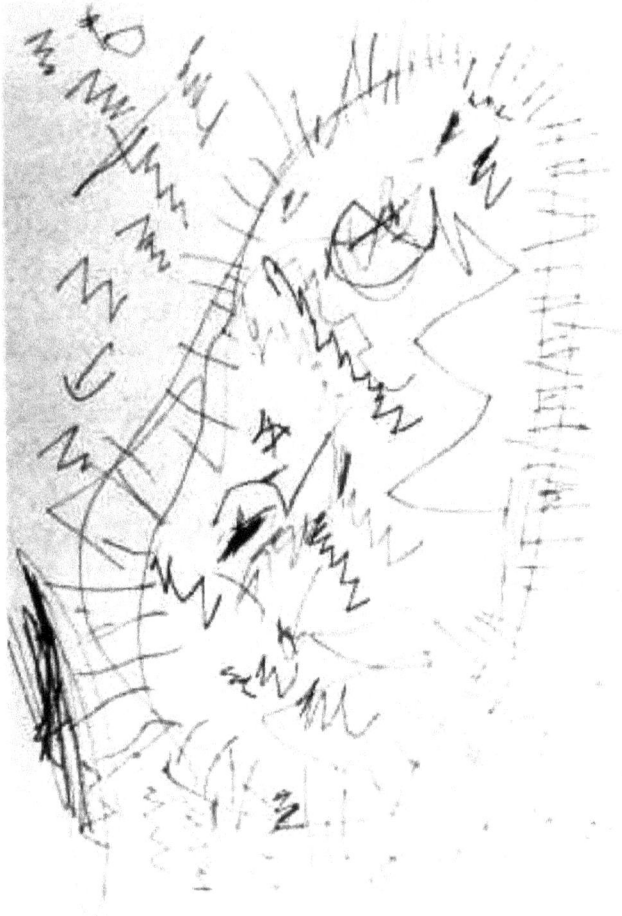

Figure 2

Ghost drawing (subject 15, 3;8 years) illustrates the inclusion of much irrelevant "static" which is not present in the same child's figure drawing

The data on body representation do not replicate the 1965 findings of Shapiro and Stine. The earlier study showed that only 4 of 18 children fewer than 46 months old drew mouths, while 27 of 36 children more than 46 months old drew mouths. In the present study, 13 of 16 children fewer than 46 months old drew mouths. In the earlier study, one-third of the subjects were from a lower socioeconomic group. Our study, by contrast, draws on subjects from the upper and middle professional class. Nonetheless, all 3 subjects who did not draw mouths in the current study were in the youngest segment. Thus, the earlier study remains suggestive of significance because, clearly, chronological age alone does not determine the emergence of sequential landmarks, but maturation and social input together create a significant combination of factors, which would account for a stepwise progression of development. Clarifying studies controlled for class are required to determine the validity of the earlier results.

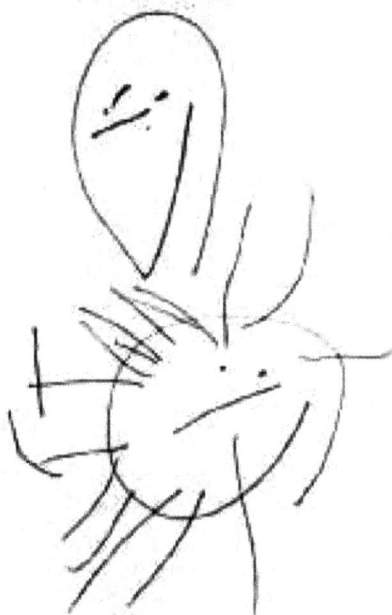

Figure 3

Figure drawing (subject 15, 3;8 years)

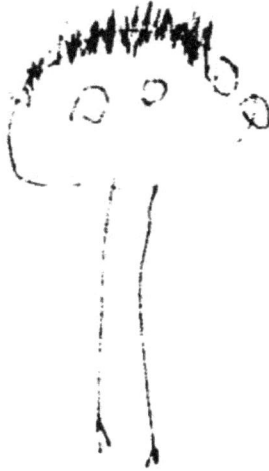

Figure 4

Figure drawing (subject 23, 4;1 years)

More pertinent to this study are the features that characterize the representation of a frightening figure, a ghost, to young preschool children. As mentioned, Freud's particular concept of the latent meaning of a ghost as a representation of the child's vision of mother floating into the room, as though without legs, seems inaccessible to direct observation. Moreover, this concept may also be culture-bound; indeed, the image of a floating white figure is probably Victorian. In the modern home scene in the U.S., the mother will have shed her white nightie for other covering, or it might even be the father who is taking his turn at baby care.

There is still another problem. The moment one designates the name of a creature, that creature enters a region of popular understanding and becomes a part of the denotative pool of other people's conceptions. There is no other way for a child to learn how to designate a class of objects except by an adult telling him that word "A" corresponds to object "a." Thus, to ask a child to draw a ghost is not to ask him about his conception of that night visitor (which might unconsciously correspond to mother), but to ask him to tell us about the meaning of the word ghost as he has been taught it. Therein lies the flaw in any study that attempts to look at latent content through manifest content. That notwithstanding, we can learn something from such a study.

For example, by comparing the representations of ghosts to the same child's human figures and verbal descriptions of the two, we may see if they are concordant or discordant. Eyes, nose, and mouth appeared much more frequently in the figure drawings of the younger children than in their ghost drawings, but there was no significant difference between the characteristics of the figure drawings and the ghost drawings of the older children. This suggests that the younger age group considers the ghost to be a figure analogous to the human form, but much less elaborate. On the other hand, there is a clear tendency for arms and legs of the ghost drawings to be deleted by older children. Verbal productions also paralleled the pictorial representations, lending some veracity to the conceptual backdrop for each production. The selective omission of the lower limbs from the ghost drawings indicates that the child in his fourth year has a differentiated view of a ghost distinguishable from a human figure. The sorting-task results show suggestive concordance with these data. In both age groups the least ghostlike card is the figure with the legs. While a sorting task may not be wholly trustworthy in such young children, this concurrence is highly suggestive. Thus, these children's concept of a ghost includes lack of legs as a distinguishing feature from human beings.

Figure 5

Ghost drawing (subject 23, 4;1 years) showing sparseness of representation as compared to the same child's figure drawing

The 64% who suggested that ghosts were uniformly scary added yet another attribute ("scariness"), which became part of the characteristic of ghosts. However, 22% of the children were able to designate ghosts as friendly, which might represent part of the contamination of the current social-reaction formation exemplified by such endearing figures as Casper, The Friendly Ghost. Despite this tendency toward friendliness, 50% claimed to have dreamed frightening dreams that included ghosts. The tendency to designate ghosts as bisexual in almost half the group was complemented by an equal group who saw them as masculine. Only 12% saw them as clearly female. This early bisexual vision attests to the lack of sexual differentiation of the children themselves, or to the fluctuating ambivalence toward the objects of fantasy toward whom they direct their anger.

We may conclude that while a study of this sort may not help us arrive at the latent content of the representations of human figures and ghosts, the results do tell us something about how children consciously think about ghosts—what features are present or omitted and how that varies from their capacity to represent the human form. If, as life goes on, the fear of ghosts gives way to fear of other frightening figures with specific features—such as the toothiness of a Dracula or the brute strength of a Frankenstein—we must assume that the later manifestations gain prominence by their resonance with phase-related concerns. That is, each stage has its individual dynamic forces which then receive expression in the discharge channels made available in the imagery of a particular culture (Hartmann et al., 1951). This surmise awaits empirical confirmation.

The word "ghost," of course, carries with it varied adult connotations, such as return from the dead or spirit. When one adds "holy" to "spirit" and "ghost," it becomes translatable into one member of the Holy Trinity which has positive rather than negative connotations to a large group of Christians in the community. The notion of ghosts being linked to the dead, however, is something which our sample of young children only dimly appreciated and is reflected in only one response suggesting a ghost's relationship to a dead grandfather. Graphic representation and concretization of such spirits appear in paintings and other media in human form variously as translucent figures, human subjects wearing sheets over their heads, or as ephemeral creatures lacking many features. Sometimes they appear as fully transformed figures such as the dove in some medieval and Renaissance paintings. Similarly, the older children studied represented ghosts with a deletion of the number of features, even as they began to show more detail in their representations of human figures. Other frightening objects such as robbers who enter the thoughts of 3-year-olds as night anxieties or as animal figures in dreams are equally as frightening and, indeed, may have more elements of the relevant latent variables of Oedipal figures. The translations into earlier remnants of unconscious residues must be seen with respect to each child's capacity to transform his or her own anger into representational objects who will do varying things to him or her which, indeed, must bear some elements from the child's experience (Freud, 1926).

It is curious that among the group of frightening figures that besiege children in the magic years, the ghost is not an eater of adults or children, as are so many of the later-night visitors. That ghosts are frightening; that they seem to have a diminished number of parts; that their locomotion is less likely to be on ambulating legs—these findings seem to emerge from the current study. These figures are then relatable to the Victorian night visitors that Freud postulated. In summary, the study appears to confirm the notion that young children's representations of ghosts result from an admixture of learned conscious ideas regarding ghosts and an ill-defined part, which is based upon primitive unconscious ideas about the unknown stranger and the mysterious images of earlier nightly visits from mother and father.

REFERENCES

Bender, l. (1946). The Good enough test in chronic encephalitis in children. *J. Nerv. Ment. Dis.* 91:277–286.

Cohen, R. (1953). Role of body image concept in patterns of ipsilateral clinical extinction. *A.M.A. Arch. Neurol. & Psychiatry* 70:503–509.

Freeman, N.H. (1973). A systematic study of a common production error in children's drawings. Read at the Experimental Psychology Society, Cambridge.

——— (1975). Do children draw men with arms corning out of the head? Nature, 254: 214–217.

Freud, S. (1900). The interpretation of dreams. *Standard Edition* 5:403–404.

——— (1926). Inhibition, symptoms and anxiety. *Standard Edition* 20:87–172.

Frosch, J. (1977). Notes on the floating ghost. Read at the Denver Psychological Society.

Goodenough, F.L. (1926). *Measurement of Intelligence by Drawings.* New York: Harcourt, Brace, & World.

Hartmann, H., Kris, E., & Loewenstein, R.M. (1951). Some psychoanalytic comments on "culture and personality." In: *Psychoanalysis and Culture,* ed. G.B. Wilbur & W. Muensterberger. New York: International Universities Press, pp. 3–31.

Jersild, A.T. (1946). Emotional development. In: *Manual of Child Psychology,* ed. L. Carmichael. New York: Wiley, 2nd ed., pp. 833–917.

——— & Holmes, F.B. (1935). *Children's fears. Child Development. Monogr. 20.* New York: Teachers' College, Columbia University.

Machover, K. (1949). *Personality Projection in the Drawing of the Human Figure.* Springfield, IL: Charles C. Thomas.

Marks, I. (1969). *Fears and Phobias.* London: Heinemann.

Nagy, M. (1948). The child's theories concerning death. *J. Genet. Psychol.* 73:3–27.

Schilder, P. (1935). *The Image and Appearance of the Human Body.* London: Kegan Paul, Trench, Trubner.

Shapiro, T. & Stine, J. (1965). The figure drawings of three-year-old children. *The Psychoanalytic Study of the Child* 20:298–309.

SokaL, R.R. & Rohlf, F.J. (1969). *Biometry.* San Francisco: W.H. Freeman.

Spitz, R.A. & Wolf, K. (1946). The smiling response. *Genet. Psychol. Monographs* 34:57–125.

Stern, D. (1974). Mother and infant at play. In: *The Effect of the Infant on Its Caregiver,* ed. M. Lewis & L. Rosenblum. New York: Wiley, pp. 187–213.

Adolescent Language: Its Use for Diagnosis, Group Identity, Values & Treatments

(1985). *Adolescent Psychiatry* 12:297–311.

A colleague told me that, when his son was about to go off to college, he wished to impress upon him the importance of using more varied language and a broader vocabulary than he had employed during his high school years. There was no issue or topic that his son had not evaluated as either "awesome" or "gross." Finding the apt moment, the father addressed his son, saying, "I want to say something to you, Johnny, that I hope you will take in the right spirit. Before you go off to college, I wish that you would consider not using two words; they are awesome and gross." The young man looked at his father patiently, waited, and responded, "Go on, what are the words?"

I begin this presentation in this way to illustrate that adolescence is not only a segregated period by virtue of a child's entry into puberty and the formation of separate groups with their own lore and customs, but because there is a wide linguistic gulf that develops rapidly. That gulf is designed to signify the separateness of the adolescent culture from the adult culture and the independence of the adolescent from his home; and at the same time it represents an abiding group cohesion which distinguishes adolescent from child and grown-up.

To be sure, the initial example cited has its ambiguity too, because the grammatical form (though adult and appropriate) is such that it is difficult to know whether "awesome" and "gross" are appositive to "the two words" or were in some ways adjectival evaluations of "the two words" that were yet to be stricken from the young man's vocabulary. Nevertheless, the young man believed that his father was describing the two words that he found so offensive. They had become so natural to him that he did not bat an eyelash when his father used them as though they were a part of father's vocabulary. The kind of confusion that emerged makes for humor. However, there were other times when an adolescent never would have imagined that his parents would use such words, because the wish implied in creating a new language (strictly speaking, a new sociolect) is to dissociate parents from the new group. "You don't belong to my language group, and I don't belong to yours!" is the message.

Another, now archaic, example from the past approaches separateness, but in the other direction. It comes from a young man from the 1940s who spontaneously responded to a shocking statement by his mother: "No shit! " His mother turned around and said, "What did you say?" Of course the latter example was from the 1940s and not the 1980s, highlighting a central problem in practical linguistics. Both language and social practice change rapidly over short time spans. These diachronic shifts make for difficulties in understanding among people.

These events are important in daily life, in common family situations, and in therapeutic situations. Those of us who do psychotherapy or psychoanalysis with adolescents understand that it is a mutual enterprise between therapist and patient, both of whom are engaged in a quest for meaning (Shapiro, 1979). It is not a simple matter to discover what someone is thinking about by what he says, if we are not acquainted with the referential system he is using and the particular vantage point from which his words emerge. Thus, we ought to know something as therapists about how meaning-organization comes about in adolescence and what the rules of transformation are, so that we can make appropriate and significant interpretations of what is being said. Only later will we be able to plumb the significance of what is said in regard to wishing and defensive operations directed toward not exposing. Thus subtleties of new sociolects would allow that an utterance used can obscure as well as reveal.

Let me address the matter of the meaning of adolescent language initially in terms of its most general psychological function: if we accept the vantage point of the dynamic psychotherapist or even a sociologist, we would have to say that entry into adulthood, adult responsibilities, and responsibilities for raising a family have been time-segregated from physical maturity and biological preparedness for procreation. That gap between biological readiness and social acceptance into the adult world is called adolescence. In modern times, the time gap is augmented by prolonged periods of education and training before one enters adulthood. In intrapsychic terms, the struggle to remove one's thoughts from Oedipal themes, or, in ego-psychology terms, the revival of separation-individuation struggles in adolescence, becomes a central problem. Using a number of strategies, adolescents endeavor to take on psychologically new and significant roles in the community, and in their own minds, which lead to increased self-esteem and peer esteem. One can make a simple parallel from a transindividual vantage point of adolescence to that which has been described for ethnic cohesion.

Following the First World War, the artificial creation of new national boundaries that created countries such as Yugoslavia also created internal problems among Montenegrins, Croats, and Serbs. They all had to band together for their new national interest, but they also announced their separateness by maintaining their own sense of uniqueness as a people and pride in their own dialects. The latter continues to be a marker of their ethnic, rather than national, cohesion. Similarly, Eastern European Jews clung not only to their ways within the Diaspora but to the Yiddish language. That language marked them as separate, though they were diffusely disseminated among a variety of nations marked by political boundaries. It always guaranteed recognition among them as kin, no matter where one found another. Adolescent language or sociolect has a similar function with regard to the wish to maintain psychological and social separateness, as a means of group identification within a sea of other individuals who belong to varying categories or groups—whether professions, work groups, unions, or even family circles. Coping with the problems of this period of life is done much better by the normalizing influence of being able to share with others in a similar situation. The shared problems of this developmental stage are better transmitted in a language that signifies and carries meaning in a manner that is not available to others. There is also a creative joy in messing with words that others do not understand—a sense of belonging to a unique social body with group separateness. I would not like to venture that this strategy is new or that it is consciously purposeful; Rather, that it grows naturally in accord with the normalizing function of adolescents' having common goals, common problems, and common needs. Distinctive social group dress as well as ethnic dress also provide group cohesion and separate identity, as individuals migrate hither and yon.

Certainly the notion of the melting pot in the United States seems idealized and mythic from our vantage point in the 1980s. It is erroneous to think that only in the Bronx or Brooklyn or on the south side of Chicago is ethnic cohesiveness maintained. In the northern towns of Minnesota or in the hills of Kentucky, original languages and dialects hold on, as well as original practices; sometimes even ethnically distinct dress continues. People maintain their languages and cultural heritage not because they are sequestered from larger communities, but because they wish to be separated and individual. The adolescent is similarly disposed. He is not welcome in all adult places, and he is also suspect in terms of the usual adult sense of what is good clean fun. In addition to these larger social issues, psychotherapists must be alerted to idiosyncratic languages, because sometimes a new language may not be a group phenomenon shared by a peer group. It may be an individual phenomenon and signify pathological separateness and even loneliness. The prepsychotic youngster, for example, who makes up neologisms, or the borderline who lives by and uses a personal code, does not want others, peers or adults, to understand what is going on in his inner thoughts and feelings. Without digressing too far, we may say that poetry may be another special way of coding the emotions—thus, poetic idiom often becomes an adolescent indulgence too. Such romantic visions sometimes encourage the adolescent to cast his thoughts and feelings in a potentially creative idiolect that may in rare instances become popular. More often than not, it remains personal and opaque.

From the vantage point of traditional linguistics, there is some question of what that science may have to say about the developmental event called adolescence. Yet there may be some contribution that psychologically sophisticated linguists can make to these considerations. Prior to exploring the matter directly, I would like to run through some of the traditional vantage points of linguistics, in order to indicate the modes of language study that have been employed. Clinicians will have to see if they can be useful as an application of a method that permits better understanding of patients.

Traditionally, the linguist looks at grammar as the relation of words to words and form or structure. Semantics usually refers to the elaboration of meaning and more specifically to reference. Pragmatics is a shorthand notion of the dialogic aspects of getting things done, viewing language as a useful tool with special regard to affecting other people. Grammar or syntax takes as its study the invariance in form of groups of words in sentences. It considers how that invariance interlocks with semantic aspects of language, but only in regard to how well-formed a sentence seems to our grammatical intuition. Well-formed grammatic sentences are easily understood and express relationships, but similar invariances may be found in dialogic rules between and among people, and also may be studied in terms of the formal aspects of how one sentence relates to another and how one person's remarks elicit another's utterance. In adolescent argot, we can sometimes find new grammaticisms, but by and large I think the study of form in terms of individual sentences is not very much different from the study of form in average sentences spoken by nonadolescents. Thus, in a strictly linguistic sense, they do not create or use new languages, but variant sociolects. What does happen sometimes, however, is that adolescent argot employs a unique use of words which might not find their way into sentences in the grammatical slots available in usual good usage.

Chomsky (1957) provided us with an interesting commentary on the latter theme in the phrase, "colorless green ideas sleep furiously." His argument was based upon the fact that every one of the words in that sentence is well suited to its position if we consider grammatical requirements, but the words are ill-placed considering their function as signifiers and carriers of meaning. Thus, we could have good grammar but poor reference or semanticity. Poetry does it sometimes too—"Spring is like a perhaps hand," wrote e. e. cummings (1926). The latter jars us just as "colorless green ideas" does because "a perhaps hand" seems poorly placed in the sentence. Grammarians use a concept of feature analysis of words to signify that the mathematical formalism of grammar requires that only certain insertions are appropriate within the strict parameters of the grammatical form. For example, what is disruptive in "colorless green ideas" is that, although colorless and green are adjectival, they are nonetheless semantically antithetical. Moreover, ideas are not colored or colorless except metaphorically, nor do they sleep, and therefore the verb form is not appropriate as an action-describer for the particular noun. An idea is inanimate and incapable of somnolence.

Let us contrast the latter with another sentence which was popular in the 1960s. "I dig my head." It carries some of the same problems as in "ideas sleeping." It is not that the sentence is incomplete; it has a pronoun, a verb, a possessive pronoun, and an object. However, how does one "dig" a "head"? The feature analysis again has been disrupted, and the sentence is jarring unless one has accepted a broadened usage for "dig," a new polysemy for a single homophone.

A similar problem arises in the language of adolescents of the 1980s. I cite an example from Valley talk (Val Speak), where there are ellipses and omissions as well as new usages. For example, the young ladies of the Valley might say, "like no biggies," which translates to "I'm telling you that it is not a big problem for me"; or "you gross me out"—that is a use of what now has become a commonplace expression that has drifted into the larger community. However syntactically disrupted it is, it indicates that "You make me puke." "Fer suure, gag me with a spoon!" qualifies as an exclamation of surprise. We will return to Valley talk and also to street talk of the 1960s and other adolescent linguistic forms later, but now I would like turn to another aspect of feature analysis, as it comes into play in therapy, employing a semantic vantage point.

The instance to be cited is the use of the opposite of the word signified. Freud's (1910) paper on antithetic meaning of primal words addressed similar issues, in his historic analysis of a common mechanism of dream work in the light of the linguistic theory of his day. He would have had a heyday studying modern adolescent productions for they tell each other that they are "bad" when they mean that they are "good." Or say that something is "bitchen," strictly speaking a neologism, when they mean it's "the best." Or when they suggest that they are interested in a young man—they describe him as "wicked," meaning "real good," or "tubular," the origin of which is "out of sight."

Bateson (1956), in one of his more whimsical moments, provided an interesting example of the problems of class inclusion of words and how the principles can be utilized in the service of play and cultural differences in carrying messages. He asked a group of scholars to imagine the universe of nameables and to make classes out of them. For example, he offered the word "chairs" and then asked the group to name a number of "not chairs," namely, to sequester a separate class. The volunteers in the group retorted, "tables," "dogs," "people," "autos." Bateson then placidly introduced "tomorrow" and arrested their attention by noting the discomfort in saying "tomorrow is not a chair." He then introduced the notion that there are two senses of not—a proper sense and an improper sense—so that there are two classes of objects which are not chairs: "proper not chairs" (tables, dogs, people) and "improper not chairs" (tomorrows). He then judged that similar reclassifications are at play with regard to normalization processes within communities, with respect to rituals, and how outsiders may not immediately understand such forms in use.

Aborigines who do not eat kangaroos may not have a confusion between kangaroos and fathers who are not to be eaten, but they may utilize signifiers in categorization to designate nonedibles in a different formal system of negative classes. They nonetheless recognize fathers as cognitively non-kangaroos. Similarly, adolescents, by using words the way they do, may come up with associational pathways that wholly disrupt our formal sense of order. Now, how is the task of the therapist changed if he has to decipher whether an adolescent is ill or just a part of a new and different linguistic group? More important, how can therapy proceed on a common ground of understanding if separateness and group cohesion may be confused with madness or perversity?

The final area concerns the social or pragmatic aspect of language, language as a tool to get things done, that is, language as an area of study that helps to understand the effect of words on people. It should be clear that to do this type of analysis and understand what is said fully, we need additional information to supplement grammatical and semantic information. Let me provide an example by making a statement. "Ronald Reagan is the greatest liberal president we ever have had in these United States." To understand that sentence based only on semantic and syntactic grounds,one would have insufficient information. We must add social knowledge, one must know my politics, my state of mind, and even to whom I am addressing my remarks, to know that I am speaking ironically. Similarly, in the case of antithetic meanings, the social, pragmatic, message-carrying aspects of the words become important. A philosopher, Austin (1962), introduced the notion that there is a class of phrases and words that perform acts: "I do" is one, "I promise" is another. Perhaps every sequence of words to someone is a performative, say some. There is a significant body of knowledge to indicate that how and in what sense something becomes a performative is dependent upon social convention. The irony intended in my initial sentence about Reagan might not be as apparent in 2084 as it is in 1984. Diachronic shifts make small differences trivial. I am sure scholars who read Aristophanes struggle with his humor, insofar as it refers to local and temporally bound politics. Similarly, the humor of Swift's *Gulliver's Travels* may be apparent in 1984, but the political references to English-Irish politics are lost to most.

The social conventions and practices of the adolescent constitute an area laden with problems, because adolescents may be accustomed to a set of usages in groups that are not easily transferred to therapy, and their social customs change rapidly. Knowledge of those social and pragmatic rules of dialogue is very important in treating adolescents—even if language were not an issue. In order to provide a runthrough of the formal aspects mentioned, let me contrast the pragmatics of two recent forms of adolescent argot that have made some dent on adult consciousness. The white-community adaptation of black adolescent slang and the modern import from California, now prevalent on Long Island also, called Val Speak, provide apt examples.

A historical note is warranted: Before we had the argot of the black ghetto adolescent, we had the special lingo of another

532

outside group, that is, the jazz musician, and then the more popular adolescent mode, the bobby-soxer of the 1940s, and finally, in the 1950s and 1960s, the adaptation of a particular subset of dialect that borrowed from black adolescents' language was transferred into the dialect of the white city adolescent. Much of the content of this era had to do with the drug culture, but also with mutual insult, raw frank sexuality, and irreverence to parents. The ease with which it penetrated and exposed that which was traditionally hidden in polite society is an interesting example of how a sociologically distinctive group, adolescents, became the exhibitionists of our unconscious and preconscious preoccupations, making everything that had been unsaid conscious, raw, and honest, showing the hypocrisy of the repressed polite adult world while embarrassing it.

The controlled formalized exchanges between black youngsters called sounding or trading dozens is a prime example that has been studied by linguists—such as Labov (1975). Trading dozens or soundings have a characteristic pattern and a set of invariant rules, he says. Insults have never been so elegantly and carefully delivered since Oscar Wilde—but in a unique language form. Not only are they insults but there are audiences for the insults, and there are rules of not jostling or hitting as the exchanges bruise sufficiently, while also testing wit. Cleverness and finally the acceptance by the group involve a careful understanding of the rules for exchanges to take place. What is permissible and what is clever are central. Labov notes, for example, that it is important to distinguish what is said from what is done. He notices that from a grammatical viewpoint there are only a small number of sentence types, which are simple in form but reveal an imaginativeness with respect to the ease of their expression—they sometimes even employ rhymed couplets. On the other hand, there is a paucity of variety in the actual words used. And there is a telling preoccupation with the central and basic themes of human dependency and sexuality. Most of the remarks center around insulting via offensiveness about one's mother. The raw aggression in relation to ritualized exchanges reveals a fusion of aggression and sexuality in a way that is unprecedented, except perhaps in the recorded curses of the Arab cultures and their extensions into Spain by Moorish invasion. An example of a ghetto couplet:

> I don't play the dozens the dozens ain't my game
> But, the way I fucked your momma is a Goddamn shame.
> Or,
> I hate to talk about your mother—she's a good old soul
> She got a ten-ton pussy and a rubber ass hole.

Labov (1975) analyzes these as consisting of disclaiming or retiring first lines; the second lines are contradictions. The format then is not dissimilar to other poetic forms. On the other hand, some of them are not as imaginative. They use common similes and begin with lines such as "Your mother is like," or "Your mother looks like," or "Your mother is." The dialogic rules of the exchanges between people are also well documented, and the returns and refrains do not allow for too lengthy a filibuster. For example:

> J1: Hey [whistle]—that's your mother over there [in response to a lady passing].
> J2: I know that lady.
> J1: That's your mother.
> J3: Hell, look at the way that lady walks.
> J4: She's sick in the head.
> J3: Walks like she's got a lizard neck.

This dialogue indicates not only the raw preoccupations of adolescents in regard to what others avoid, but also the counterphobic exposure of aggression and sexuality in relation to the adolescents' mothers. It has been institutionalized in a way that is shocking to grown-ups but pleasing and amusing to the teenagers. These are the expressions of poverty-ridden ghetto youngsters who hang together in groups in order to find some support outside of their homes, which are often incest-ridden and violent. They expose to their peers the things that may be commonplace at home. So why not express them openly— why not seek group counsel, if you will, and group support, without having to bash heads between groups or even seek out an alien therapist—and bring what was personal and frightening to a peer forum in order to make the associated anxieties less potent? It has been determined that, although there is much intragroup cohesion by virtue of these sociolects, there is also cross-group adolescent migration or linguistic drift of such practices. Take, for example, the fact of transmission of some of these dialect examples into the white community.

The white upper- and middle-class adolescent community during the 1950s and 1960s adopted many of the forms and phrases of groups their parents would not permit to live next door. There is no doubt that some of the language came from blacks and the poor, just as the transmission of jazz had come that route before. However, it was not only in the talk of the adolescent of this period that we recognize the identification with the poor and the black, but also in their dress. Indeed, our modern adolescents still dress in blue jeans and denim, originally the cloth of workers and laborers. Such trends in style provide an apt example of how identification with the poor became a symbolic counterattack on affluent parents of adolescents. It was the adolescents' way of saying we are not yours—we want something else in life—we don't want your money—we will shame you by an avowal of your own shameful lost past.

Individuals like this who belong to good cohesive groups do not frequently enter therapy. Linguistic drift in this group paralleled the dress, until there was a drift to inarticulate vagaries that were also common in the 1950s and 1960s. Phrases like "I feel," "like," "I am uptight," "like, man," and "you know"—all disguised a mass of inarticulateness and nonexpressibles of adolescents of the white community that was not found in a more glib usage of the black community. This occurred despite opportunity, middle-class education, and encouragement to good speech. It paralleled a negation of the adult community and perhaps even had its parallel negation in the movement toward varying cults that also disavowed the affluence of the larger parent groups. With this in mind, we can understand better phrases such as "After all the shit went down I had to cover my ass, because I was sure he was going to lay it on me." That phrase seems almost understandable and commonplace in the 1980s to adolescents' therapists who have had time to adapt. But imagine having just learned standard English and having to decipher it. As though a testimony to the rapid changes of adolescence and the tendency for linguistic drift, too, we now have yet another new sociolect to consider that represents new identifications and yet another sign of new adolescent values different from those which were espoused earlier.

This new talk is beset with a further negation of that which adolescents affirmed in their admiration of the poor blacks. The following are a few phrases from the newer language:

1. Lets greg on the white zone—I hear there are a bunch of Debbies there who are complete Martians.

Yet one more:

2. *Bite* the ice Melvin—like, I am so sure! That grody tale about that bitchen dude barfed me out. So bag pipe it—I'm gonna buzz the nab and mac out.

The first one represents the surfer's indicating that he would like to get together where the waves are good, because he understands that there are a number of sexually stimulating, naïve girls there who are from other parts, like the Midwest. The second one translates, "Get lost, you weird person—There is no way that I will believe that awful story about the best guy we know. You make me puke. Forget it—I'm gonna leave and get some pizza."

Let's try another one:

3. Fag your face, airhead—you're blitzed and crispy—I'm gonna look for a wicked dude with a cruisemobile. [Get lost, stupid, you're drunk and a drug burnout. I'm gonna look for a real good fellow who has a terrific car.]

I do not think it is just California that created the Valley girls—although it certainly was the waves that created the surfers. However, recent evidence suggests that, with mass media, the drift of the new argot to teenagers in the East is complete. With this behind us, how does the analysis of the language of the adolescent help the psychotherapist? Essentially, it helps because we must understand that the devotion to a particular language form does not preclude bidialectism or bilingualism. Just as a two-year-old who is brought up bilingually seems to know rather quickly to whom he should speak in which language, the adolescent takes a clear stance in relation to the therapist when he or she chooses to use adolescent separatist tongue. If he insists on his adolescent argot, he is challenging the therapist to commitment regarding which will be the language of therapy. If there is a shift in linguistic form during a session, one may be able to look toward the defensive use of either the argot or the therapist's language when the shift comes about. The question for most therapists is whether to intrude or empathize with the presentation by showing we understand the adolescent language nuances and by encouraging use of the language that is closest to his feelings. We are between a rock and a hard place. If we intrude on the talk by suggesting that we do not understand, or if we confront by suggesting that they do not want us to understand, we are offering a challenge. Yet the establishment of a therapeutic contract demands that both parties obey the pragmatic rule of sincerity that an exchange is about to take place. But how is it that we can establish the bargain and the empathy for the problems of the adolescent and indicate that understanding takes more than linguistic jousting?

The adolescent use of new languages is by design a signifier of the difference between the therapist and the adolescent that is similar to the distance that the adolescent has established between himself and his parental group. It may be a designation and statement about his separateness that are ego-syntonic and not to be penetrated. On the other hand, we could interpret the form of the language in terms not only of the sexual obviousness in the themes that recur, but of the fact that the adolescent group concerns that are expressed in a separate code sometimes sexualize more than is necessary. This may parallel the tendency described by Blos (1962) to look for a solution to anxiety in masturbation. The soundings of the 1950s, 1960s, and 1970s made an adjectival form out of the word for intercourse (fuck). They also made "mother" half of a curse word. They constantly bring the individual to the emotional peak of protection, or flying in the face of that protection, of his family bonds by insulting family. The need to be cool in both the 1960s and the 1980s has taken on the form of new identifications, first with poverty, and then with a kind of resounding immersion in decadence, laughing at the parental straight-and-narrow. Yet sexual activity still seems to be the common object of the conflict that it always has been. While dudes are on girls' minds, Joanies are put down, and dresses are shorter than ever and more flouncy and feminine—there is also an ample amount of latency-age play around anality in disgust, grodiness, and that which is awesome by virtue of its smuttiness.

Grown-up attention to being attractive takes on a caricature form—just as the bobby-soxer in the 1940s disguised sexuality by wearing long baggy shirts and in the 1960s by wearing work clothes, the Valley adolescent has invented a chic that is pure kitsch and even little-girl pristine. And yet the evolution has come about and the forms change. The advertising industry also has resexualized denims in the ads for designer labels. While the therapist's stance takes cognizance of the group identifications and their function in the psychological life of the adolescent, serving to keep the adolescent separate from the adult, the therapist also recognizes that the language helps the adolescent to belong and provides a normalizing experience in sharing concerns with peers. Thus, as a therapist, I would not recommend an assault on this identity which, because of its ego-syntonicity, seems natural to the adolescent—nor should the therapist treat adolescent lingo as a cute curiosity, because narcissistic injury and anger are sure to be aroused. Thus, our temptation to interpret what we understand as a subcultural phenomenon may have to be kept in abeyance until the symptom is ripe for lancing.

The adolescent may see early interpretation as inappropriate and an uninvited transgression. But to not understand is to be too removed. Thus, therapy must proceed within a balance between being able to listen and infer, and being able to accept differences and say, "please explain."

As one gets to know the particular adolescent, one will be able to interpret when the language is used defensively and when a wish has become preconscious. Do not be fooled by the constant reference to sexual and aggressive themes, as if the surface language automatically signified deeper latent content, because too rapid an interpretation at a depth level may be the last thing needed. Just as there are no primitive tribes according to anthropologists, because current practices in other cultures have gone through a long evolutionary change just as those in more cultured groups have, the unconscious is not more easily available just because the language seems more primitively referential. The layers have to be peeled in a different direction. The Valley speaker, the jive speaker, the hip speaker are no less conflicted about Oedipal and other themes than the polite speaker of standard English, and the ritual language may be less explicit than we imagine. The words may not carry the impact and emotional valence to the natural speaker that they do to the alien auditor. For example, the therapist may be provoked by a short dress or tight jeans, but the interpretation of provocation as an intention must first be dosed and built up by carefully worded preliminary interventions. Mutual regard and therapeutic alliance may permit confrontation, in that group practice may coincide with individual wish only once the preliminary work has been done.

What about the individual who comes with a more unique kind of vocabulary? A young man, for example, told me that he wrote poetry and translated it into a secret code because he does not like others to read his poems. This represents a less social form of language, an idiolect. Another patient said he felt "scarable."[should this be scarable or scareable?] That was clearly neologistic and, indeed, idiosyncratic. There is no group behind such secret and individual references. They are private, and there is no evidence that the individual authors are about to normalize their creations by easy sharing with peers. It may be the call for something personal, unique, and special, and, while group languages must start with individual creativity, they must similarly become popular. There is no such community for these individual users of their own language. These are the more schizoid—sometimes even preschizophrenic—alone and isolated, seeking restricted understanding, sometimes from a therapist with whom such secrets may be safe. Frequently such practices lead to further isolation and are reflective of the fear they feel for larger communities. Indeed, the normalizing process of sharing both a language and inner secrets during adolescence seems to me to be an extension of a need for community and the potential sign of health that Sullivan (1953) saw in the more limited chumship. When this cannot come about because one's inner secrets and thoughts are so private or considered to be so noncommunicative, then we may be dealing with more serious pathology.

In general, care must be taken in regard to what we know about adolescent language and language use, and special attention should be paid to the task to be done. We must turn always to the pragmatic function of our exchange. If the pragmatics is to hide from the group or isolate the adolescent, it is a more serious defense than that of using a special dialect. If the pragmatics is to share with a community which is narrower than the larger community, then language takes on a highly specialized function which is part-and-parcel of being an adolescent in the first place, but not the only requisite.

Conclusions

The therapist must be aware of a number of facts about language to proceed with this ethnically distinct developmental period. Language usage changes over short time spans, but even as it changes it provides a unique possibility for understanding the ideas and values of each new wave of adolescents. The group expression, however, is not immediately connected to unconscious wishes, no matter how raw or primitive the utterances seem. Therefore, the therapist should be alert to the new argot as a defensive intrusion as well as a potential royal road to understanding. That fact should make us alert to the bidialectism of every adolescent who lives in at least two subcultures, his group and his family. We may be able to follow our transferential significance by virtue of how we are addressed and which language is accompanied by emotion-laden themes. Tolerance of uniqueness of tongue is as much an adolescent challenge to our tolerance for his individual status as a part of a separatist movement. However, the therapeutic contract ultimately requires signs that trust and information are to be exchanged in the service of potential change. That change is, after all, the aim of the therapeutic talk in the first instance. In the last instance we may have to agree that the exchanges even build toward yet a third language—the language of therapy where, we hope, each party has a new two-person code enabling growth.

REFERENCES

Austin, J.L. (1962). *How to Do Things with Words.* New York: Oxford University Press.

Bateson, G. (1956). In *Group Processes: Transactions of the Second.* Josiah Macy, Jr., Foundation Conference. Madison, NJ: Josiah Macy Foundation.

Bios, P. (1962). *On Adolescence.* New York: Free Press.

Chomsky, N. (1957). *Syntactic Structures.* The Hague: Mouton.

Cummings, e.e. 1926. *Collected Poems. New York: Harcourt Brace.*

Freud, S. (1910). Antithetic meaning of primal words. *Standard Edition* 11:153–161.

Labov, W. (1975). *Language in the Inner City: Studies in the Black English Vernacular.* Philadelphia: University of Pennsylvania Press.

Pond, M. (1982). *The Valley Girls' Guide to Life.* New York: Dell.

Shapiro, T. (1979). *Clinical Psycholinguistics.* New York: Plenum.

Sullivan, H.S. (1953). *The Interpersonal Theory of Psychiatry.* New York: Norton.

PART V.

TALES FROM OUR CULTURE

Culture, including the specific language of our culture, features myths and popular stories that engage the imagination of children, adolescents and adults alike. These stories are taught and recited again and again from early childhood into adult years as religious readings, cautionary and heroic tales, epics, and novels. They carry themes that have found their way into stories that engage problems of everyday life and narrative solutions to universal themes of birth and death and mourning, among other conundrums that trouble the human psyche. They are universal, existential problems that have found their way into early recitals of sagas, tablets, scrolls and later books, and most recently into films and serial narratives.

This section comprises three selections that apply to such issues: I employ the tools of scholarly and psychoanalytic analysis. The first contribution is about books themselves, their contents, and how we use them during our lives. The second is a variant on the Santa Claus story as it appeared in a child's fears and its relevance to a cultural examination Santa Claus' roots as St. Nicholas who was rescuer, gift-giver and night visitor. The third concerns the power of a name in history, across religions and in grasping the role of learning to name in childhood. Naming helps to master overwhelming forces in everyday life and its application in later years to understand inner life is represented in fantasies. I engage the issue of naming in the Rumpelstiltskin tale.

Each paper was written for an occasion—"On Books" was a challenge provided by an overstock of book reviews when I became editor of *JAPA*. In this essay, I address the difference a book makes in finding themes that preoccupy the individual mind and the book as a source of intellectual esteem of hidden secrets and sexual arousal during adolescence and after. The content and themes may be replaced, for the bibliophile, by the book itself as fetish, sign of wisdom, and finally may attain economic value because of rarity, its uniqueness, or its mint condition. How we manage these varied emotional and practical investments can be studied via how we treat books.

The second paper, never published, arises from a dilemma of a three-year-old, who feared Santa would steal her gifts, rather than give them to her. As observer, I thought that concern was a curious transformation for a child and looked into the historical evolution of the Santa myth, only to find a compelling story of St. Nicholas in past narratives as a benefactor and rescuer, but also as a counterpart thief. Later cultures present him as a split image—as giver and punisher—and then a unique transformation in the new American characterization known as a "jolly" Santa Claus, who is specifically anchored to our New York Dutch ancestry. Most important to this presentation is the continuous interplay of personal fantasy regarding children's night visitors, and the public zeal to retain this age-old myth within the modern family in newly acquired garb that satisfies early 20th-century taste even as it is related to earlier Euro-Middle Eastern myths.

The last contribution was written as a *Festschrift* tribute to an Italian colleague (Jacqueline Amati-Mehler), who has written most intelligently about language and psychoanalysis. The theme concerns the power of naming, across cultures and specifically as a children's story, "Rumpelstiltskin," first appearing in an oral tradition which was then recorded as one of *Grimm's Fairy Tales*—The tale maintains a curious appeal over time and also is a favorite of children. There are many secrets wrapped into guessing the name of the elfin rescuer of the king's new wife, a maiden, tricked by her own father, who despicably boasted of her powers to spin straw into gold. The overlap

547

of the unnamed benefactor and the power of naming is a symbolic trope to be discovered by the reader. It is an age-old problem of children concerning multiple developmental puzzles, such as where babies come from and a symbolic puzzle for psychoanalysis to be understood as a transformation of a childhood myth into an appealing repeated folk story that somehow heals by repetitive reading. The language code, speech, is acquired in its specific form at the mother's knee, while the rapidity of acquisition seems certainly to be a universal biological miracle. The stories that are told in the mother tongue also draw on universal themes that occupy humanity; when translated into local myths, they soothe the mind.

On Books

(1983). *Journal of the American Psychoanalytic Association* 33(Supplement):3–10.

There is no intellectual enterprise in which the gathering of new knowledge and information is important where the reading of books is not a central activity of its practitioners and students. This holds true for psychoanalysis as it does for the humanities, the laboratorysciences, and all the learned professions.

This supplement is a first—an entire issue of the *Journal of the American Psychoanalytic Association* devoted to books—yet it is but an extension of a practice already prevalent in the intellectual world, as evinced by time-honored book review sections of newspapers and literary supplements. Although the *Journal* has always published book reviews and book essays, there has been an increasing time lag between the publication of a book and its review in the *Journal*. This supplement is an attempt to catch up and to provide our readers with the latest information, so that we can hereafter offer a more timely guide for selecting and reading books pertinent for psychoanalysis.

In our modern world, even reading book reviews can become a problem, although the intention of reviewing is to make the task of combing the literature easier. Like the compulsive, we become ever more removed from the primary drive and intention and focus on a displaced behavior. On the other hand, reviewers try to make our reading choices more pointed, insofar as they tell other professionals and scholars what there is to be read, and they tell their tales from a vantage point that is personal and creative. A book review offers color and opinion and judgment, in addition to a recapitulation of the text in summary form. We can admit to being readers of reviews as well as readers of books, without shame.

Being a reader of reviews is considered easier than being a reader of books, because there never has been a time when so many books were published in so many languages on so many topics at one time. Modern technology permits an outpouring of volumes unimaginable to those who were exposed to the early marvels of the printing press. In the United States alone it is estimated there are 50,000 new publications each year. Whereas Erasmus (Huizinga, 1957), living in the 15th and early 16th century, could maintain a naïve belief that he had read every book then in print (only to learn there was a library in Alexandria that had burned with other volumes he had not seen), such a boast would be unbelievable for a 20th-century man. An even earlier scholar wrote: "Of books there are many and study is a weariness of the flesh" (Ecclesiastes, 12:13). It seems that as far back in written history as we can travel, books have occupied us for the pleasure and, alas, for the pain they provided. Of course, the books that were available in the Biblical world were studied and restudied as a daily enterprise that was seen as a testimony to religious belief. It is not for nothing that Judaism was called the Religion of the Book, that Moslems refer to the Koran as a source of all knowledge and strength, and that Christians look to the Word for guidance. While the modern secular reader may claim a broader and perhaps harder road, because of the number and great variety of books to be mastered, he nonetheless may not read so much in depth or so redundantly as his religious predecessor. No one can doubt that the modern reader does have a larger terrain of wood pulp and ink to scan.

The largeness of the enterprise cannot undo the fact that study still is the royal road to increasing knowledge and to satisfying curiosity. But satisfying curiosity raises a further issue of how to understand the excitement some experience in reading. What makes reading enjoyable? What is the source of its pleasure? Could it be that the pure aim of seeking knowledge and satisfying curiosity about things in and of the world, and of ideas is sufficient to drive us? Is the aim conflict-free? Nunberg (1961) reminds us of the infantile origins of curiosity. He suggests that the basic questions to be answered are: "Where do babies come from?" "What is the difference between boys and girls?" and "What are father and mother doing together?" These developmentally vibrant queries should not lead us astray and permit us to light upon a simple explanation that reading is *nothing but* the satisfaction of infantile curiosity. Although such satisfactions may drive us all in some part, mature adult aims should also be considered. New vistas are opened in a world yet to be discovered. Keats (1818) refreshingly reminds us that his world had never been so broad as when he first looked into Chapman's Homer, and "heard Chapman speak out loud and bold." The awe described and the capacity of that translator to create the experience of travel anew was likened to discovery, as if Keats were a "watcher of the skies" or a "stout Cortez" staring at the Pacific, "silent upon a peak in Darien." The sickly R. L. Stevenson draws upon the book as an image to carry himself, a homebound youngster, to foreign lands. The elderly Kant, who never left Königsberg, noted that reading Hume awakened him from a dogmatic slumber that permitted him to create his most innovative works after his 60th birthday.

Freud (1900, pp. 169-173) also drew on the image of a book, a "botanical monograph," to indicate how the dream may utilize the book as a symbol to understand unconscious wishes, in this specific instance, competitiveness. Knowledge-seeking and learning thus may serve negative and positive Oedipal aims, as well as aims of infantile forbidden looking and knowledge-seeking. In describing his associations to the monograph, Freud (p. 172) further directs his reader to his own past—to childhood events in which he and his sister were given a book to tear apart. He moralizes that such permission is "Not easy to justify from an educational point of view!" Despite the demurral, Freud claims this childhood activity led in his later life to "a passion for collecting and owning books, which was analogous to my liking for learning out of Monographs: a *favorite hobby*... I had become a *book-worm*." Considering both the infantile and more developed behaviors described by both Freud and Nunberg, we can see that books provide us with access to lost and forbidden languages, secrets and early memories, as well as permission to enter awesome lands full of new excitement. Words become the conveyors of meanings which then lead us into our own unconscious drives and backwards to our past, but also permits the ego mastery enabling us to deal with the world that has come to be through another's creative vision.

Words said and printed may not only be utilized for information and knowledge, but also may become sacred, holy, and ritually significant. The magic of words in prayer and benediction permit us to consider a class of words that substitutes for actions! Passwords, secret words, secret texts, words said only in holy places and the average ceremonials of life, such as promising, belong to this class. The word collapses with the action that it signifies, betraying important pragmatic values as its utterance performs functions. Austin (1962) has given such words the designation of performatives. Words become actions or action equivalents as signifiers of mutative events in life. Consider the effectiveness of stop signs, "Do not open until Christmas" notes on a gift, or "poison" on a bottle—all written words that guide behavior. Psychological treatments such as psychoanalysis also require that words have power. People who change in psychoanalysis see themselves as having been brought to new levels of insight and consequent changed actions, through words. Similarly, books have an enormous influence on those who read.

Analysts themselves may interpret differently after reading this or that clinical theorist and change an entire stance as an interpreter. Again, the Book takes on larger powers as a vehicle for mediating both the changer and the patient who receives the words. The active-passive dichotomy implied in the latter does not do real justice to the interactive aspects of the reader and author or patient and analyst; the exchange is the thing to be considered. The reader is not only influenced, but brought into a dyadic exchange as the mind is engaged by the text. But the text is also enhanced by the reader, for he too brings his past and unconscious to bear on the text by interpretive reading. Recent analogies of this sort have been exploited to reconsider how we read Freud (see Weber, 1982) in varying historical contexts.

It is no wonder in light of this background that the cultivation of the intellect is a major aim of publishers. We spend time in universities and institutes enlarging our minds and we hope that bigger thoughts will emerge. Just as Luther Burbank cultivated new hybrids, we cross-fertilize our minds by varied and intensified reading in hopes of hybrid strength and new vigor. The words, the *bon mots*, in well-written books are pointed and carefully selected to augment understanding. This process has been called, by some, the phallicization of the intellect, in instances where the aim is confounded by pregenital influences. Psychoanalysts are no less victim to this hoped-for aggrandizement and augmentation than are others. Freud, in his "botanical monograph," provides us with such a proposition in the confessions exposed in that text. The aim of the dream was a competitive justification. He had to justify not having brought his wife flowers, as she would have loved him to, even though she regularly treated him to his favorite flower, the artichoke. The oral analogy to reading as an incorporative enterprise is not strained. He also points to his competitiveness with peers, especially concerning a specific monograph that did not lead to the fame for which he longed. Thus, Freud's difficult feelings about Köhler's discovery of the anesthetic uses of cocaine were pictured in a dream that used a monograph, a book, as the vehicle of reference. Others have pointed to the book as representing the female genital with its delicate "leaves." Overdetermination permits many more derivative inferences, too. The image of a book or the thought of a book can represent more than the simple referential extensive object composed of cover, binding, illustrations, and pages. The book is suffused with meanings that are both culture-specific and personal and also idiosyncratic.

We know well that there are people without specific reading disability who develop reading blocks. The development of an overall reading block in relation to books as places of discovery is not difficult to understand. These blocks frequently occur secondarily once reading has been achieved as a skill, frequently in adolescence. The conflict-free sphere of intellectual development through reading may be encroached on because the adolescent discovers that books can be sources of sexual arousal. They may contain illustrations that are sexually explicit or may have texts that describe vividly or suggestively practices the adolescent has never seen or heard of and only fearfully imagined,causing rising excitement and giving impetus to autoerotic or interactive wishes. Some of those same adolescents become trainees and students in analytic institutes. Here again the conflict emerges: to read or not to read? The problem is frequently compounded because some supervisors suggest that to read too much while one is being analyzed creates a defensively resistant intellectual barrier against personal discovery. Intellectualization of the analysis itself is not the aim of self-discovery. On the other hand, it is broadly agreed that to be a psychoanalyst requires the accumulation of a large base of knowledge that can only be gathered from books. As one supervisor told me as I was approaching analytic training, "You had better get used to reading a great deal daily if you want to be a good psychoanalyst." What might have become a weariness of the flesh in my past education would have to be turned about and changed in sign to a pleasurable activity in the pursuit of a new career. How could this be done? How could this sublimation of old and forbidden curiosities be turned toward a conflict-free aim of discovery and enhanced competence?

In search of the latter aims, a strange turn of events may occur that represents a variant of misplaced concreteness. The love of knowledge and learning—originally *philosophy*, is converted into the love of books—*bibliophilia*. Analysts as well as others become collectors. For analysts it begins with the excitement of investing in one's first acquisition of the *Standard Edition* of Freud. We are easily turned into estheticians of books; we love to handle first editions of Freud and then of volumes written by others. We take on new nonpersonal objects and adore beautiful volumes; we display the handsome typography and illumination of old texts; we collect everything from Vesalius to autographed first editions of Freud. Sometimes we even obey the rules of romantic love—we admire at a distance and never let adoration come to fruition by entering into a relationship by reading the admired text. As noted earlier, Freud himself indicated that when he became a student he had developed a passion for collecting and owning books. He wrote, "I had recognized that the childhood scene [that of tearing the book with his sibling] was a 'screen memory' for my later bibliophile propensity." Then, with some chagrin, he noted that his early passion would turn to sorrow at times, because when he was seventeen he had run up so large an account at the bookseller's that his father "had scarcely taken it as an excuse that my inclinations might have chosen a worse outlet" (Freud, 1900p. 173).

Freud's propensity is repeated in subsequent generations. When we walk into the study of an analyst, the large library displayed forces us to wonder how much of what is there has been read, how much is but a show, how much the big library is the concrete symbol for big knowledge. Indeed, some turn not only from loving knowledge to loving books, but displace the aim further to loving knowledge about books. The bibliophile can tell you the price of books, the dealers who have books, the sources of books. They can tell you about who owns the rarest volumes. Books become valuable in themselves and not for the knowledge they hold. Kant's warning about the limits of knowledge, expressed in his declaration that a thing-in-itself is essentially unknowable, turns our heads toward knowledge about things. Books as sources of ineffable knowledge are transformed to valuable possessions that outlive the reader, as though they did not share the same mortality as the reader. They also become equivalent to security because they are negotiable as money. To the analyst, however, money entails unconscious significance that is less than complementary to its temporal value. Ferenczi's (1914) Latin quote *pecunia non olet* may be apt. Although money does not smell, it can be held, hoarded, and cherished, very much as books are substantial and able to be held, fondled, admired, and passed on for value. For that matter, books smell as little as money does. Those who make knowledge about books and possession of books an end in itself are surely not following the central propositions of the analytic aim of self-knowledge. Similarly, those who look into books only to find out what is the difference between the sexes, where babies come from, and what is going on between mother and father are obeying infantile urges. The bibliophile may be serving a false god. Nonetheless, the true seeker of knowledge may also enjoy books and collecting without fear that all is regressive, or too much lingering in the foreplay. Perhaps it is the foreplay of reading that enhances the pleasures of the mature aim and therefore is not to be shunned, but savored as a remnant of our infantile past.

For a psychoanalyst not to read is unthinkable. However, we read only a small portion of what is produced and printed. Book reviews and book essays by respected colleagues provide us with a kind of annotated menu for our intellectual appetites and permit us to direct our limited attention appropriately. While the review is never a substitute for the book, as the book is no substitute for its content, some books may not be worth our time so much as others. Direction is needed in a busy week that contains the treatment of patients, study, and family. The most contemplative life is never wholly contemplative, but every life should contain time for savoring books, augmenting understanding, and comparing ideas. It is toward guiding the pursuit of these aims that this issue of the *Journal* is directed.

REFERENCES

Austin, J L. (1962). *How to Do Things with Words* New York: Oxford Univ. Press.

Ecclesiastes (12:13). In *The Dartmouth Bible* ed. R. B. Chamberlin & H. Feldman. Boston: Houghton Mifflin, 1950.

Ferenczi, S. (1914). The ontogenesis of the interest in money. In *Sex in Psychoanalysis* New York: Dover 1956.

Freud, S. (1900). The interpretation of dreams. *Standard Edition* 4. Huizinga, J. (1957). *Erasmus and The Age of Reformation* New York:

Harper Torch Books

Keats, J. (1818). On first looking into Chapman's Homer. In *The New Oxford Book of English Verse* ed. H. Gardner. New York: Oxford Univ. Press 1972.p. 602.

Nunberg, H. (1961). Curiosity. New York: Int. Univ. Press.

Weber, S. (1982). *The Legend of Freud* Minneapolis: Univ. Minnesota Press.

Santa The Robber

Previously Unpublished Paper.

Introduction

Once upon a time, not so very long ago, there was a little girl. However, she was old enough to say what was on her mind. In fact, she was barely one month shy of three years old. In anticipation of Christmas and the coming of Santa Claus (without religious trappings), her excitement suddenly turned into a worry that instead of bringing her much-wanted presents, that Santa would steal her toys—that he would be a robber instead of a gift-giver. Now, this little girl was an ordinary little girl and not a patient, so that her ideas did not come to me within a context where I could be assured that further understanding was possible. What was I to make of this—was it normality or perversion?

I thought of Job's comforters and their explanations of his plight and wondered what intervention could soothe the worry. Had she done something when she was younger? But how young and how bad could she have been to warrant such a transformation of pleasurable anticipation into a fear? Had her father or grandfather done something that this could be interpreted as a visitation of their curse unto the 3rd generation? I did not believe in phylogenetic memory or the sins of the father visited unto the child—so I discounted that one. Perhaps it was something beyond my understanding!

On the other hand, there had once been a time when I had read things other than my professional volumes, and I remembered that Santa Claus (whom everybody recognizes as a distant relation to St. Nicholas) had some unique roots in both early mythology and early Christianity that might help us to understand our young friend's plight. Indeed, St. Nicholas among his many patronates related to rescue and children, is also the patron saint of merchants, pawnbrokers, and, by extension, thieves. I asked myself how a little girl, not more worldly than she, could arrive at a personal psychological preoccupation that corresponded to a cultural myth and its changing historical revisions as well. How could her personal Santa Claus, at three, find such an easy parallel with the long history of St. Nicholas? Since, as noted, I do not subscribe to a notion of phylogenetic memory, nor did I have evidence that this little girl had closet experiences in the busy market place (there was no evidence, for example, that her favorite dolls or play jewelry had ever been pawned; no pawn ticket was to be found among her belongings) my thoughts wandered to the notion—not such a rare notion for a anthropologist or psychoanalyst—that there is something in the structure of myths and the structure of mind which warrants our attention because of their symmetry. The Structuralist vantage point advanced by Levi-Strauss (1966) espouses such a view, but Freud (1907) also wrote about it early in his career in his description of the parallels between religious ritual and obsessional neuroses. Jung (19__) certainly was devoted also to the notion of a collective unconscious and universal fantasies and the tension of opposites.

The other thing I thought, being a child psychiatrist, was: How interesting it would be to see if I could find, in my clinical work, dreams representing Santa as a robber, or normal developmental data to suggest that "polar" view of our little girl that led to her representation of Santa as a robber rather than as a gift-bringer. An additional area of interest that also titillated my thought was the relationship between the age-and-stage anxieties of children of three with respect to night visitors other than Santa Claus.

The latter is most easily dealt with. Robber anxiety and fears of being kidnapped are common during the 3-to-6-year-old period. Moreover, Gesell (1946) and more recently Beltramini and Hertzig (1983), who reviewed the New York longitudinal study data, suggested that delays in going to sleep are as frequent as 20% in 3-to-5-year-old middle-class children, and more than 30-minute-long bedtime routines are found in 25% of 3-year-olds and 44% of 4-year-olds. Wakening is as common as 45-50% for 3-5 year olds. Other night visitors are also rampant in the lore of childhood. Night concerns are as common as daydreams. The tooth fairy (Kanner, L., 1928), the sandman, prayers concerning dying before waking, and prayers that some supernatural being take one's soul if death ensues are embedded in our culture.

I would like to pursue the latter popular myths and childhood concerns in relation *to Santa Claus as a robber* by discussing some of the mythic and the changing tales about "the Santa Claus idea" and show the relationship of these to current practices and to normal developmental anxieties about night visitors to children. But first I will provide some clinical examples of similar transformation, using an adult dream presented in the course of an analysis and children's fantasies and responses to Christmas gift-giving that correspond to the worry presented by my small friend, as they were related in therapy.

CASES

Number One

A five-year-old, in therapy for a variety of phobias, stole various small objects from her therapist over a three-month span. These included pens, checkers and other small items. The stolen items were not returned, but incorporated among her own toys at home, which she kept under her bed. Her mother referred to this *cache* as a "junk pile" or a "mess." Periodically, the youngster would bring attention to the fact that she was taking these things by saying, "You're not going to look in my lunch box, are you?" indicating that there is where the sequestered items were hidden and apparently provoking the therapist to punishment or external control. She did not comply.

When the issue of *Christmas giving* arose in the therapy a reasonable present was agreed upon, though the child's wishes were unbounded and extravagant. Prior to that time, she had left drawings with the therapist indicating that once Christmas arrived she would take the drawings home and cease giving. Thus, she was giving while thieving, and Christmas was to be a demarcation when taking or receiving would be permitted and she would no longer give.

When the present was given at the session prior to Christmas, the youngster also brought a gift for the therapist bought by her mother. However, the child wanted to take the wrapping paper from her mother's gift, but more to the point, she did not wish to accept or open the gift given to her. She showed no enthusiasm when she finally did open it and was ambivalent about taking it home. Taking and giving were fraught with danger of obligation and guilt about her own avarice and thievery. The subsequent themes in the therapy concerned time and money and their value. Ambivalence about wanting to stay in therapy with the therapist forever was countered by the realization that sessions were limited in time, and she felt she had to steal time as well as things and not give completely, but take back that which she gave. Getting and giving were impenetrably woven together for this five-year-old.

Number Two

A ten-year-old in therapy told the following tale about his 5-year-old brother: He was concerned about receiving gifts on Christmas morning. He mused about how Santa Claus would get into the house and developed a compulsion about checking all the locks in the country house where they spent Christmas, to make sure that the doors and windows were bolted. He thus revealed the linkage in his thoughts between Santa Claus' arrival and his belief that route of entry would determine the authenticity of the good visitor. One locks up for robbers who enter doors and windows, but not chimneys. The acid test of legitimacy of Santa Claus was the appropriate route of entry, but we should note that the concern about robbery was aroused in a setting of wishes to receive.

Number Three

A young man in his 30s was in analysis for one year as we approached
Easter. He described a discussion with his father, who was going
away on one of his frequent trips. He wanted to meet with his son to
discuss his future plans, and also to encourage the young man to visit
his mother (from whom he had been divorced) for the holidays. The
patient recently had told his father that he had entered treatment.
His father hinted that he could save him a lot of time and pain
by discussing his past with him, rather than with an analyst. He
indicated that it was typical of his father to be intrusive in his life,
but did not mention his father's implied anxiety that treatment costs
money and that he might have to contribute.

He then reported a dream: "I was in my father's office and his
entire staff was there. There was a big canvas bag filled with boxes of
presents, like for Christmas, and Santa Claus was to give the gifts.
I felt a great deal of envy. Then an intruder knocked on the door
and tried to enter. I slammed the door and put on the chain latch
as though he was a thief. The robber pushed and I kicked at him in
self-defense.

He associated that he had been exercising, and he felt stronger
and more muscular. The intruder reminded him of his father, though
he was also Santa. Closeness to his father had frequently turned into
angry disappointment. He then said that he really wanted to meet
with his father in order to *try to get him to supplement his sister's
therapeutic costs.* (I noted that while he reported keeping the intruder
out, as author of the dream he also invited him to enter).

After a silence, the young man said that he had been thinking
about the presents—he still wanted his father to do things for him.
He then countered that such wishes were inappropriate for someone

of his age and maturity. That very morning, he had ruminated about a call from his sister, who described difficulties with her impotent boyfriend. He then noted that at sixteen, sex was on his mind all the time but that he couldn't even imagine impotence. He described awakening in the morning with a prolonged erection. Curiously, he asked his father about the new experience. His father responded that when he got older, he wouldn't have erections for so long. Then he noted gratuitously that his father had *always brought presents when he returned from a trip*. He also hit him with a hairbrush when he was bad, and then would kiss him, saying that it was for his own good. The patient added ironically, that long trips, too, were supposedly for his own good. In fact, when concerned about the young man as a boy, his father had consulted a psychiatrist, who told him that if he didn't stay at home more, his son would have difficulties later in life. Again, he added ironically, that both his parents had rationalized their harsh divorce as well, as a means of making men out of boys. Despite that avowed intention, the patient remembered how devastated he had felt when his father left home as his parents finally separated. He then commented on other and varying disappointments, and parenthetically said that he had asked his father to *bring a gift back* from this trip, knowing from past experience that he shouldn't expect anything.

I noted:

(But he was Santa Claus in the dream). The patient added quickly that the presents were not for him! I asked if when he asked his father about subsidizing his sister's treatment—if he also thought it would be nice if his father paid for his treatment too. In that sense, the analyst might be the intruder stealing his father's money, among other things, from him, while he altruistically surrendered his own desires and wished for gifts for his sister. He remembered that he thought of asking his father to pay for his treatment, since he felt the father was the source of his problems, but he knew that I would never get his money if that were the case. His father was so unreliable. Indeed, his father had asked the patient about a month ago what would be the one thing that he would want as a *gift*. With some chagrin, he admitted that he did not say psychoanalysis.

He noted that his prior therapist had indicated that it would be inappropriate to have his father pay for this treatment. He thought that his current analyst would share his prior therapist's opinion and agree that restraint in wanting too much was good for his treatment and character. At the same time, he resigned himself to the belief that he would *not get* or that *what he wanted would be taken from him* because he was not compliant.

The image of father-as-giver to others, stimulating altruistic and selfish wishes, is evident in father-as-Santa. However, the thief is also the father, and the young man's appearing as the protector against the robber represents the ego's mediating restraint. One can only imagine who I was to be, and to become, *as giver, intruder and punishing robber* in his assigned role as restrainer of the patient's wishes during the remaining therapy. Again, the intertwining of desiring and stealing is evident.

Historical Review

St. Nicholas has been associated with a variety of patronates (DeGroot, A.D. 1969), many of them relating to rescue and children. However, it should be noted that the St. Nicholas of history, who was the nexus around which many mythic tales are told, is a far cry from our current image of Santa Claus. In order to approach our theme, a long-term review of what is known and what has been promulgated is necessary—for such knowledge will provide an important avenue to understand how our current practices of giving at Christmas time could have been distorted in the dream and provoked anxiety of our patients in clinical settings, as well as in our young friend, whose anxiety stimulated this investigation.

Prior to a full discussion, it should be noted that St. Nicholas has been a long-time favorite in Eastern Europe, Asia Minor, and Italy as well. Nicholas was one of the more popular of given names among people who belong to the Eastern and Greek Churches, and these areas boast many shrines and churches in his honor. The fact that there was a proposal to drop St. Nicholas from the Roman Catholic Canonic lists as sainted is a curious turn of events, given the popularity of a more secular Santa Claus in our current life in the West.

Historically, St. Nicholas was a fourth-century Bishop in Myra, a city now in Southern Turkey. His life was full of good deeds, and he showed very early promise as a pious and potentially successful saintly figure. As mentioned earlier, his patronates were many and his good deeds were sung far and wide. Patronates that were related to rescue encouraged his becoming the patron saint of sailors and merchants, the patron saint of penniless virgins, and the patron saint of gift-giving and pawnbrokers and, by extension, thieves. By the sixth century, he was probably one of the most popular saints in the Eastern Church. In fact, his popularity had spread so far that by the 11th century Italian sailors pirated and removed his bones and deposited them in Bari, in the south eastern portion of Italy, where the holy relics still reside. (Slide AB) By the 12th century, the legends of his feats had spread northward within Europe so that Austrian-

and German-speaking people through to Scandinavia began to adopt him as their saint of giving.

His first patronates in saving sailors are depicted in a number of medieval and Renaissance paintings. The Florentine Lorenzo Monaco depicted a highly formalized life, with storm threatening a city, and with anxious sailors awaiting the arrival of the good saint. Images of Lorenzo di Bicci and the illuminated scenes of the *Belle Heures* of Jean De France, Duc de Berry (see Figure 1) show Nicholas aloft, also rescuing sailors from the tempestuous sea.

In case one wondered about the origins of our modern flying superheroes, we can see in these early depictions that they had nothing on St. Nicholas, who from his earliest representations was able to transport himself as a rescuer on high, with red cape flying. The scenes of rescue at sea, of course, permits an easy transposition to concepts of birth and rebirth, also found in the frequent imagery of the sea as the transformed amniotic environment of the fetus prior to birth. Botticelli's Venus born on the waves is but one version of birth, consonant with our theme.

The birth motif has given rise to a number of interesting cultural practices, such that on the Saint's Day, December 6th, in the northern countries of Europe such as Holland, lovers give "St. Nicholas cakes" and they implore that St. Nicholas pray for them (*Dem Klose Beten*) so that barrenness might be relieved and a baby be conceived. This relationship to birth merges into other forms of rescue that are central to St. Nicholas patronates and also suggest that children are among his more special charges.

The second most popular theme of rescue concerns a nobleman who was blessed with three daughters. However, he fell on hard times, and without appropriate dowries his daughters might remain spinsters or, as was the custom, even be sold into prostitution. St.

Nicholas again appeared and saved the day. This story became very popular and was represented in images and in paintings during the Renaissance: they can be seen by a master of the 14th Century Veronese school,and by Lippo Vanni (14th c Siena), Pisanello (15th c Pisa), and Ambrogio Lorenzetti (14thc Siena) (see Figure 2). They show the saint anonymously giving three bags of gold through a window to a desperate nobleman and his daughters. Emphasis on anonymous giving of the three bags of gold became the focus of the iconography that took hold later, in the cultural drift relating to St. Nicholas' rescuing function. Fra Angelico also painted St. Nicholas in 1437 for the Church of San Domenico in Perugia, in an impressive three panels depicting scenes from his life. This Triptych was removed by Napoleon and then returned to the Vatican in 1817, and was shown in the Papal Collection at the Metropolitan Museum of Art in New York during the 1990s. Three bags of gold were then transformed into three balls of gold and depicted with the Saint in Bishop's mitre with a shepherd's staff, in a painting on display in Vaduz, Lichtenstein. This later composite representation is essential to understanding St. Nicholas as pastor, rescuer, and giver. The 3 balls that represent his gift were incorporated afterward into the iconography used to represent merchants.

In order to grasp the latter fact, a slight academic digression is warranted: In classical times, Hermes was depicted as having stolen cattle from his older brother Apollo. N.O. Brown (1947) looks at this as reflecting an aspect of the mores of primitive pastoral tribes involved in crafty business. He argues that businessmen and wandering herdsmen required a patron who would and could deal with stealthy action; and thus the sly trickster was looked to for idealization and comfort. Hermes is portrayed as one who put others to sleep—i.e., he could cloud their consciousness sufficiently so that something could be taken that was essential to survival. In this light Hermes is considered to be a friend to mankind, and in Homer's *Odyssey* and in Plutarch's writings he is recognized as a giver of good things to enjoy. Thus, the culture hero as a trickster has roots as far back as early Greek civilization. His qualities as shifty, cunning, and thieving even on the day of his birth are described in the Homeric ode to Hermes of the 6th century B.C., according to Brown. The reader should be alerted to the role of sleep in this tale as a means of representing out of awareness events of gift giving and thievery. The many night visitors represented in children's lore are similar.

There are parallels to this story among other pastoral peoples such as the Hebrews—Laban's tricking Jacob by having him work seven years for the wrong bride is noteworthy, as is Jacob's stealing Esau's birthright and taking advantage of his father's blindness with the aid of his mother. These themes were given expression in medieval times in the cunning of the merchant, who was frequently a seaman. Indeed, it led to the practice that merchants carried with them a "thieves' thumb" as a talisman, or in the story of Renard the Fox, a culture hero in animal disguise. Later representatives of such figures are seen in B'rer Rabbit stories from the American South. St. Nicholas' transformation from the Saint of Merchants to the Saint of Thieves does not seem as fantastic when viewed from the vantage of historiography. The link of such patronates is carried down into modern practice in the image of the pawnbroker as trader and merchant, who takes as his icon the sign of three balls of gold—the same 3 balls that St. Nicholas used to rescue the virgins (Figure 3). Interestingly enough, these same balls are incorporated also into the coat of arms of the Medici, a family of merchant bankers whose symbolic shield also signifies their allegiance to St. Nicholas. Here they are depicted in 1751 by Hogarth in *Gin Lane Beer Street—*.

(Figure 4) allegories of London debauchery and prosperity with the thriving pawnbroker during the 18th century. (Figure 3)

One cannot leave the concept of St. Nicholas as rescuer without alluding to his other patronates. The concepts of the trickster hero and rescuer of children are evident in thinly disguised form in the idea of the child's outwitting the parent in his struggle for independence. Such a transformation of the commercial trickster is not so far from the mark, in tales of children's being carried off and achieving when away from their parents. A story is told of a child *Basilios, who was kidnapped from Myra by Arabs*. During the period of absence he served as cup bearer to an Emir. His parents longed for his return, however, and that return was accomplished miraculously on St. Nicholas Day by the good Bishop (see Figure 5 painting by Signorelli [1444–1523].) Thus, the story succeeds in incorporating St. Nicholas' association with rescue of children, and the gift of giving a child to bereft parents or barren parents on his day. Signorelli portrayed the entire event almost as if in a single dream image, with the child serving the Emir and the Saint swooping down from above to return him to his parents, who are shown kneeling gratefully in front of him. The parallels to Ganymede as cup-bearer to the gods in Roman mythology and family romance fantasies will not be belabored.

Rescue is not remote from reconstitution of that which has been dismembered. St. Nicholas' "patronate of clerks" is based on interesting story that includes treachery while asleep and thievery: Three clerks, or divinity students, were on a journey and stopped at an inn for dinner and sleep. As they slept, the innkeeper and his wife robbed them and in order to hide their crime, dismembered the youths and stored them in barrels of brine. Seven years passed, until St. Nicholas happened on the inn and requested a meal and specifically instructed them to turn toward the barrel of brine. He reconstituted the clerks magically and the innkeeper and his wife were saved by repentance. These events are portrayed both in an altarpiece in France by Lorenzo diBicci and a north European wood cut (Figure 6). The latter story indicates the introduction of thievery while asleep and rescue from death, dismemberment and sleep. St. Nicholas is also portrayed as resuscitating a child directly by Ambrogio Lorenzetti (Figure 7) thus rounding out his role as gift giver, rescuer and life giver. A stone base relief at Bari depicts the haloed saint amidst panels that designate his holy acts, as does a 17th century Russian icon (Figure 16).

Practices in Northern Europe surrounding St. Nicholas are of special significance to our discussion. In Holland the Krampus is a jolly joker not unlike the trickster. He accompanies St. Nicholas on the Saint's day, bedecked with articles for punishment as well as presents. Father Christmas, Kerstman, is the early representation of Santa Claus who brought presents to some families. However, the real Sinter Klaas was the important figure. F. Red L.(1965) claims there were no such double figures of St. Nicholas and companion in Austria on Christmas day of his youth in the early 20th century. Instead, the myth of the Christ child as bringer of Christmas presents took on greater importance than St. Nicholas as gift bringer in that predominantly Catholic community, and the split image was reserved for December 6th. This transformation was clearly an attempt to focus on the sacrificing image of Christ in this Catholic country.

I have been able to uncover some more arcane and historically early but persistent practices that still exist from an area of the Southern Tyrol which are almost the same as pictured in a 19th-century Dutch illustration showing the Bishop with mitre and staff and Black Peter (or Krampus) behind him (see Figure 8).

In Bad Mittendorf in Styria, Austria even today, there remains a pastoral tradition that probably goes back to ancient times and is repeated yearly, that has a strange similarity to the earlier split between Santa Claus the giver and Bartel, or Black Peter the punisher. It is likely that, as winter came on early and severely in that area, there was insufficient fodder to sustain domestic animals. They had to be sacrificed and then preserved in a setting where cornfield demons had to be mollified. Currently, on St. Nicholas Day's eve, St. Nicholas and his companion, carrying faggots very similar to Bartel's march down a snow-laden street amidst drawn shutters as the sun sets (Figure 9). They then trudge to a central square as cornfield demons with rattling chains, emerge). Children are paraded in front of St. Nicholas, who asks questions in a similar fashion to that described by Redl in his tales of Austria. He inquires if prayers are said nightly, and he rewards those children who are good with gifts. There is also the ever-present threat of punishment, or even kidnapping by the more demonic-looking companion. The next morning, fruits, nuts and pastry are found at the door of the house, either in shoes or elsewhere, to inform that St. Nicholas has overcome the devil and that the winter will be a successful time. (Note parallel to hanging stockings in North America). In France, too, children must first pass muster of Père Fouettard (Father Spanking) before they can receive rewards from Père Noel,.

Turning now to American practices, one has to seek the roots of our modern promulgation of the Santa Claus story in three historical figures, Washington Irving, Clement C. Moore, and Thomas Nast (Ebon, M., 1975). It is said that Washington Irving may be the most important influence on our current image of Santa Claus. His is an interesting example of storytelling that became history. There is good evidence that early Americans had little or no toleration of Roman

Catholic saints, because of the Puritan revolt against Papism. Indeed, even though New York was settled by the Dutch, who enjoyed the saint, there is very little evidence that St. Nicholas' practices were ever present in the New World until after the American Revolution, when there was a return to the emphasis on the Dutch heritage of the colony. These practices served as a counterpoint to early British influences and became a deterrent to the continuity of Tory pride. During the early colonial period in the Massachusetts Bay Colony, Christmas reveling was prohibited. There was no Christmas day celebration and work went on. Wassailing and other wandering from home to home emerged later and was considered a heathen legacy. Washington Irving provided post-revolutionary New York with the false *History of New York* of "Diedrich Knickerbocker," who told of the origins of New York and set in motion a series of visions which were later transformed.

He described the Goode Vrow, the boat of early Dutch settlers, which arrived in New York with a figurehead that represented St. Nicholas. In the history of New York, he indicated that the Saint was honored and followed. A broadside executed at the behest of John Pintard, the founder of the New York Historical Society (Figure 10) shows St. Nicholas dressed in toga, flanked by a beehive as a sign of industry and a dog to indicate loyalty. In the inset of the Broadside there is a hearth with a child crying, holding the faggot that was used to beat him, with an opposite image of a good child joyously holding nuts and fruits in her skirt. This early broadside suggested the links to a Dutch heritage of reward next to punishment and interest in the Saint promulgated by the group known as the Knickerbocker Society. It also depicted the ambivalent relationship of the Saint to children, both as gift-giver and as righteous punisher. It also follows a lore that boys are nasty and girls as nice. Jan Steen's painting shows a similar mixture of blessing and punishment (Figure 11) The Metropolitan Museum of Art collection includes one of 6 renderings of a painting by the American painter, Robert Weir (1837) that portrays an impish Santa gesturing in front of a fireplace with tiled façade, one of which shows the iconic three balls, bedecked with 3 stockings. Santa is carrying a bag of toys and attached switches, while iconic representations of the Dutch culture are strewn in the foreground, a clay pipe and an orange . (Figure 12)

In 1822 Clement Clarke Moore, a minister and Head of the Anglican Church's General Seminary in New York's Chelsea area, wrote a poem for his children that has become the famous "Night before Christmas." It was heard by a visitor and later published and attained fame. It personifies Washington Irving's image of Santa Claus in words. However, it was not until 1863 that Thomas Nast, a German-born artist and political cartoonist, transformed St. Nicholas into Santa Claus as a jolly elf climbing down the chimney on a snow-driven evening. A later representation (1876, Figure 13) also shows a naughty child lurking around the chimney to watch, though he should be asleep.

There are varying transformations of Santa represented in early American Christmas tree ornaments (Figures 14,15) where Santa Claus, not yet fully the jolly imp, but somewhere in between. The Saint is pictured holding the good child on his lap and kidnapping the bad child in a sack. While the current emerging image of Santa Claus in modern times emphasizes the giving of gifts and aspects of commercialism and has roots in the early Saint, the punishing rejecting images have disappeared. However, in Austria even in the 20th century, practices continue that remind us of the Saint's dual role. Somehow the double psychological significance remains indelibly written in awareness and depicted clearly in some cultures, less so in others, and only personally in the unique fears of children and others.

Finally, it should be noted that gift-giving is not uniformly practiced throughout the world on St. Nicholas' Day or even on Christmas Day or Christmas Eve. There are cultures where the 12 days of Christmas are still respected, as in the well-known carol, for it was on the 12th day or Epiphany that the Magi brought gifts to the Christ child. In Latin countries, such as in South America, gift-giving takes place on Epiphany, featuring three ships sailing in from across the unknown world, presumably to greet the newborn Christ child. Boxing Day, a Victorian tradition, was usually the morning after Christmas, when those in service came upstairs to receive their gifts and receive the further gift of permission to watch boxing matches. In Greece, gift-giving is on New Year's Day and not associated with St. Nicholas but with St. Basilio. However, there are practices in both Southern Italy, Sicily and Greece as well where loaves of bread are baked with symbols of rebirth, such as an egg, and the gift of St. Nicholas is represented in a coin baked into the bread. The lucky person who gets the slice with the coin receives a gift associated with the Saint. The French feature the King's Loaf . It also has a coin baked into it with the lucky slice as a reward.

The emphasis on childhood, of course, has its sources not only in St. Nicholas' attention to children, but in Jesus' birth itself. The Feast of Childermas was a commemorative mass to honor the holy innocents slain by Herod, as he attempted to eradicate the yet-to-be- born and prophesied Infant Jesus. The linkages to the Oedipus myth are easily made. The King tried to put off the prophecy of his death and succession—by sending the infant Oedipus away to be slain. The tale of Passover is also interwoven with rescue of the Baby Moses from the waters and his family's story and ultimate rescue of his people. Thus, the anxiety about the massacre is also somehow imbued with the joy of the new birth, and again, the ambivalent and conflicted aspects of the symbols employed in myth-making become evident.

Discussion

Attitudes towards Christmas and Santa Claus vary as greatly as does the giving and taking that I have suggested are so intimately intertwined in the psychic life of children and adults. One could point to the 1659 Puritan decree that imposed a fine on the celebration of Christmas, because of its ties to Papism, Dickens' Scrooge (1847) and the more recent *Grinch who stole Christmas* as examples of the tendency to deny giving or steal rather than give. Scrooge, of course, involves happy conversion on the basis of an early form of the "primal scream therapy" in his visit with the Ghost of Christmas Future, which leads the child, Tiny Tim, to finally extol the graciousness of the old once-grudging bachelor.

Psychoanalytic literature during the early '40s reveals a similar debate between the poles of Christmas giving. Jules Eisenbud (1941) described two cases of women who were very distressed each Christmas, based upon the frustration of infantile wishes and disappointments in Santa Claus, who never satisfied their wishes (for the derivatives of the paternal phallus.) Sterba's (1944) counter-argument elaborates the joyous relationship of Christmas to birth-rebirth fantasies and expectations, as he reviews the analogies in iconography of Christmas to features of expected anticipation in pregnancy, Santa's bag full of presents, and speculations about Santa's routes of entry and exit as they relate to impregnation derivatives and the culmination in the joy of birth. At the end of his discussion, he notes that in Belgium and Holland, December 6th, St. Nicholas Day, is much more a day of gift-givingfor children than is Christmas, and that it has been only during the past 300 years that there has been a postponement until Christmas itself. He further suggests that St. Nicholas has turned into Santa Claus, (*Knecht Ruprecht* or *Weihnachtsmann*) during this evolution and merged fully in the United States in our Santa Claus.

Late 20th-century empirical studies of children (Prentis et al.,1979), show diminishing belief in Santa Claus as causal reasoning increases: while 85% of four-year- olds in a Southwestern, upper-middle-class, Christian community believed in Santa Claus, only 25% of eight-year-olds continued to believe in him wholeheartedly. Despite this, parents reported that 85% of six-year-olds and 75% of eight-year-olds continue to leave food, drawings, etc. for Santa Claus at night and 90% hung stockings which correspond to the same 90% of the parents who strongly support the myth as "good exciting fun." Thus, while reason has its sway with maturation, the heart surely prevails in practice; or is it greed and gluttony?

These facts are in sharp contrast to the spoilsport attitude of some who suggest that the myth supports unrealistic expectations and hopes and that the celebration is marred by unpleasant memories; and children should not be seduced by romantic visions of sugar plums when hunger prevails in the larger world. Whether it is good clean fun and supportive of optimism or indeed, a bane on our pocketbooks and a commercialized form of merchant's deceit and seduction, it seems that Santa Claus' popularity rests on something deeper than the happenstance of history or a moment-to-moment exploration of what individuals feel.

I have tried to suggest that the evolution of the myth of St. Nicholas is a most apt starting place to understand children's irrepressible imaginations. Much as a cultural theme may be incorporated into individual fantasy, individual mental growth also adopts appropriate cultural forms for mental reworking, in accord with maturing cognitive structures. The developmental correspondence of increased difficulties in falling asleep, the beginning sense of responsibility and guilt, with the lifelong mental preoccupations of how much one should wish for and how much one should be rewarded or punished find useful expressions in the Santa model. Other night visitors of 3- and 4-year-olds involve giving and taking as well. It is not only the robber who threatens the preschooler and steals or kidnaps, it is the tooth fairy too, who in our culture takes away only to provide a return in money for that which she takes. Kanner (1928) notes that there is a high degree of commonality cross-culturally throughout the Western world regarding loss and regaining of teeth (not yet transformed into a night myth as in the United States). One throws a tooth over one's shoulder for a mouse to retrieve, while the wish is offered in rhyme that he bring a new tooth.

The polarization of giving and taking as an early characteristic of thought processes, with varying transformations in accord with responsibility and guilt, may be reported in later psychopathological forms as expressed in the dream presented by my patient. Scrooge too, while a disappointed man, without the reader's sympathy became a guilty man with fear of retribution on "Christmases yet to come"— He converts to a gift-giving Santa substitute in his beneficence to Tiny Tim's Cratchit family. Similarly, the more recent Grinch is thwarted as a selfish thief, and in the end children and the spirit of giving triumph.

The varying patronates of St. Nicholas run the gamut of all the phases of anxiety, as suggested by Freud in *Inhibition, Symptoms, and Anxiety* (1926). There is the anxiety attached to themes of helplessness and wish for rescue and rebirth in the patronate of sailors; the anxiety of separation is seen in the story of kidnapping and ultimate return and reunion; the anxiety of body dismemberment and castration and reconstitution features in the story of 3 students; and finally, we find the anxiety related to superego guilt and gratitude in the responsibilities of coming to marriage prepared to give and to raise children. Even before the early 20th century, when Freud explicated these stages in the development of the signal for anxiety, it was written into our cultural history in the St. Nicholas patronates. The systemization of these myths did not address the issue from the vantage point of marveling at the human mind, but surely are representative of the potential for its various forms and expressions as they are transformed generationally and also in individual development.

In the words of the famous *Daily Sun World* editorial, "Yes, Virginia, there is a Santa Claus," but we must add an admonition not to become too excited, because he may exact something from you as well as bring you something.

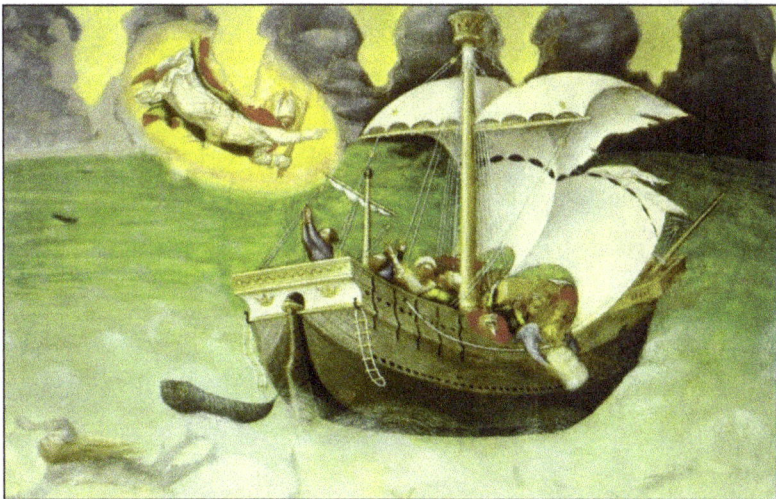

Fig. 1. St. Nicholas Illumination from Belle Heures of Jean de France, Duc de Berry. 1414. Metropolitan Museum Art

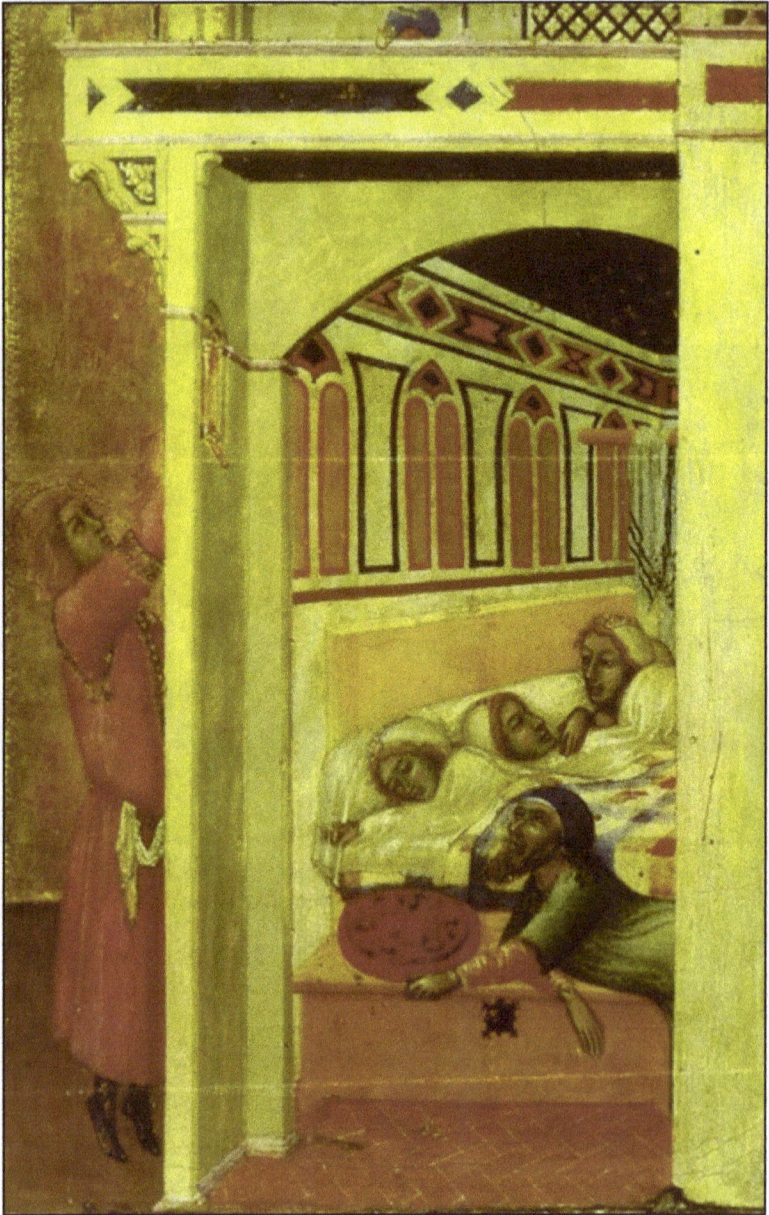

Fig. 2. St. Nicholas and the three virgins:
Ambrogio Lorenzetti 1300s. the Louvre Paris

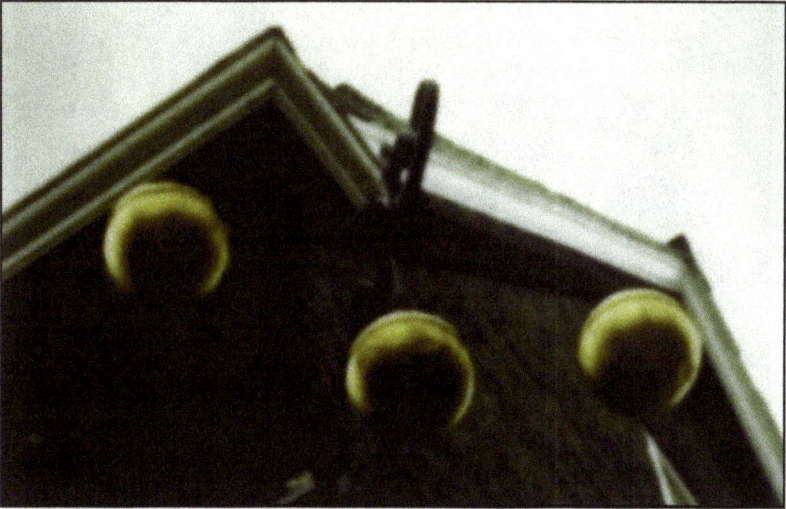

Fig. 3. Pawn shop, England. Phtograph

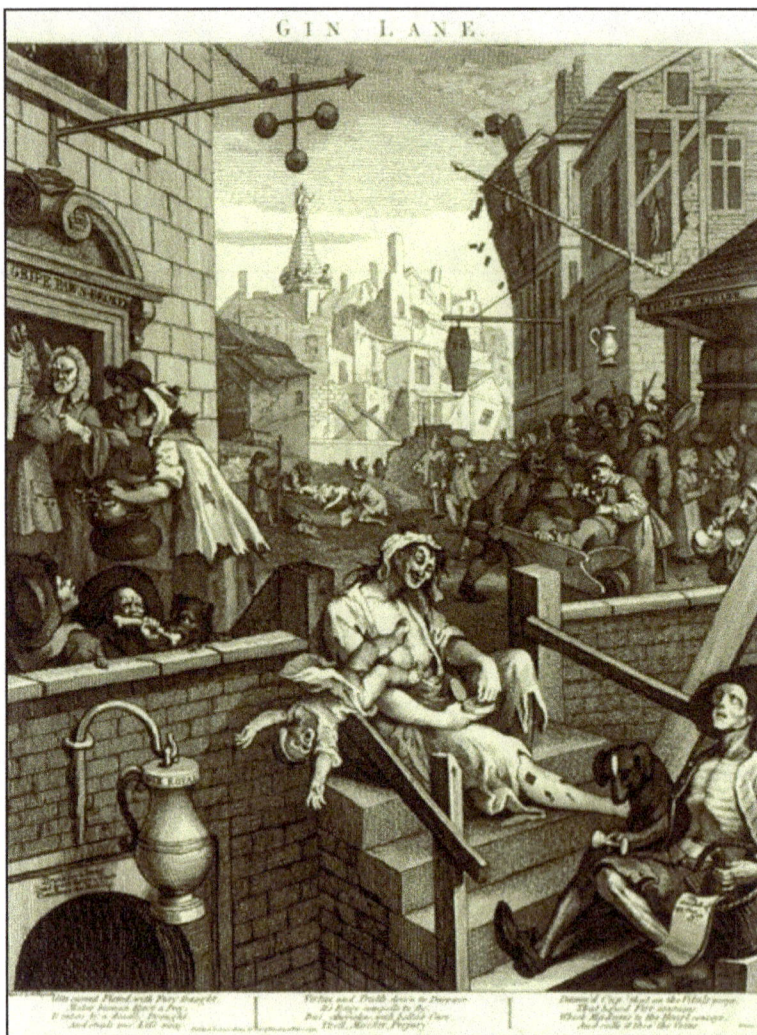

Fig. 4. Pawn shop in Gin Lane etching, Hogarth,
18 C. Metropolitan Museum NY

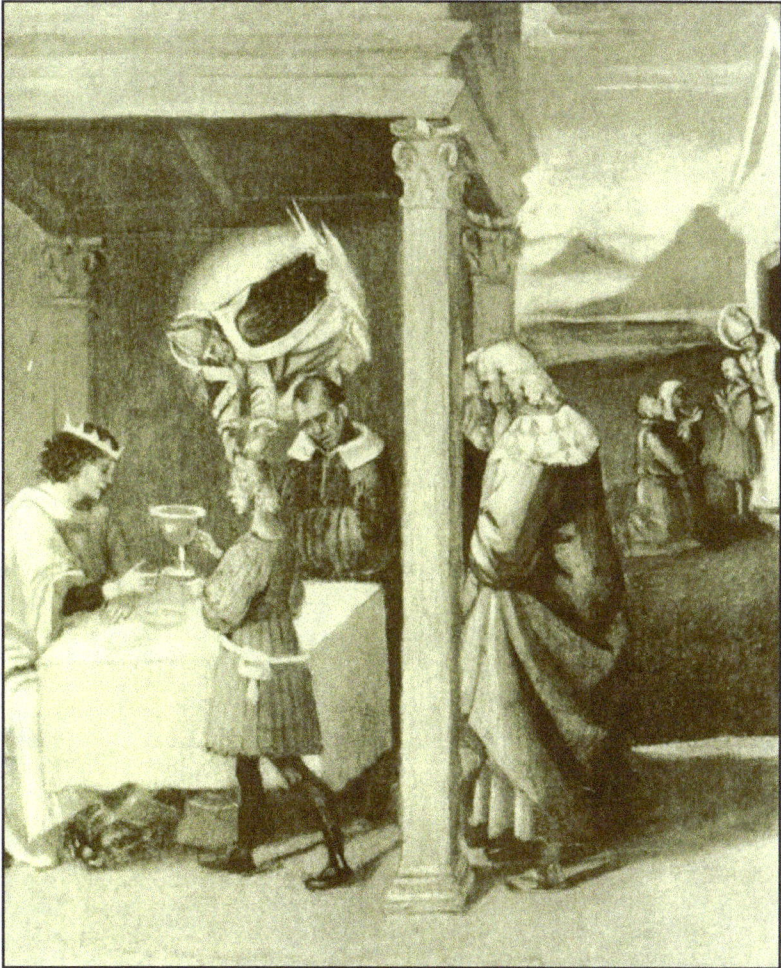

Fig. 5. Three Aspects of St. Nicholas:
Rescue of Kidnapped Child, Signorelli 1441-1523

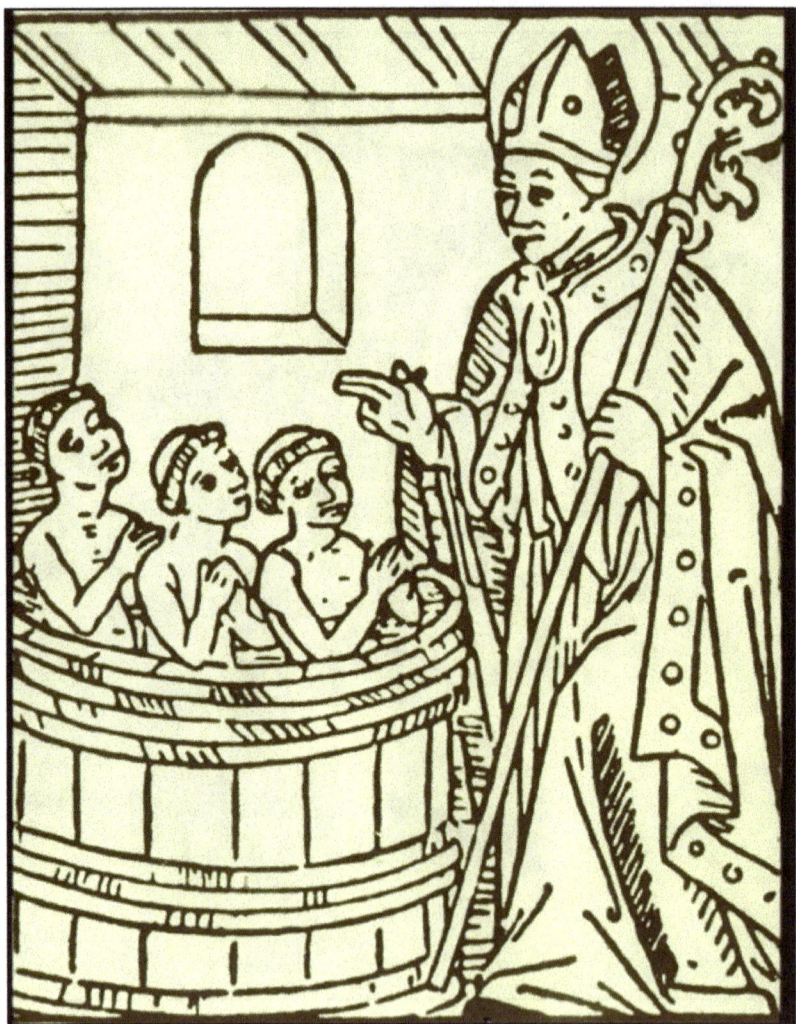

Fig 6. Reconstitution of 3 Clerks. woodcut,
Middle Ages, artist unknown

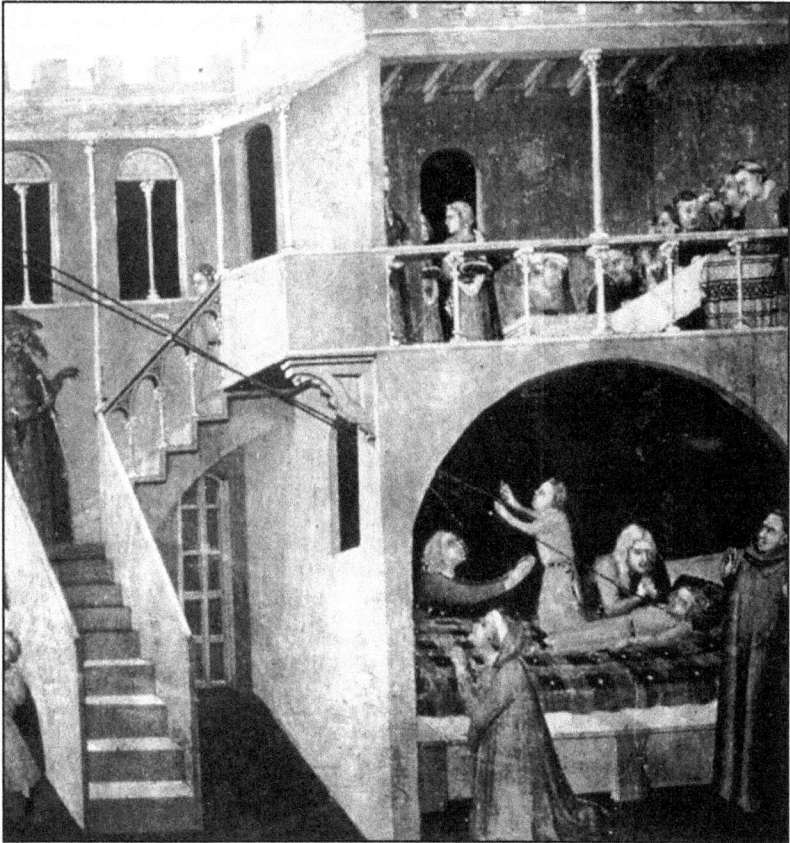

Fig 7. St. Nicholas Rescusitation of Child,
Ambrogio Lorenzetti 1300.

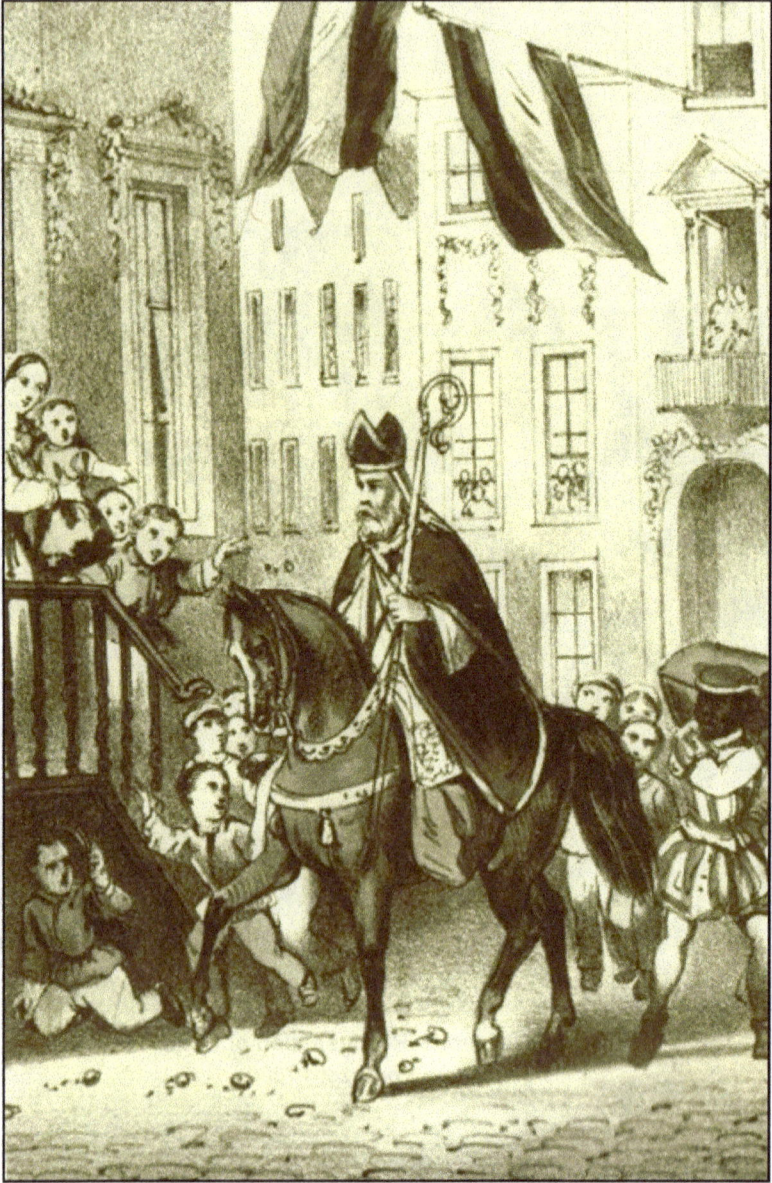

Fig. 8. St. Nicholas and Bartell,
19th Century Austrian Representation

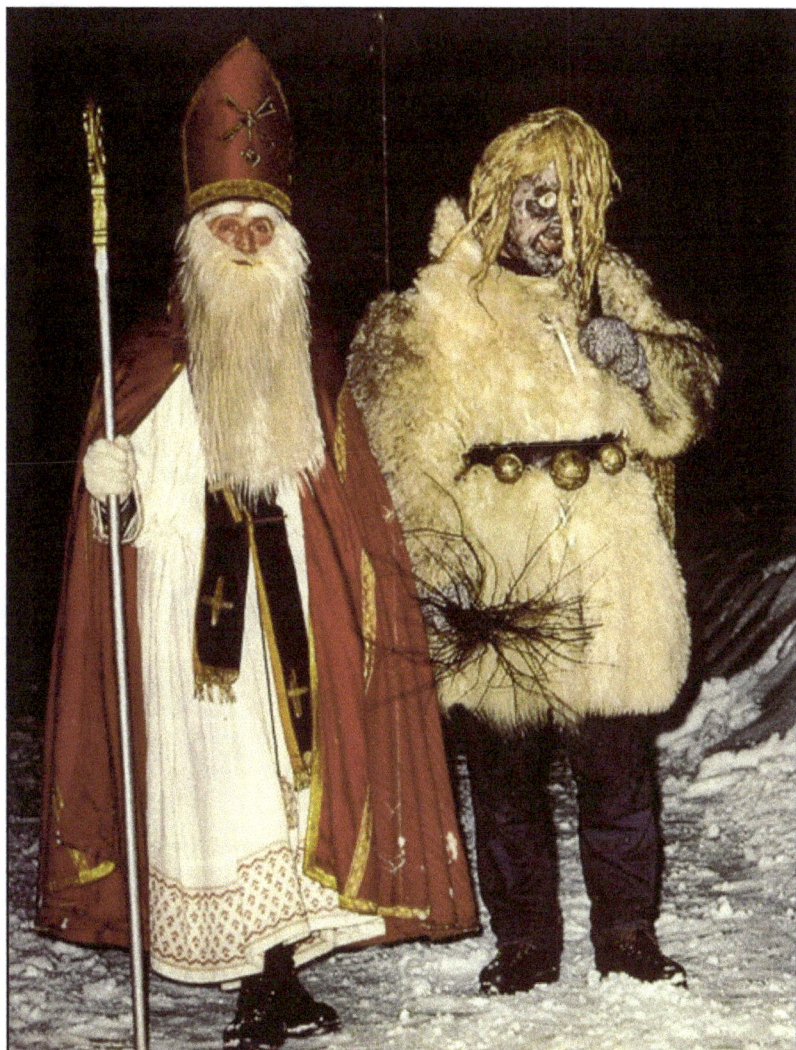

Fig. 9. St. Nicholas and companion Bartell,
Photo: Bad Mittendorf Austria, *Natural History* Magazine

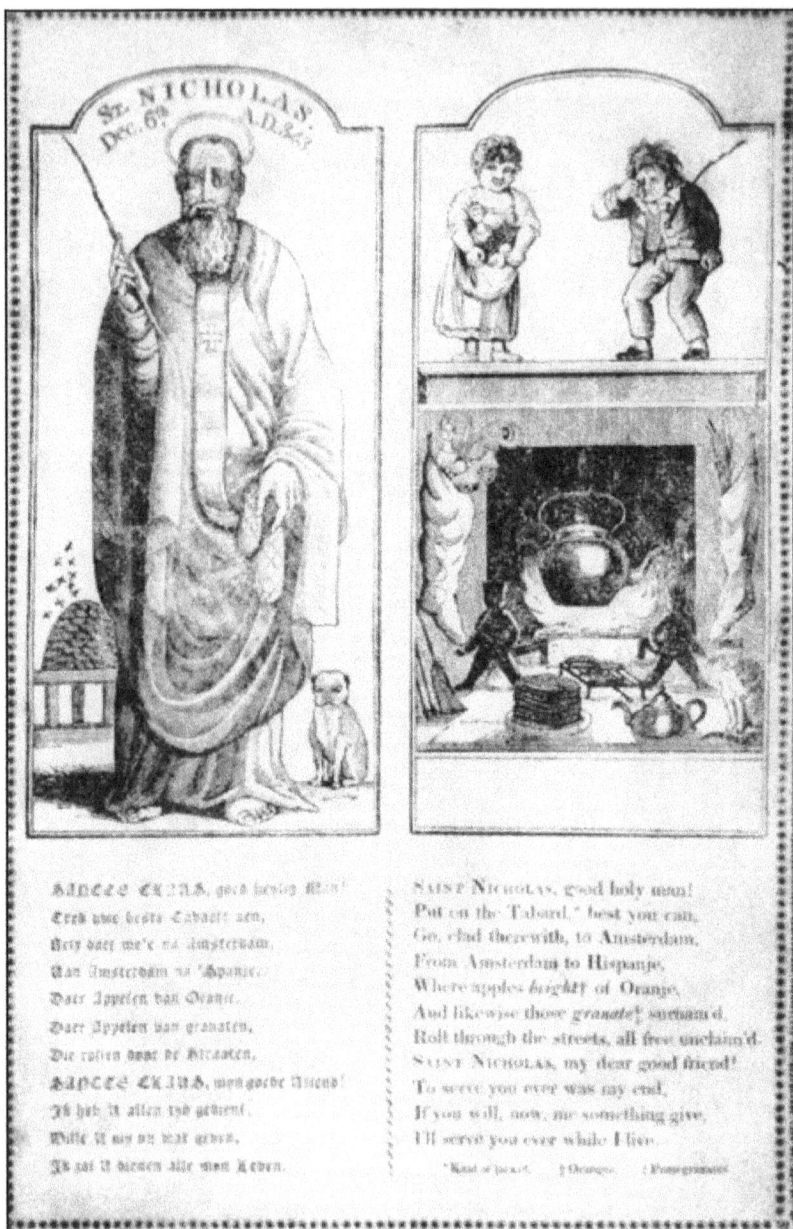

Fig. 10. Broadside (NY Historical Society,
Alexander Anderson 1775–1870)

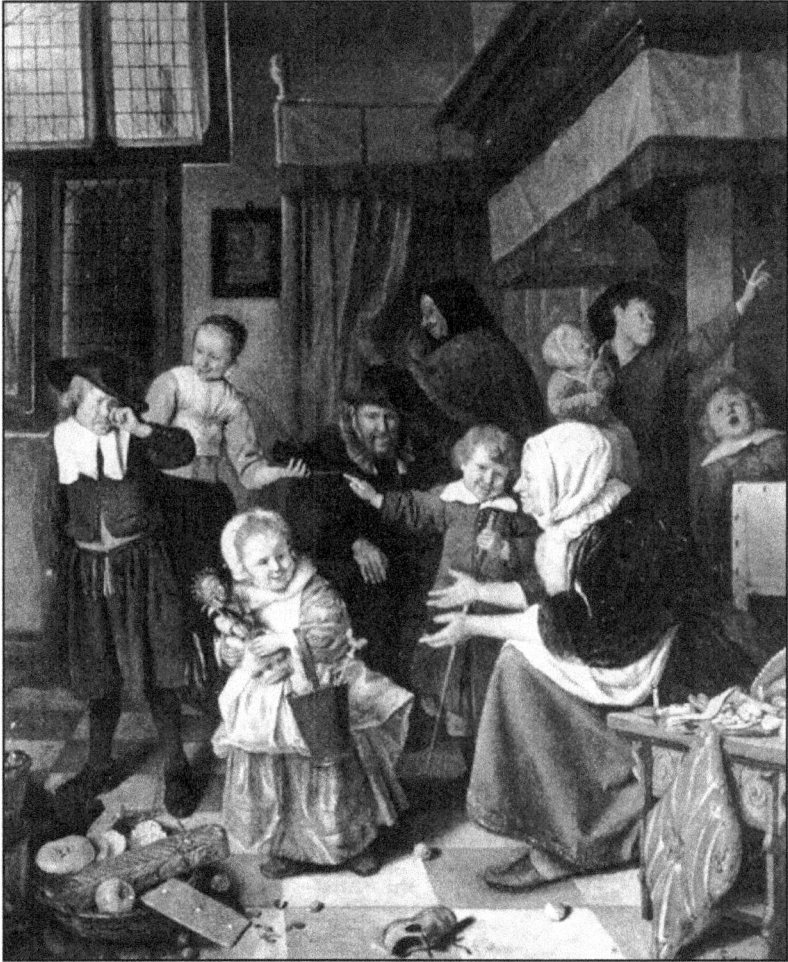

Fig. 11. St. Nicholas Day. Dutch, Jan Steen, 1600s

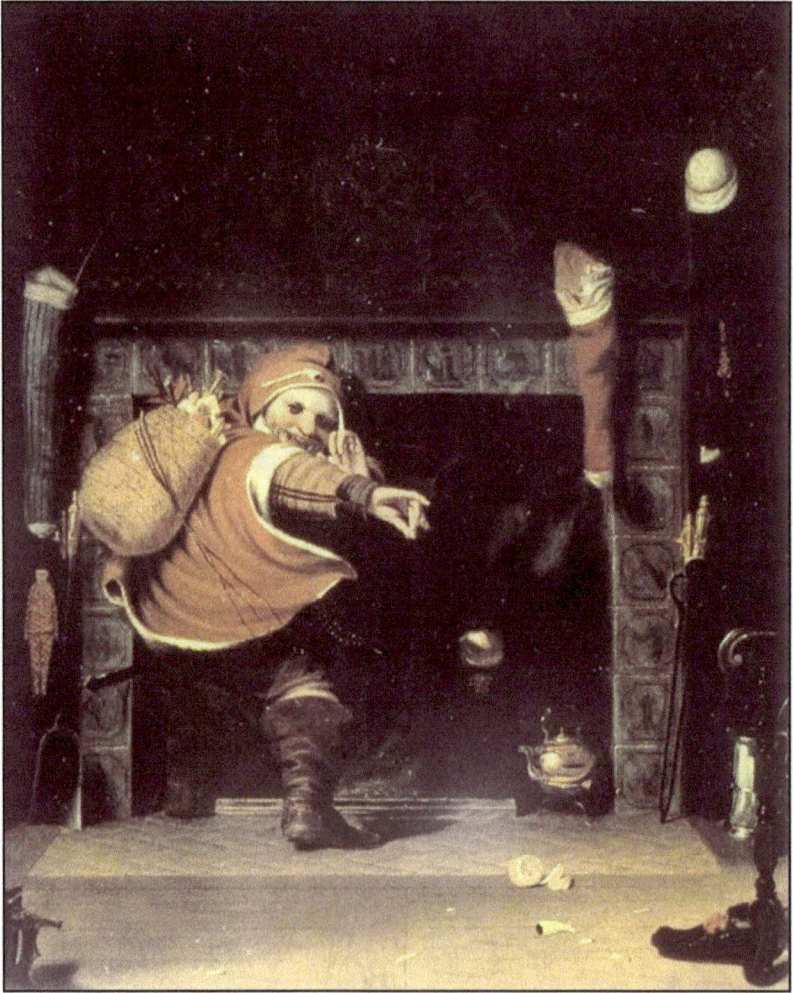

Fig. 12. Santa Claus, Christmas Eve. Robert Weir
1837. Metropolitan Museum NY

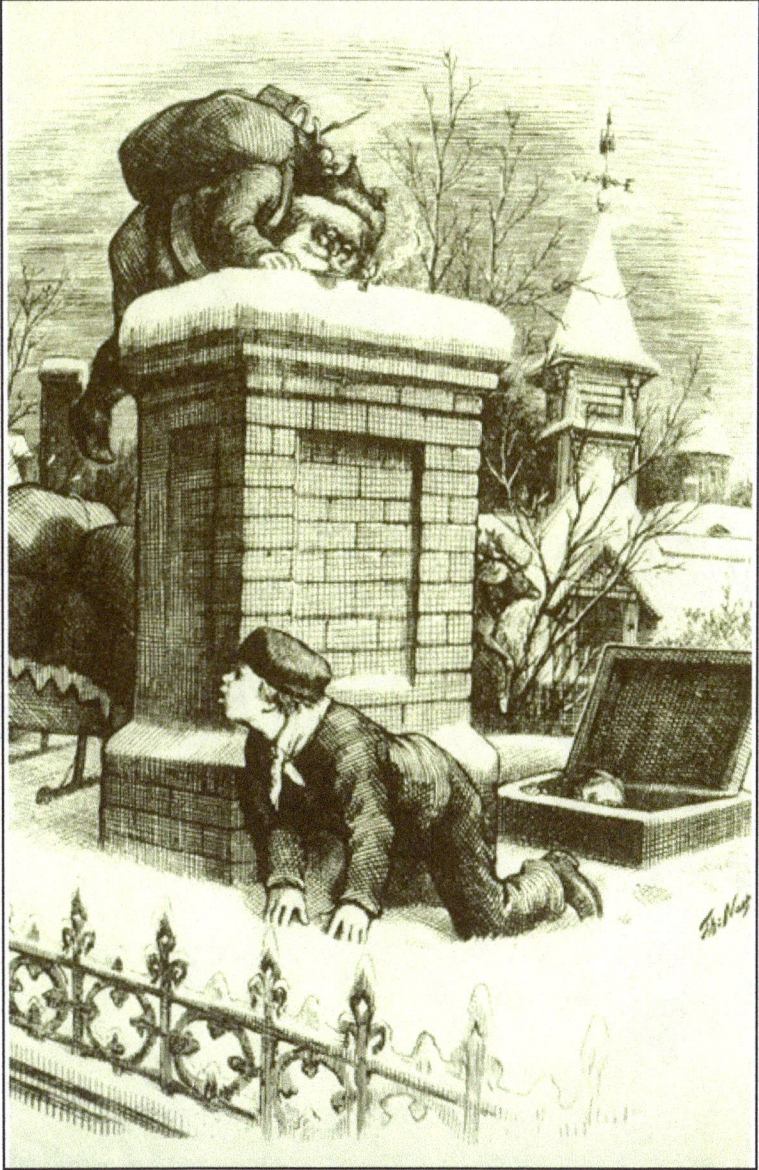

Fig. 13. Santa on Roof. Thomas Nast,
Harpers Weekly, 1/1/1876

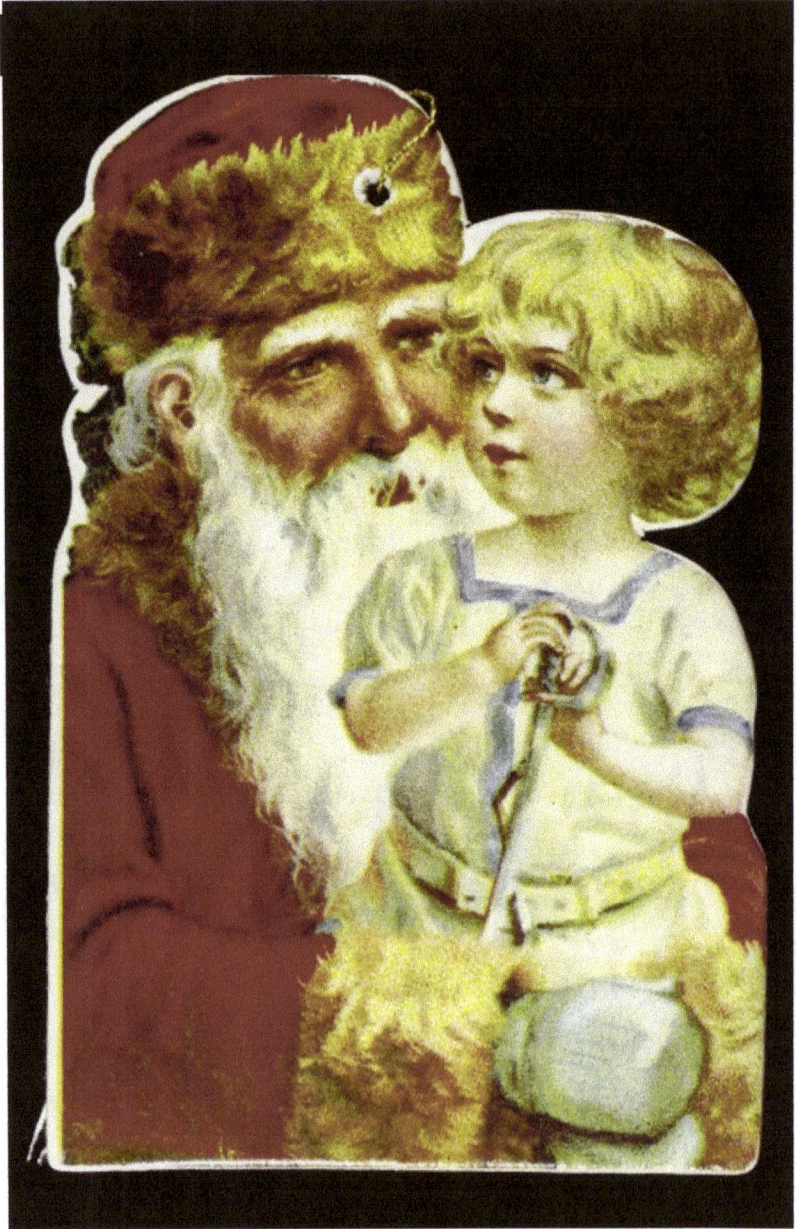

Fig. 14. Christmas Ornament, early 1900s

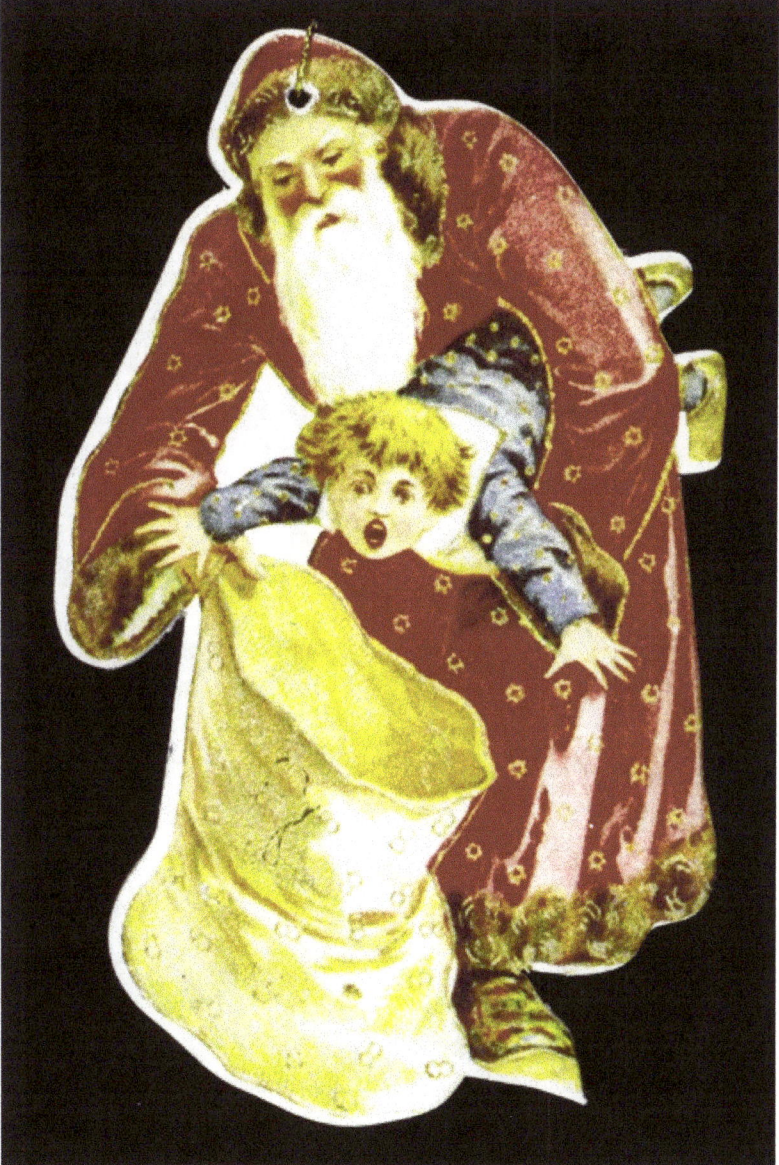
Fig. 15. Christmas Ornament, early 1900s

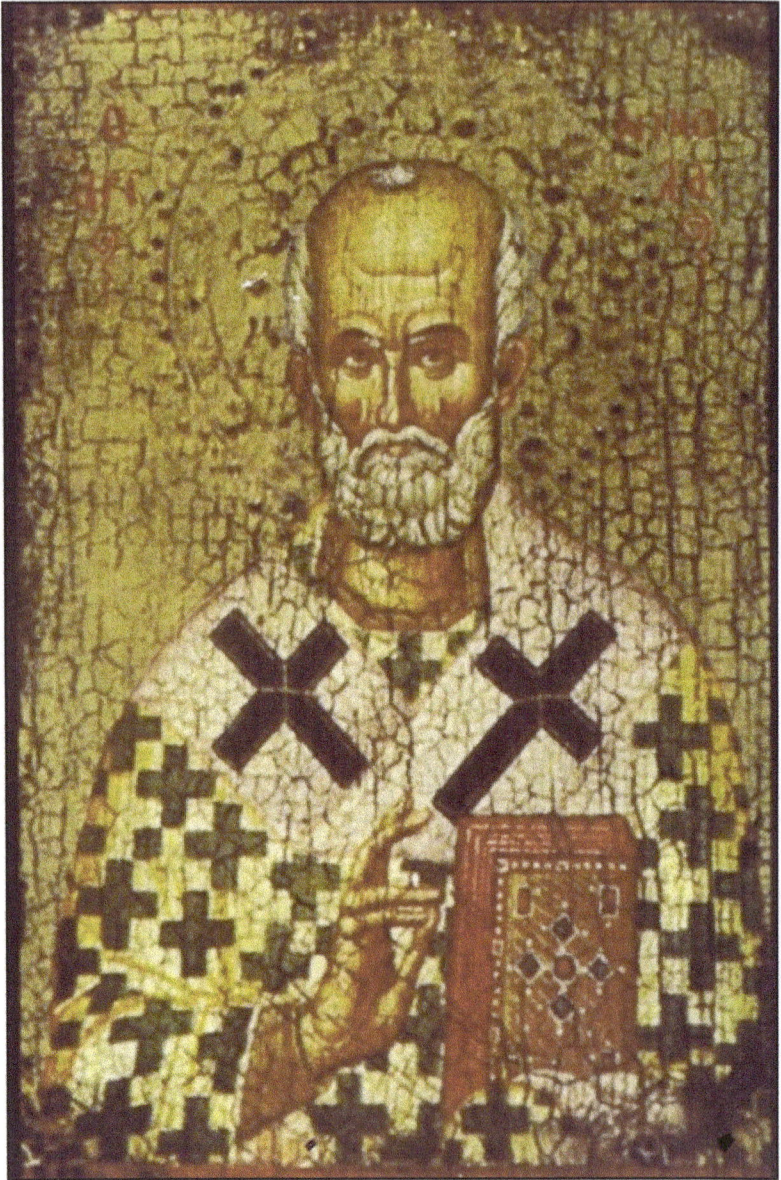

Fig. 16. Ncholas, Orthodox Icon

The Mystery of the Unsaid Name

(2007). In *Language, Symbolization, and Psychosis*
(eds. Ambroso, GS Argentieri, & J. Canestri).
London: Karnac Press, pp.166–186.

Commonalities between God and Rumpelstiltskin

The subtitle of this essay may seem provocative insofar as I have juxtaposed God to an elfin benefactor in a Grimm fairy tale. Nonetheless, each text concerns cautions about naming. We are admonished not to utter the name of God in vain in the sacred text which contains the Ten Commandments. Furthermore, God is most frequently named indirectly as "the Lord" or in a similar paranomic device, lest we be accused of sinning. Such prohibitions to the naming of god also exist in non-Judeo-Christian religions and cultures as well and with even harsher retaliatory consequences. Curiously, in Judaic practice, celebrants of the Lord have gone further in obeying the prohibition against saying God's name insofar as supplicants do not even utter "the Lord"(Heb.*Adonai*) but rather "the Name" (Heb.*Hashem*) when practicing prayer or in discourse about benedictions. Thus, they are now twice removed from the proper name of God.

In addition, it is well known that among certain African, Amazonian and other tribal peoples the use of proper names or taking photos by a stranger is prohibited, for fear that the stranger will actually take control of the person by possessing the representational image that is produced or uttered. Thus, the signifier or name of mortals as well as gods is also infused with power.

The tale of Rumpelstiltskin includes some similarities to the prohibition described in naming God and the power of the representation. This fairy tale, gathered among others by the brothers Grimm during the early 19th century, presents a central elfin figure as the nightly visitor and benefactor to a maiden, married off to a king, who was told by her greedy father that she could spin straw into gold. Rumpelstiltskin, hearing her plaint, assists her in her chore for small rewards in the form of trinkets, such as a bracelet or ring, until he strikes a final bargain that her first-born child is to be given to him as a reward for his super- alchemical feats (turning a nonmetal fiber into a precious metal). The forfeit for the bargain can only be broken if the young Queen guesses the nightly visitor's name. Thus, the designation, or naming, has the potential to break the secret bargain that up to now has empowered the Queen, but its final iteration will force her to give up her first-born. In both instances, the sacred and profane, naming takes on magical power with consequences to the speaker. There are many instances in our sacred texts and literature where similar references are made to the power of naming and its importance. It certainly is not by chance that one of the first tasks of newly created man in Genesis was to name the beasts of the field and the flora as well. The New Testament Gospel of John initiates with the phrase," In the beginning was the Word and the

Word was with God." According to Jones (1914) the Annunciation, too, is an impregnation via audition. Odysseus' encounter with the Cyclops ends with the protagonist's response to his blinded victim that his tormenter was "No Name." These uniquely Western texts are matched across cultures by similar stories that employ empowerment by words as creative acts and gestural equivalents.

The magic words "Abracadabra" (Aramaic for "It will be done as I say") is but one example of an incantation that is filled with unexpected power for action, moving far beyond mere saying.

These historical and cultural examples have been incorporated into the modern study of language which reaches beyond the labeling power of words. Many modern linguists have declared the ascendancy of pragmatics over semantics and syntax as a means of deriving the core feature of signifying, and now they study how we "do things with words." Austin (1962), Searle (1969) and Lakoff (2003) have explicated the power of designating as performatives and speech acts in which the utterances have active consequential effects on the surround. Within such a system, naming God or Rumpelstiltskin represents more than a casual designation.

How can we understand these narrative gestures unless we address the significance of naming, itself, both culturally and from the vantage point of psychoanalysis? Or better, how can we use our psychoanalytic perspective to illuminate these disparate cultural phenomena? There is a long tradition from Freud on, to extend our interpretations from the couch to culture. There are pitfalls in this venture, but many scholars have utilized the psychoanalytic method to illuminate and enrich understanding of texts by using ample convergent data to support their conclusions. This proviso in place, I will proceed.

Within psychoanalysis, we examine the power of the word, designated both in classical Freudian linguistics and in more recent Lacanian designations such as "Le Nom du Père," which stands for more than the name of the father. It designates a whole constellation of signifiers pertaining to power and the triadic Oedipal constellation.. Freud's (1919) explication of the "uncanny" brings home the idea that unconscious repressed derivatives are called up by a word that links experiences with repressed constellations. The sense of awe is linked to the "uncanny" because it depends upon similar depth factors that are associated to the audible word. Indeed, the German word for uncanny is *unheimlich* which is related both to the familiar, home, and secret, eliciting dual meanings. I, (Shapiro 1976) and then others, have referred to the very act of interpretation as a naming event that illuminates the patient's thoughts and actions by representing what they do and what they say in a linguistic system that can be considered in consciousness. More recently, Fonagy and others (1998) suggest we pay attention to the "mentalization" of unconscious constellations as a significant factor in our work as psychoanalysts.

A most general proposition in linguistic terms is that every utterance in words is an interpretation in so far as the choice of words binds the concept represented to a limited range of denotations and connotations within a code, i.e., it has a definition that excludes other dimensions of meaning. Psychoanalysts in practice listen carefully to usage as a clue to selective meanings. Similarly, psychoanalytic scholars attend carefully to texts for clues to better interpretations.

This brief review of the commonalities among linguistics and psychoanalysis and textual analysis suggests that we can approach the "unnamed" from the vantage of the consequential power of "uttering a name." If we explore the power of giving something a name we will then be able to contrast it with what we avoid when we prohibit naming. Two suggestive literary texts come to mind that exemplify this point. One is from Lewis Carroll's *Through the Looking Glass* in which Alice meets Humpty Dumpty, and the other derives from a play by Tom Stoppard, *The Invention of Love:*

> When Alice encounters Humpty Dumpty he says: "...but tell me your name and your business"
> My name is Alice, but..."
> "It's a stupid name enough!" Humpty Dumpty interrupted impatiently. "What does it mean?"
> "Must a name mean something?" Alice asked doubtfully. "Of course it must." Humpty Dumpty said with a short laugh: "My name means the shape I am-and a good handsome shape it is, too. With a name like Alice you might be any shape, almost." (Carroll, L. The Annotated Alice, 1960, pp.263)

In the Stoppard play we encounter A.E. Housman, the poet, in Hades meeting a friend who describes a group he belongs to, where they have been defining the then gay community, insofar as it could exist in England during the time of the restrictive Indecency Laws:

> "Chamberlain:... We belong to a sort of secret society, The Order of Chaeronea,like the sacred bond of Thebes. Actually it's more like a discussion group. We discuss what we should call ourselves. "Homosexuals" has been suggested.
> AEH: Homosexuals?
> Chamberlin: "We aren't anything till there is a word for it."

These fragments provide us with examples of the significance of words in binding, not only the cognitive boundaries of thought, but also the affective features of the words we employ in language. Speech is the main vehicle of linguistic expression and the spoken word carries not only referential power, but as noted earlier, performative power. The link between references to God and Rumpelstiltskin will, I suggest, provide a means to grasp the depth meaning of the unnamed and the affects that accompany the prohibitions in naming. I will approach the matter of the unnamed from the converse side by studying naming and its role in culture. I will also make some further suggestions regarding the difference between negating and the "unnamed." Then I will examine the Grimm fairy tale as it may illuminate the prohibition of uttering the name of God. Let us begin with the linguistic texts that are relevant and proceed to the psychoanalytic contribution to our topic.

Linguistics and Naming

The early 20th-century literature addressing naming and its fuller themes in the science of Semiotics was influenced by Ogden and Richards (1923) who showed clearly that names or words do not simply reference singular things and objects, but refer to concepts or class categories. Taking a somewhat Platonic stance, they show that words, except perhaps proper nouns, refer to ideas and concepts. Each word delimits the referential frame and segregates categories. Earlier in the century, Saussure (1911) wrote about signifier and signified to address the mental form of designating as a linguistic task. It took the later innovative work of Austin (1962) to initiate the more recent interest in the performative aspects of naming, i.e.

their functional and pragmatic role in intentionality which Searle (1969) elaborated as speech acts. Words could never again be simple labels, but would from then on be seen as initiators or stimuli of intended action. Semantics expanded from the study of defining and designation to encompass rhetorical intent. The text could no longer be analyzed and understood without knowing the context of its expression and perhaps the intent of the "sayer."

Wittgenstein's (1953) first foray into this realm also involved the idea that words took on significance only in sentences and therefore were contextually determined. While this early idea was later modified, others used the concept to advance the pragmatic effect of narratives. Lakoff's (1986) work in this area best explains the categorizing function of the mind. He sees this function as the central tool by which we master the idea of the world within naming categories homed in specific cultures. Names call up rather delimited and specified concepts that then are the stuff of the mind's "filing system" within any culture.

Following an exhaustive review of the relevant literature on designating and categorizing (including some of the authors noted above), Lakoff suggests a number of features that must be included to afford a complete description of the categorizing function that establishes word boundaries. These include: family resemblance among a class of words, centrality and gradients as we enlist more connotative extensions in use, metonymic reasoning, where the word itself stands in for a concept contiguous to the word,(e.g. Crown for King, White House for President). He also reminds us of generativity and polysemy, allowing for a dynamic extension of connotative significance of words to new meanings and usages.

He argues that the structure of thought is characterized by a limited number of cognitive models. Some categories are scalar with degrees of membership in a category, while others are classical with rigid boundaries; some are metonymic, some are centrally organized, emerging as spokes deriving from prototypes. He then notes that categories are not simply arbitrary, as semanticists of the past suggested, but may be empirically derived from experience, which includes bodily states and socially defined extensions of meaning, in accord with the models listed above. These latter notions should be particularly trenchant for psychoanalysts and will be addressed in the following sections.

He continues that concepts are not transcendental, i.e. that reason is not just the mechanical manipulation of abstract symbols. Nor do concepts merely provide internal representations of external reality. The mind is not simply a mirror of nature, but is limited by the needs of any language culture. These assertions are tested functionally by the following examples. Various cultures designate colors in accord with their needs, even though the objectively measured wavelengths of colors can be detected independent of the designations. The perspectivism implied by these choices do not deprecate or trivialize the indexing systems of each culture. They merely suggest that designations are intimately limited by the specified requirements of each linguistic group and are linked to core experiences.

Among the simplest examples I can cite is the Lévi-Strauss description of an Amazonian linguistic system where flora are simply divided between edible and not edible, compared to our elaborate multinamed empirical Linnaean taxonomy and functional biological systems.

While linguistic systems are shared by needs of a culture, they also can be shaped within cultures to influence power distribution and the interest of subgroups. In a recent book, Lakoff shows the powerful impact of words on politics. Slogans and word clusters

604

(2003) influence our "frames of reference" in construing the way we see things and as a result have powerful pragmatic effects. Thus, the defining features of a word prescribe limits to meaning; but they also convey affective power in use. The name of God perforce must have pragmatic power as it is uttered, or else it can become an empty icon chanted in ritual phrases.

These considerations direct us to the unnamed: If the "named" is trapped by various dimensions or features within a category, it cannot be boundless in its signifying references and function. There is an injunction not to utter the name of the deity, because there is no name we can employ that does not have specified features that constrain it. A name limits our conception of God.

Nonetheless, some religions have seen fit to permit embodiments of God in various forms to make the deity palpable in human terms and accessible—as more than awe inspiring; as more than an ineffable boundless enigma that monotheism, in its purest form, requires. Parenthetically, the Old Testament does designate the name of God (Heb. Yahwe, Elohim) only to suggest later that when we see the tetragram signifying his name, we say instead, "The Lord." We also have the multiple incarnations in the Hindu religion, and we have the incarnation of Jesus in Christianity and the referential metaphor for God as father and "all powerful." These variations do not exclude the more mysterious and the "not to be named" third element of the Trinity, the "Holy Spirit," or the god who appears as a burning bush in the Moses text, simply asserting in a humanly audible voice "I am that I am." We preserve the unnamed in these variations as the special quality that determines the deity. In this vein, Lakoff introduces the common occurrence in culture of the expansion of prototypic names or basic categorization to extended or family words. We may look at the various designations of an incarnation as an aspect of the deity.

They are symbolic extensions of the prototype of the most abstract representation of God.

Continuing the argument as it bears relevance to designating aspects of God, contiguous features are represented in classical Christianity as Saints, or in the Old Testament as prophetic voices. Indeed, it is here that the spokes from the prototypic idea of God reach into polysemantic concrete representations. This need for concrete representations derives from religious groups' need to turn to a deity for comfort and justification of suffering. The notion of one ineffable God may at times be too abstract and difficult to grasp as a disembodied object of prayer. The demand for signs of presence and visible power require new representational qualities. We long for a name or an image to be magically uttered or seen. The Christian credo (*Credo in Unum Deum*) and The Hebrew "Sh'ma" (Hear oh Israel, the Lord is one) remain awe-inspiring but remote abstract concepts without flesh. Such remote power is the counterpoint of the concrete representations preferred by various believers.

Although the "one God" credo is abstract and remote, there are a number of attributes which have been used to characterize the Godhead—all knowing, just, omnipotent, loving and most central possessing the power to create. Creativity as an essential feature of God's power has been central to theological and social dimensions of belief. God is a force that creates. One Old Testament narrative showing the primacy of God as creator is exemplified in the Book of Job. The afflictions suffered by Job lead to a curious confrontation in which God reveals his essence by asserting his creative power. The voice in the whirlwind that represents God appearing to Job is humbling: God intimidatingly asks, "Where were you when I created the universe"?—thereby suggesting that Job's querying his personal pain is trivial in the face of the magnitude of the deity's works. The boundlessness must be referential not only in his ubiquity, but in his unending creative works. A name cannot encompass such power.

In modern times, the religious anti-evolutionary movement has countered the Darwinian chance natural-selection hypothesis with the idea of a Creative Intelligent Designer to account for our evolving to a state in which we can even consider this matter intellectually. Thus, the believers add "intention and intelligence" to the deity's work plan in evoking creation and grand design. The idea of intention in creativity provides yet another metaphor that anthropomorphizes God in the form of a dialogic partner in a speech act. The notion of an abstract force's guiding history without intent or special consideration for man is too unnerving and intolerable for those who wish to maintain awe of the unique order in the non-artifactual world. Parenthetically, we have not even addressed the referential analogy pointed to by feminists in the practice of referring to God as a HE. Even the pantheists cannot bear the idea of an unembodied "it."

The linguistic analysis of the various dimensional and emotional constraints on the features of our defining God takes us this far. I hope to enhance understanding by adding a psychoanalytical point of view that explores the unconscious factors that enrich meanings of our subject. I will attempt to link the unnamed Rumpelstiltskin to the conundrum of the unconscious significance of God as our unnamed Creator.

Psychoanalysis and the Unnamed

"The Unnamed" may be seen to have unconscious roots and significance that can be discovered by a psychoanalytically oriented probe.

First I will review Freud's and later psychoanalysts' forays into linguistic issues.

Freud (1900) was fascinated by problems of representation. Dreams, symptoms, and parapraxes all required transformational rules for their emergence into consciousness. These rules, similar to the tropes in narrative analysis, were invoked within a symbolic system that he believed were built into the mental apparatus. Freud's topographic theory was most closely allied to the Saussurian linguistic model, accounting for the French Psychoanalytic School's continuing devotion to this earliest model. Lacan's (1956) devotion to Saussure and his specific employment of linguistic tropes also are found in the topographic model. Freud's use of thing and word presentation model permitted a split between the system *ucs* and the system *pcs*. He required that thing-presentations be attached to word presentations in order to pass from ucs through pcs to system *cs*.

Freud's linguistics initially concerned interpretation in words as a means of rendering the unconscious conscious. The Oedipus complex, primal scene, etc. are but a few of the deeper unconscious constellations that lie at the basis of derivative social structures that are rendered in language. These complexes are transformed into designative units that are used to structure human relationships and narratives. I (T. Shapiro, 1979) have written that the structure of drives and wishes is syntactically arranged in a form akin to sentences with a subject, verb & object thus allowing for naming as a narrative statement.

Each verbal or symptomatic expression requires mental mechanisms or as linguists say, transformational rules, to establish their relationship to base or core meanings. Thus, there is much overlap between the idea of "dream work" and literary linguistic "tropes" such as metaphor and condensation. Indeed, Lacan's work draws heavily on this aspect of Freud's thought as it also directly references Saussure.

In rendering unconscious constellations linguistically, we *name* the yet-unknown deeper constellations. We also tame the affects that are bound to formerly unconscious ideas, permitting us to wrestle them to awareness. Metaphoric interpretations also show us that understanding entails rich physicalist references that reach to affects as well as to bodily features of definition (see Grossman, W. & Steward, W.A. 1976). Lakoff too, from a non-psychoanalytic vantage, makes prominent reference to the bodily origins of many metaphoric structures, paralleling Freud's idea that ego was once body ego. Freud's bold statement merely addresses the idea that our infantile preverbal experience of the world does not transcend the subjective body-centered experience, because the declarative form of experience is not available. Later linguistically based concepts are grafted onto these earlier templates and are recast as words (declarative memories) characterized by limited features for definitional clarity.

My own work at the interface of linguistics and psychoanalysis has been directed toward the importance of naming as interpretation. Rendering in words that which has been unconscious is a moment of recognition for a patient. The newly informed patient can then deal with a conscious verbal formula that references action dispositions toward others that can be applied to life experiences, understood, and modified since we are now dealing with a mental event. (I have already noted Fonagy's mentalization as but another variant form of the same process).

Freud also made other forays into linguistic issues in his papers, "The Antithetical Meaning of Primal Words" (Freud, 1910) and "On Negation"(Freud 1925) to name but two. The Antithetical Meaning of Primal Words is especially cogent for this discussion, because Freud analogizes the discovery by cultural anthropologists that our earliest words may represent two antithetical meanings. Thus, one word initially pointed to both divergent meanings. Freud exploited the discovery to explain the idea that any word or sign may be used defensively to represent its opposite. In our current discussion of God's powers, we have revived the old Manichaean heresy that suggests a co-existence of forces of evil as equal to and opposite to God's power. The postulated dual power was disruptive to God's singularity and the monotheistic credo during the period of scholasticism. It raised the issue of existence implied in negation .

Negation differs from idea of the unnamed and will be addressed here as an addendum. Freud (1925) and the linguists agree that negation is a type of semantic designation that includes designation of the entity, which is then denied by special markers such as *not*. We must first assert "X" for it to be negated. This is not only so in symbolic logic, but in the psychoanalytic recognition that negation is a form of lifting repression and of recognizing an entity only to then verbally reject it in consciousness. Thus, negation requires expression of a word with all the constraints that apply, plus a formal sign that denies. It is therefore different from the unnamed.

In religious terms, the Devil is recognized as "the force that negates" according to Goethe (1953). While the devil asserts God's power by his opposition, he also contests it and tempts and exercises a counterforce to the assumed all encompassing good of the deity. This "entity as counterforce" is not the same as the "unnamed" God. The Lord's name (unnamed) remains the intellectual abstract representation of the Godhead as in the Credo. Believers keep it abstract and unnamed in order to maintain awe and abstract remoteness. We will return to the paper on antithetical meaning a it applies to Rumpelstiltskin and to God as I argue the unconscious meaning of the unnamed.

Rumpelstiltskin & God

I will make extensive reference to a scholarly article regarding Grimm's story as a starting point for my argument. Harry Rand's (2003) paper "Who was Rumpelstiltskin?" provides a significant gloss on the fairy tale and a route to our expanding understanding about why the name is to be evaded and its meaning shrouded in mystery. In elaborating Rand's arguments, I will also offer some modifications and addenda that I believe will render the fairy tale more understandable and permit a more comprehensive understanding of the unnamed. In so doing, I will also extend the argument about what the "unnamed" god represents. What would knowing or saying his name do to our faith and our awe?

Rand comments on the many variations of the folk story which is available in a number of languages, and then settles into a discussion of what clues the name Rumpelstiltskin means from its etymology. His approach is designed to expand understanding of the deeper meaning of the tale. He also finds significance in the circumstance of the creation of this orally transmitted tale. The tales were created in medieval *Spinnstuben* or spinning rooms, that were occupied by women who gathered to spin together. They amused themselves by telling creative tales, likely with negative and mocking references to men. The Spinnstuben may be compared to men's leisure-time company in bars and pubs. The tales are significant in their intent to both entertain and narrate the plight of women during the Middle Ages. Thus, we can expect some interpretive passages and themes in the tales that serve the social and political aims of this "spinster" (also derivative of the spinnstube) group.

Approaching the tale in this manner allows us to conjecture about the negative roles of men in the tales. In *Rumpelstiltskin*, a father uses his daughter as a means of raising his stature by marrying her to royalty and lying about her magical skills; the King wanting the maiden to satisfy his greed and his procreative powers for a son are each prominently featured. Rand suggests that the only benign male in the tale, and its tacit hero, is Rumpelstiltskin. The little man lends his powers to facilitate the novice Queen's desperate plight and requirement to satisfy the King's greed by spinning straw into gold.. Rand's etymological analysis of the name, Rumpelstiltskin and its relevance to the story line is revealing.

Rand describes six essentials features about the night visitor: 1. He is male;2. He is short but not described as one of the traditionally designated trolls or other "wee-folk"; 3. He accomplishes vital work that seems magical; 4.His magical powers notwithstanding; he still wants a living child; 5. No one has ever heard his name "it is outside her vocabulary." 6. When the Queen utters his name he shouts "The Devil Told You!" and either disappears or self-destructs in a number of ways by splitting himself in two or into many fragments according to which text is read.

Rand then breaks the name into stems and segments. This approach, incidentally, uses a particularly Germanic feature of constructing words from various stems which are agglutinated into a single compound word. Words such as *Mundtuch* or napkin are constructed from mouth and cloth; another is *Tischtuch* (tablecloth). In this instance, we learn that the root, *Rumpel*, designates shriveled or rumpled and that the root, *stilts,* is related to the English word stilt or stiff, and the name ending *kin* may be a condensation of skin or kin as in tiny—as in the French suffix *ette,* or *kin* as in munchkin or manikin. Rand then indicates that from this analysis the little man is a "flaccid penis." He continues that such a little man, despite his powers, is rather benign and not aggressively harmful and the only male in the story who is sympathetic to the young Queen.

At this juncture I suggest that his conclusion is puzzling, because this is a powerful, indeed magical little fellow and the stem for stiff is just as prominent as the stem for rumpled. I contest the conclusion that the penis is flaccid by applying a similar analytic method. Indeed, "the little man-penis" has features that would make the reader think of him as erect and potent. This change will become important to our understanding about why he has to be "unnamed," and why his name has to be discovered and then uttered to alter the bargain with the Queen.

Etymological analysis of the name reveals the dual aspect of the little man's binary state, erect and rumpled. Freud's analysis of primal words offers a psychoanalytic means to understand the unconscious meaning of the dual opposing word stems. Thus Rumpelstiltskin, by virtue of his name, is represented as both erect (stilts) and flaccid (Rumpel) and thus, personifies the nature of the penis itself, which exists in nature sequentially in both forms. The categorical features of each word root indicate the limits of meaning within a purely linguistic construal, as described by Lakoff. There is further reason to suggest phallic power from this narrative as well as the name itself. The power to create gold from straw is indeed a transformational miracle, suggesting magical power that is only matched by the miracle of conception and the transformation of the sperm and egg to a human form. The story redundantly expresses Rumpelstiltskin's wish to have the Queen's child as the price for the miracle performed. This wish is shared by the King or any husband. Thus, the new bride is expected to bear a child not only for Rumpelstiltskin, but for and by the King. It is not of passing consequence that at the time of creating this tale, child-like wives belonged to the male leader of the household as chattel.

There is also unexploited symbolism in the tearful bride's waiting for her husband's entry or "sexual intrusion." She must do the impossible, make gold from straw (a baby from intercourse), without understanding the role of the penis in the task. The tale suggests that the novice bride relies on childish images of romance and sexuality without knowledge of coition. The apprehension concerning the King's anticipated entry is relieved when the elfin creature bursts into the room, unasked for, but welcomed particularly when his miracle is performed. Her apprehension about the magnitude of the task of spinning straw into gold is alleviated by the amiable elf. Psychoanalysts are familiar with the body-penis equation in which the part stands for the whole, as in metonymy. The little man, as penis, also serves as a complement to the small gifts from the queen at each evening's end. They are each circular feminine enclosures, a ring and a bracelet, which are not hard to decipher in this context as female genitalia. Thus, both the very entry of the little man into the queen's space, and the nature of her gifts, are graphic symbols of the King's nightly sexual intrusions. In the end, we have to accept the erstwhile maiden's grasp that the creative little man has produced the pure gold, a baby, to be born at a future date.

Intercourse and procreation are not linked by temporal contiguity, but by new knowledge of the relationship of conception to birth. It is a surprise for the nubile girl to learn that the baby has not grown *ex nihilo* in a mother's womb, but that it is in part a product of the work of the little man who enters nightly and magically and figuratively spins straw into gold. The tale is about discovering the creative power of the male, and the role of the phallus in procreation. It tells why the male has a claim on the baby born nine months later. This is simultaneously an age-old tale of primal learning and personal coming of age.

Once told in this manner, we have a suggestion why the little man is unnamed. His name is not known or voiced because of the phallus' awesome creative powers. The maiden's repression and lack of knowledge move hand-in-hand as self-deception and also to support the awe of magical creation. What should be a miracle of the gods is in fact a material product of the work of the human corporeal penis and figuratively of the imaginative phallus. A more homely interpretation might be read as follows: the innocent maiden, victimized by her greedy father, enters the marriage bed not knowing about the means of procreation and its link to intercourse. The phallicmanikin bursting into her room is discovered to be the creative force of life itself—once the name of this intruder is discovered, some mastery occurs by new knowledge. The name helps the young woman to assimilate and adapt to marriage, intercourse and procreation by its signifying function of linking an idea to an experience in life. Naming again comforts, by the acquisition of new knowledge that both reveals and contains the boundaries of the unknown. Like a proper interpretation, it elevates the repressed into words to be contemplated in thought.

Let us recapitulate. The tale of Rumpelstiltskin is a metaphoric restatement of the act of mental assimilation by the pre-nuptial girl, signifying that the intrusion of the male penis is not just an exploitation of her virginal body, but the means of creating a child. The Oedipal girl's sense of despair and exploitation by the father in giving her to another man is gradually overcome by the bride's anticipation of the gift of a child. The additional theme in the story of the girl's outwitting the little man, represents a bit of feminine politics where the passive is turned into the active. It is a reference to issues that were salient during the Middle Ages. The Queen triumphs over the "King and his little man" by prospectively winning her child. Ownership in the Middle Ages, of course, was a masculine privilege, and this triumph could be seen as the potential preemptive power of motherhood, even in the face of the "Droit du Seigneur"(See Jones, E. 1925).

The Spinnstuben women were very likely delighted by the young Queen's outwitting the small man, as well as the inclusion in the story of his self-destruction when his name was uttered. His cry that the Devil was the source of the discovery puts us in mind of the counterpoint between the natural forces at work in the story. The imagery of the nightly entry of the small man into the "Queen's room" in association with the circular gifts is unmistakably a representation of intromission. It also reminds us that the worry about an evening visitor with the intent of intercourse might also be related to other regressive anxieties of young children regarding a variety of night intruders—robbers, kidnappers, sandmen, etc.

In light of the interpretation above, we can see that the unnamed creative body part was not named, because then the awesome nature of procreation would be delimited to a mere physical act. Nominalization curtails the imagined fancied power of the male member. Say it and it is! Abracadabra! Shazam! The magic of words as performatives and speech acts becomes apparent. We do indeed do things with words. We also can magically pretend things do not exist if we do not say their names.

Now I will pull together the various strands of my argument. I have juxtaposed the prohibitions against uttering the name of "god" and the challenge and forfeiture game that centers on discovery of the name of the elfin night visitor to the Queen of a fairy-tale kingdom. One situation involves a prohibition against uttering a name, while the other affords power to reverse a bargain by she who discovers and says a name. These are clearly somewhat different, but both affirm the power involved in naming and saying. Each narrative is an example of attempts to delimit the meaning of the object by representing it in a word that constrains it in a cognitive frame. Each also provides the listener with a sense of the power of utterance, when considered from the vantage of a performative in which "saying" is a form of "doing." The more magical and awesome aspect of the experience has been explained by the Freudian analysis of the sense of the uncanny that belongs to the repressed from which the "unsaid" draws its affective power.

How do these two stories fit then? In the Rumpelstiltskin tale, we find it is an allegory of the procreative, or simply creative, power of the penis. If I were to employ a more abstract Lacanian interpretation, we might say the phallus is the imaginary representation of the power relationships among humans. There are many similar culturally bound symbols to point to. The Greco-Roman "Herms" which adorned the front courtyards of our Western ancestors are concrete reminders of domestic phallic power and guardianship. These stone steles were intimately tied to the protective power of the phallus as well as creative representations of fertility. They are but another historical representation of imagery parallel to the tale of Rumpelstiltskin.

In the case of the unnamed god, I have argued that this is a similar reference to an abiding and unfettered creative force. The syllogism presented could be solved as follows: The meaning of god is the phallus or in body language, the penis. The regression from abstract to bodily derived words that represent corporeal flesh and blood

617

is not new to psychoanalysts or to linguists. I have elaborated the body-phallus equation and the many more abstract representational references that represent regressive human forms. The linguists, too, show that body language, metaphor and metonymy abound in our daily word play. Freud's quip that sometimes a cigar is only a cigar, of course is the Urpsychoanalyst denying his own theoretic position.

Contrariwise, 'God the creator" is represented in abstract terms that are remote from representation of the body, especially in monotheism. Such tropes permit us to place our fate outside human hands in an abstract awesome force. Many monotheistic believers, gathering at times of need, retain the awe reserved for the mystical by not saying God's name. However, if the responder to our prayers is not to be seen as a sham, making him more distant secures awe. The Wizard of Oz, of course, comes to mind, insofar as he is discounted to be "just a man" and the pyrotechnics around him are humbug. Nonetheless many religions also alternate between the awesome abstract and the concrete, as exemplified in various practices that bring God to flesh and human representation, while others do not even say his name.

This duality of need is visible even in cultures supporting Christianity, where the "Word has become flesh." The theology maintains the mystery of the Trinity with a Holy Spirit in reserve for awe. The plea for *Imitatio Christi* is a flesh- and- blood model in the form of a human, but the spirit remains in the background. Similarly, the Hindu incarnations and the prophetic anointments of the Old Testament use a force that is unnamed. In human terms, we return to my syllogism: the name of God is equated to the creative power of the penis. It is a symbol of the procreative force within and across generations.

This force is a powerful image that is not immediately obvious empirically. The procreative power of the phallus has to be discovered, insofar as there are nine months between intromission and conception to birth. This linkage had to be discovered not only by the Queen in the tale, but by primal peoples as well. The discovery may have displaced some of the awe reserved for the deity as progenitor, establishing a power vacuum that our ancestor males took advantage of to become the kings and possessors of power over women. Socially and politically, the power grab down-played the role of the female as a procreative force, even though many generations of diverse cultures honed fertility images and practiced rites solely devoted to the generative power of women.

From the purported awesome impregnation by polytheistic gods, newer cultures elevated men to thrones and a new hegemony by showing they were doing God's work.

There remain many representations of female goddesses and more recently female saints followed by beatification of the Virgin Mary. Indeed, since males could not reproduce without females, the creative force is in fact a dual responsibility. This fact is symbolically stated in the tale of Rumpelstiltskin. Every Rumpelstiltskin must have his bracelet or necklace to exercise his creativity. The key to the relation of Grimm's tale to God rests in the unknown name. Once the name is discovered, its utterance frees the maiden from her bargain, and the little man's awesome gift is no longer necessary in the face of the greater miracle of birth.

I am sure that the male-dominated culture at the time of the Spinnstuben created feminine unrest and envy. We of the 21st century hopelessly repeat these same religious (Can women join the clergy?) and social (Should women in the workplace earn as much as men?) conflicts by the continuing argument between the sexes.

This does not make the argument regarding the symbolic significance of the "unsaid" less cogent. There is a need to bring our human condition under the sway of higher forces, such as deities, who fill our need for the ritual experience of uncanny awe and belief.

The "unnamed" protects us from the banality and confined humanity of the named. Any name entails limits and constraints because it has restrictive categorical meaning—but the abstraction is not the thing. Nonetheless, linguistic analysis shows that each abstraction can be analyzed into baser corporeal references. Our use of a psychoanalytic method of analysis, in turn, helps us to understand the roots of awe that are also features of our symbols. The discovery of the creative power of the genitalia is relived in each adolescent in the recognition that sexuality is related to procreation, just as our primal ancestors uncovered the same fact of life that helped elevate men to thrones. The awe accompanying the worship of God is based upon repressing the deity's powerful attributes. Moreover, we do not casually utter the name of God, because to say his name is a speech act that represents an enactment of that awesome power.

REFERENCES

Austin, J.L. (1962). How to do Things with Words. New York: Oxford University Press. Carroll, L. (1960). *The Annotated Alice: Alices Adventures in Wonderland and through the Looking Glass.* USA, Clarkson N. Potter.

Fonagy, P., & Target, M. (1998). Mentalization and the changing aims of child psychoanalysis. *Psychoanalytic Dialogues* 8:87–114.

Freud, S. (1900). The interpretation of dreams. *Standard Edition* 14:5, London: Hogarth Press, 1953.

——— (1910). The antithetical meaning of primal words. *Standard Edition* 2. Hogarth Press, 1957.

——— (1919). The uncanny. *Standard Edition* 17. London: Hogarth.

——— (1925). On negation. *Standard Edition* 19. Hogarth Press, 1961.

Goethe, J.N. (1953). *Faust in the Permanent Goethe.* New York: The Dial Press.

Grimm, J. (1944). *The Complete Grimm's Fairy Tales.* New York: Pantheon Books. Grossman W.I. & Stewart, W.A. (1976). Penis envy: from childhood wish to developmental metaphor. *Journal of the American Psychoanalytic Association* 24:193–210.

Jones, E. (1914). The Madonna's conception through the ear in essays. In: *Applied Psychoanalysis Volume II* (pp. 266–357).

Lacan, J. (1956). *The Language of the Self: The Function of Language in Psychoanalysis.* Translated by A. Wilden . Baltimore: The Johns Hopkins Press, 1956.

Lakoff, G. (1987). *Women, Fire and Dangerous Things.* Chicago: University of Chicago Press.

——— (2003). *Don't Think of One Elephant?* White River Junction: Chelsea Green Publishing.

Levi-Strauss, C. (1966). *The Savage Mind.* Chicago: University of Chicago Press.

Ogden, C.K. & Richards, I.A. (1923). *The Meaning of Meaning.* New York: Harcourt Brace & World 1946.

Rand, H. (2000). Who was Rumpelstiltskin? International Journal of Psychoanalysis, 81: 943–962.

de Saussure, F. (1911). *Course in General Linguistics.* New York: Philosophic Library, 1959.

Searle, J.R. (1969). *Speech Acts: An Essay in the Philosophy of Language.* New York: Cambridge University Press.

Shapiro, T. (1970). Interpretation and Naming. *Journal of American Psychoanalysis* 18:399–421.

Stoppard, T. (1997). *The Invention of Love.* Grove Press.

Winnicott, D.W. (1953). Transitional objects and transitional phenomena: a study of the first not-me possession. *International Journal of Psychoanalysis* 34:89–97.

Wittgenstein, L. (1953). *Philosophical Investigations.* New York: Macmillan.